Pilates

Rael Isacowitz

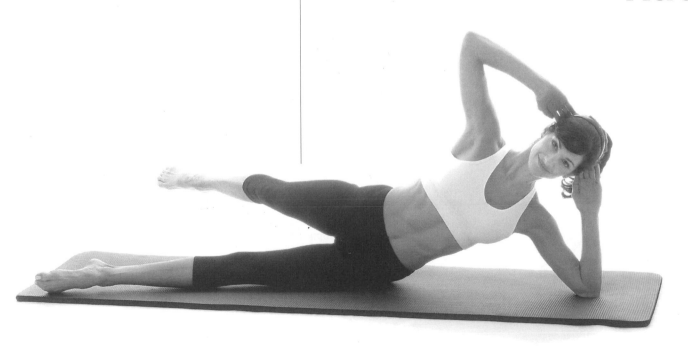

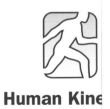

Human Kine

Library of Congress Cataloging-in-Publication Data

Isacowitz, Rael, 1955-
   Pilates / Rael Isacowitz.
       p. cm.
   Includes bibliographical references and index.
   ISBN-13: 978-0-7360-5623-6 (soft cover)
   ISBN-10: 0-7360-5623-8
   1. Pilates method. I. Title.
   RA781.4.173 2006
  613.7'1--dc22   2006007911

ISBN-10: 0-7360-5623-8
ISBN-13: 978-0-7360-5623-6

The Web addresses cited in this text were current as of May 2006, unless otherwise noted.

Acquisitions Editor: Martin Barnard; **Developmental Editor:** Julie Rhoda; **Assistant Editor:** Carla Zych; **Copyeditor:** Cheryl Ossola; **Proofreader:** Anne Rogers; **Indexer:** Nan N. Badgett; **Graphic Designer:** Robert Reuther; **Graphic Artist:** Kim McFarland; **Photo Manager:** Dan Wendt; **Cover Designer**: Keith Blomberg; **Photographer (cover and interior):** Kirk Fitzik; **Art Manager:** Kareema McLendon-Foster; **Illustrator:** Jason A. McAlexander, MFA / © Human Kinetics unless otherwise noted; **Printer:** United Graphics; **Cover Model:** Lisa Clayton; **Interior Photo Models:** Karla Adams, Lisa Clayton, Leah Turner, Kristi Cooper-White, and Rael Isacowitz.

Human Kinetics books are available at special discounts for bulk purchase. Special editions or book excerpts can also be created to specification. For details, contact the Special Sales Manager at Human Kinetics.

Printed in the United States of America   10   9   8   7   6   5   4   3

Human Kinetics
Web site: www.HumanKinetics.com

United States: Human Kinetics
P.O. Box 5076
Champaign, IL 61825-5076
800-747-4457
e-mail: humank@hkusa.com

Canada: Human Kinetics
475 Devonshire Road Unit 100
Windsor, ON N8Y 2L5
800-465-7301 (in Canada only)
e-mail: orders@hkcanada.com

Europe: Human Kinetics
107 Bradford Road
Stanningley
Leeds LS28 6AT, United Kingdom
+44 (0) 113 255 5665
e-mail: hk@hkeurope.com

Australia: Human Kinetics
57A Price Avenue
Lower Mitcham, South Australia 5062
08 8372 0999
e-mail: liaw@hkaustralia.com

New Zealand: Human Kinetics
Division of Sports Distributors NZ Ltd.
P.O. Box 300 226 Albany
North Shore City
Auckland
0064 9 448 1207
e-mail: info@humankinetics.co.nz

I dedicate this work to two people whose unwavering
support allows me to discover and rediscover every day:
Adelle, my wife, who makes the old adage *Behind every good man there is a great woman*
more true than ever, and my son, Elan, who will always be my ultimate teacher.

We shall not cease from exploration,
and the end of all our exploring will be to arrive where
we started and know the place for the first time.
—*Little Gidding, T.S. Eliot, 1888-1965*

Contents

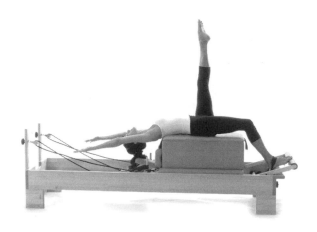

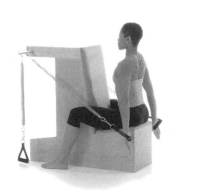

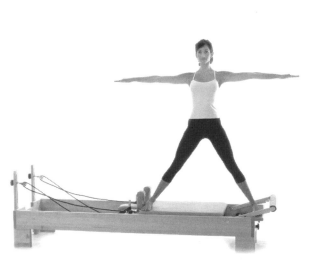

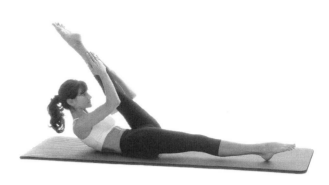

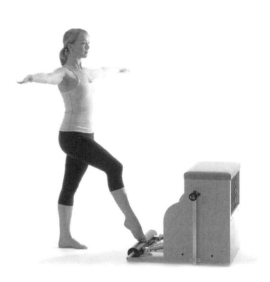

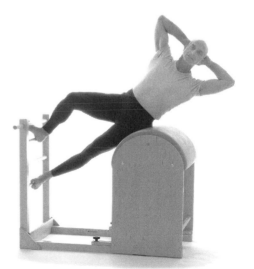

Foreword

When I first met Rael in Santa Fe, NM, in 1991 the Pilates community was indeed a small entity. Upon the recommendation of John Claude West, who had studied with me and was running his own studio in New York, I was invited to teach a workshop on the wunda chair, a Pilates apparatus that I had worked on a lot with Joseph Pilates. Until then, I had not been consulted for professional advice by the Pilates community. The gathering in Santa Fe was a breakthrough, first and foremost, in recognizing the first generation of Pilates teachers and also in the sharing of information and drawing on our collective experience and expertise.

Following a double knee surgery I was guided to Mr. Pilates by Pearl Lang, the renowned dancer and choreographer. He used the wunda chair extensively for my knee therapy as he felt I would particularly benefit from working on this apparatus. I received vast amounts of information and practiced primarily on the wunda chair for rehabilitation. I went on to develop my own repertoire and continued to use the wunda chair in my teaching at Henri Bendel from 1973 to 1988. I still use it in my teaching today, including the Pilates program I run for the Tisch School of the Arts at NYU.

When I entered the studio in Santa Fe, I was immediately surrounded by a group of seasoned professionals who had come from far and wide, hungry for information and enthusiastic about spending time with me. I noticed a man in the group, and when I asked for a volunteer to demonstrate some of the work he eagerly jumped up.

He got on the wunda chair and started demonstrating. I immediately recognized that he was an accomplished mover and that he knew Pilates well. As I started prodding and poking, making intricate adjustments to his alignment and movement, I could see a look of astonishment cross his face. The young male ego! This made me chuckle inside. He was clearly strong, but he relied too much on his strength and athletic ability rather than on his core.

We proceeded to work for several hours together as I taught, demonstrated, adjusted, and corrected. I respected his openness to learning and his humility in the presence of another teacher. That workshop was a pivotal point in the evolution of Pilates. From that point on the wunda chair, which had become all but obsolete, boomed in popularity. Rael has often expressed to me that our meeting changed his career. It set him on a path of inner exploration and self-assessment. His work changed and his teaching changed; he discovered how to work from within. Rael and I went on to become, above all else, good friends. I am now regarded as one of the Elders of the Pilates community, and Rael as a world-renowned teacher and a leader in his own right. He has developed a fine teacher training program, Body Arts and Science International, to which he invited me to serve as honorary advisor.

Back in 1991 Rael requested that I conduct a workshop at his center in Southern California. I made a promise to him that I would do it, but I could not say when.

Thereafter, on every occasion we met, he would remind me of my promise. It took 14 years for me to fulfill it. In 2005 I came to Southern California from New York to give a workshop at On Center Conditioning. Although Rael also taught, the students got to witness their mentor being guided by his mentor. This in itself was a valuable lesson, possibly more valuable than the work itself.

Rael performs the work with unique mastery, and he certainly moves from within. At the same time he dem-onstrates an ever-present youthful desire to continue learning and growing. We need to keep the lineage of Pilates alive, preserving the past and respecting the future, upholding the values and principles of this system—and few have done as much toward that end as Rael. He is the male that Mr. Pilates wished for to continue his work.

Kathy Stanford Grant
First-generation Pilates teacher, Pilates Elder

Preface

For more than 16 years I have wanted to commit my work as a teacher and student of Pilates into words, yet each time I attempted to do so the enormity of this system of physical and mental conditioning overwhelmed me. I knew that in order to offer something profound and valuable to Pilates enthusiasts I needed more knowledge and experience. So back to the studio I went, to master the repertoire of movements, to explore the work further, and to teach another few thousand sessions. This process of ever-expanding education spanned five continents and more practice hours than I could ever recall.

By 1990 I had already been doing Pilates for 10 years. I had earned a bachelor's degree from the Wingate Institute of Physical Education in Israel, danced professionally, and completed my master's degree in dance studies in England. I had been an avid competitive athlete since my youth and had practiced yoga since my early teens. Yet endeavoring to master Pilates felt like learning to crawl and walk again. This humbling process, which taught me how to move with an ease and flow that I had never before experienced, inspired me—and at times frustrated me. Apparently I had embarked on a lifelong journey of learning and practice that would deepen my understanding of movement and offer me a path to physical and mental well-being.

The time it has taken me to prepare to write this book makes the product well worth the wait. Not only has my own body of work, knowledge, and experience expanded exponentially, but Pilates has become a household name, and the number of people who practice it worldwide has grown exponentially. As a result, the demand for well-trained teachers has also increased. My educational organization, Body Arts and Science International, now conducts courses in 14 countries. Joseph Pilates had dreamed of universal recognition and growth and believed it could happen; yet even in his most ambitious dreams, he could not have envisioned the extent of the popularity of the Pilates method that we witness today. He wanted to see his method (which he called *Contrology*) taught in every school because he believed it could affect society in a positive way. He wanted the medical profession to embrace the physical and mental implications of his work on general well-being. His dream would come true in several respects. Today many of his principles and concepts are widely recognized. He has touched society as a whole in a positive way, and the medical profession is beginning to recognize the value in his system. I have always proclaimed that if everyone on Earth did Pilates mat work every day, we would live in a far better world—it simply makes you feel so good!

Joseph Pilates died, by many accounts, a disillusioned man. One need only read his book *Your Health,* in which he expresses his disdain for the medical profession and people's close-mindedness. I often ponder the tragedy that he and his wife, Clara, didn't live to witness the growth of the method to such mammoth proportions. Yet the spirit of their teaching lives on, and I feel a deep personal responsibility to uphold their work and its integrity to the highest of standards. I hope this book makes a valuable contribution to keeping the flame burning strong.

Acknowledgments

Pilates is the culmination of a career that has spanned almost 30 years, and several pages of acknowledgments would not suffice to thank all the people who have helped me along the way. Many people have taught, inspired, and guided me: students, teachers, colleagues, peers, friends, and my dear family. All have influenced the outcome of this book and all deserve my deepest gratitude.

I do want to highlight a few people who played important roles in the preparation of this book. Martin Barnard, who first approached me on behalf of Human Kinetics, always went beyond the call of duty to support me. I invariably came away from our conversations inspired and full of drive to create the best Pilates book possible. In moments of fatigue, Martin's words were like salve to the spirit. Thank you, my friend.

Julie Rhoda's editing skills played an enormous part in this final product. Her enthusiasm and positive attitude always made me feel as though my words were appreciated and my hard work was recognized. She never once signed off a letter without sending her warm regards and best wishes. Julie, you always have mine.

In the early phases of preparation, two friends, Dr. Jason Cheng and Chris Murray, spent hours drawing out of me imagery and descriptions for each exercise. They quizzed me, challenged my knowledge of human anatomy, spent hours transcribing our meetings, and offered generously of their own experience and knowledge. Jason is one of the finest osteopaths I have worked with, always searching for more knowledge and striving to grow. Chris is a colorful personality who is far too humble about his expertise in exercise, martial arts, and movement (and buying used cars).

Carol Appel is a jewel in the Pilates community and a very dear friend whose intelligent input is always appreciated. Her significant contribution to the historical overview in this book adds to its authenticity and advances the notion that education is a collective collaboration.

Kirk Fitzik, a photographer, designer, and friend, gave generously of his time, expertise, and enormous talent. He shot 2,500 pictures in the process. Kirk, I can only hope that you got as much out of the experience as I did.

It is with pride that I thank the talented models whose dedication and skill was an inspiration: Karla Adams, Lisa Clayton, Leah Turner, and Kristi Cooper-White. Each one of them has trained with me, is an accomplished teacher, is an active member of Body Arts and Science International, and is a devotee of this system. If they represent the future of Pilates, it is indeed very bright.

A hearty thank you to Lulu Lemon, who provided the clothing worn by the models in this book. Your generosity is greatly appreciated.

The staff and faculty of Body Arts and Science International, the Pilates education organization that I founded in 1989 and continue to direct, and On Center Conditioning, the beautiful Pilates studio in Southern California that I established in 1991, are the backbone of everything I do. I am proud to work with you all. I never get to thank you enough—thank you!

I am honored to have traveled this path of exploration and practice and to have encountered so many soulful people along the way.

Introduction

Pilates is the subject of many books that broach the topic from diverse angles. Yet this book is the first to take on the enormous task of providing a comprehensive overview and study of Pilates, including the full range of apparatus. It covers terrain that has previously been dealt with only in a few professional educational programs, presenting it clearly and concisely. It is my hope that *Pilates* becomes the definitive textbook for those who teach and practice the method with commitment and life-changing intent. This book is for professionals and serious enthusiasts who seek a deeper understanding of the Pilates method—from the muscle focus and action of the exercises to the far-reaching benefits. It guides teachers and students through the philosophy and much of the vast repertoire of the Pilates method.

All mentions of Pilates and the Pilates method in this book refer to the system of physical and mental conditioning developed by Joseph Hubertus Pilates. Although some of the movements differ from the exact manner or sequence in which he performed them, this text is inspired by and closely aligned with his original works. The legacy passed down by this man, whom the great choreographer George Balanchine called the "genius of the body," remains an invaluable resource. Joseph and his wife, Clara, set up the first Pilates studio in New York City soon after arriving on the shores of America from Germany in the mid-1920s. The rest is history—and an important and fundamental aspect of the method itself. Understanding the method's history allows one to understand the movements and see them in the context of society at that time, noting the lifestyle and general activities of people in the 1920s. At that time, computers did not exist to give people round-shoulder syndrome; there was no fast food hastening people on their way to obesity; fewer cars meant that people were more active; and lower back pain was not a complaint of 80 percent of the population as it is today. It was a very different world.

Pilates covers the art and science of human movement as it relates to the Pilates method. I believe that every movement of this method can and should be substantiated both scientifically (through anatomy, physiology, biomechanics, and kinesiology) and artistically (through aesthetics, inner sensations, psychological components, and the flow of energy and life force). The significant overlap between the art and science of human movement has been recognized and explored through the ages. The mind and the body share a nourishing, symbiotic relationship that brings about profound and at times inexplicable results. This mind–body relationship lies at the heart of Pilates.

An in-depth exploration of each aspect of Pilates would far exceed the parameters of this book; for instance, 100 pages on just breathing would not suffice to cover the topic. Instead I provide information about the Pilates method as a whole, emphasizing the repertoire, exercise presentation, description, and analysis. Of course a discussion of breathing is included since it is one of the tenets of the method, and a breathing pattern is offered for each exercise. Similarly the subjects of anatomy, physiology, and biomechanics are not covered here in detail, but a working knowledge of these areas of study is important for Pilates professionals and serious enthusiasts. If you require more information about a particular subject or area of study, seek out further knowledge and understanding. See the selected resources list at the end of the book for suggestions.

Brief History of Pilates

Joseph Pilates was born near Düsseldorf, Germany, in 1880. He was a sickly child, plagued with rickets, asthma, and rheumatic fever. His drive to overcome these ailments led him to explore and practice bodybuilding, gymnastics, diving, and other physical pursuits. He studied Eastern and Western philosophies and forms of exercise and was greatly influenced by ancient Greek and Roman regimens. This rich background provided him with the foundation, shaped by his experiences, to innovate a system that he developed throughout his life.

In 1912, Pilates traveled to England as a circus performer in a living Greek statue act. When World War I broke out, he was interned in a camp on the Isle of Man along with other German nationals. While there, he taught and practiced his physical fitness program and began devising apparatus to aid in the rehabilitation of the disabled and sick. A look at the apparatus of today reveals that certain pieces must have been fashioned around the frame of a hospital bed. Pilates is credited with assisting many victims of the influenza epidemic and helping others recover from wartime diseases.

After the war, Pilates returned to Germany and was invited by the German government to train the new army. Recognizing the implications of this, he decided to leave for America. (By certain accounts he was invited to the United States to help train world title holding boxer Max Schmeling from Germany.) The period before Pilates' immigration to the United States is not well documented, but he appears to have met some of the great European movement innovators of that time, such as Rudolf von Laban, Kurt Jooss, and Mary Wigman. Although Pilates was not a dancer, these early encounters may have set the stage for his profound involvement with the dance community later in his career.

On the way over to the United States, Joseph met Clara, who soon became his wife and played an integral role in developing and teaching his method. She has been described as a compassionate, knowledgeable, and kind teacher, in some ways a superior teacher to Joseph Pilates himself. In 1926 they set up their first studio in New York City, which attracted a diverse population, including socialites, circus performers, gymnasts, and athletes.

But those who truly recognized the value of Pilates' system and his inherent, deep understanding of the workings of the human body were the members of the dance community, including luminaries such as George Balanchine, Ted Shawn, Martha Graham, and Hanya Holm. They embraced the method, often integrating it into their dance technique and training, as they witnessed its positive effects on dancers' bodies in both rehabilitation and performance.

Pilates was a disciplined man, as his teaching and his physical condition and performance reveal. His work shows the influence of yoga, gymnastics, boxing, martial arts, and Eastern and Western philosophies. He taught

Pilates takes you through a range of exercise levels, from fundamental through intermediate and finally touching on the advanced level. The book's 205 exercises are conveniently organized; each piece of apparatus is addressed in a separate chapter. The exercises in each chapter are grouped into blocks based on regions of the body, and within each block are series of exercises. The description of each exercise includes its level of difficulty and a recommended resistance range. I also provide a muscle focus, objectives of the exercise, commentary, some ideas for imagery that will prove valuable in both executing and teaching the movements, and a checklist

and demonstrated his work in many environments, from the studio to his small New York apartment to the outdoors, where he seemed the most comfortable and inspired. He had the drive of a believer and the creativity of a genius. This was a man who believed deeply in his system as a way of life. He was convinced that it could affect every facet of one's being, and therefore society as a whole.

Pilates dreamed of seeing his work taught in every college and school. He believed that children should be given knowledge of the body, and that the information should be simple and accessible. He revered the simplicity of movement and the elegance of nature's design of the body, both human and animal. Many early articles on Pilates describe his passion for animals and animal-like movement, which is indicated by the names he gave to several of the exercises.

Over the course of his career Pilates developed more than 600 exercises for the various pieces of apparatus he invented. His guiding philosophy was that achieving good health means that the whole being—body, mind, and spirit—must be addressed. Pilates equipment is designed to condition the entire body, using positions and movements that simulate functional activities and thereby correct body alignment and balance. An extensive repertoire of exercises, from fundamental to master level, can be done on each piece of apparatus. Using springs, pulleys, and gravity, the equipment challenges the musculature in diverse ways, with particular focus on the intrinsic muscles. These deep layers of muscle are encouraged to work to achieve optimum movement mechanics and maintain correct positioning and alignment.

Joseph Pilates was a man ahead of his time in his approach to well being, in his creation of exercises, and in his invention of exercise equipment and its integration into home life. He arguably created the first home gym with the invention of the wunda chair, which doubled as a piece of furniture. The image of Joseph Pilates extolling the virtues of his equipment in his New York apartment, with Clara looking on, suggests that his presentations exceeded the bounds of mere demonstration. Rare footage corroborates this impression; Pilates produced a film that explains and promotes the many facets of his system, including personal health tips and showering techniques. Something between an instructional guide and an infomercial, the film suggests that Pilates was ahead of his time in his marketing methods as well as his approach to health and fitness. Years after his death, his work has possibly spearheaded a revolution in the world of fitness and led to an evolution of the wellness industry.

The Pilates method offers a path to total health. It is not merely a physical fitness regimen of mindlessly repeated exercises. Pilates is a holistic approach to well-being and a lifelong process of refinement. In the opening paragraph of his book *Return to Life Through Contology,* Pilates wrote, "Physical fitness is the first requisite to happiness. Our interpretation of physical fitness is the attainment and maintenance of a uniformly developed body with a sound mind fully capable of naturally, easily, and satisfactorily performing our many and varied daily tasks with spontaneous zest and pleasure."

of points that help ensure a positive outcome. This book does not include the most advanced and master-level work, which warrant a separate book altogether.

Over the years several approaches to the practice of the Pilates method have emerged. One approach advocates doing the work, building the apparatus, and sequencing the exercises exactly as Pilates did. Other approaches deal primarily with rehabilitation; they have created protocols for specific treatments that use the Pilates apparatus but have changed the repertoire substantially. Often practitioners do not address the original repertoire or the holistic aspect of the work; and at times the relationship to the source is very loose indeed. Still other approaches deal with specific populations, such as dancers or athletes, adapting the repertoire to their needs and, again, at times forgoing the original Pilates exercises and philosophy.

Throughout this book and in my teaching and practice I strive to remain true to the essence of Joseph Pilates' work while allowing an evolutionary process to take place. I call this approach Body Arts and Science, and out of it has grown Body Arts and Science International (BASI), an educational organization that teaches Pilates to professionals. The approach incorporates the art and science of the Pilates method in a contemporary context, along with a desire to share this dynamic system with enthusiasts and professionals worldwide.

Joseph Pilates planted the seeds of a new approach to body conditioning, yet we can surmise that he did not define or even understand many of the concepts as we do today. Computers and sophisticated research methods enable us to scientifically substantiate notions that were largely based on intuition. Therapists have long yearned for a system that could take patients from the early stages of rehabilitation to the long-term goal of a conditioned, efficiently functioning body. Athletes have searched for ways to gain an extra edge to peak their performance in competition. For years, dancers have looked for a system by which they could improve their strength, flexibility, and mechanics while maintaining the body type they are required to have. Gymnasts, figure skaters, runners, actors, circus performers, musicians, singers—and the list goes on—constantly seek to enhance their performance and extend their careers. Over time, and now more than ever, we have come to realize that the mind as well as the body should be addressed. Herein lies the true potential of the Pilates method. If the performances of world-class athletes are separated by only hundredths, sometimes thousandths of a second, more strength or flexibility will not help them secure victory; they have maximized that already. Nor will adding five hours of practice to an already grueling weekly schedule. It is tapping into the potential of the mind and its intricate connection to the body that will provide the elusive edge. Many have found the answer in Pilates.

Pilates not only offers a bridge between mind and body, between everyday life and optimal performance, between rehabilitation and healthy movement; it also offers a system that, when used to its full potential, can enhance every aspect of life. It offers a solution to those with restricted mobility and to elite athletes. It is as beneficial for an 11-year-old as it is for an 80-year-old and as motivating for men as for women. It is adaptable and diverse, and that is its magic—not that it can transform the body in a few sessions or offer a perfect physique at the wave of a wand (which unfortunately is sometimes claimed). Pilates is for the elderly who cannot find an environment, equipment, or system suited to their needs. It is for the person who wants to look and feel better. It is for someone who wants to function at an optimal level, pain free. It is for people who seek balance in life, who want to change their lives for the better. Pilates, in other words, is for anyone and everyone.

CHAPTER 1

Enhancing the Mind and Body

Is the exponential growth of Pilates—a method known by few people before the year 2000—merely hype? Why this sudden growth spurt? The reasons for the enormous popularity of Pilates lie in its far-reaching, diverse benefits, which include but are not limited to improvements in fitness and athletic performance, enhanced appearance, and a heightened sense of well-being.

The dance community has long benefited from Pilates for good reason. Dancers are supreme athletes, as measured by the feats they perform and the level of physical fitness they exhibit. But they suffer a very high incidence of injury—some studies suggest even higher than among football players. Dancers need an exceptional conditioning regimen that supplements their dance training and assists in injury prevention and rehabilitation. A dancer myself, I have often proclaimed that Joseph Pilates is the unsung hero of the dance world, given that many a dance career has been enhanced or saved by this method. Now everyone can benefit from the method that dancers have used as a form of cross-training for so many years, and, in some ways, enjoy the same results.

Athletes were the first to utilize cross-training extensively and to recognize the far-reaching rewards of doing so. Yet they are only now awakening to Pilates—and embracing it—as a legitimate form of cross-training to enhance performance and prevent injury. Many of these athletes have at their fingertips any form of conditioning they choose to improve their performance. The fact that so many elect to use Pilates is a testament to its value. It is good for the highest-ranked golfers and the best swimmers in the world; the most elite dancers, figure skaters, and tennis players; the fastest, highest

To achieve the highest accomplishments within the scope of our capabilities in all walks of life, we must constantly strive to acquire strong, healthy bodies and develop our minds to the limit of our ability.
—Joseph H. Pilates, *Return to Life Through Contrology*

jumping ball players; and a host of actors, singers, and musicians. At the same time it is also the best possible choice for people who have never exercised before and is an excellent foray into the world of fitness.

In 2000 I gave a presentation on enhancing athletic performance using the Pilates method. In preparation I informally surveyed some Olympic-level athletes, asking them what they looked for in a cross-training regimen and how they thought Pilates could help their performance. The answers varied with the person and the activity. But most of the responses included two goals: to improve core strength and to explore the benefits of mind–body control and power. These two concepts encapsulate the essence of Pilates; very few, if any, training regimens are as effective as Pilates in achieving these goals.

Is Pilates for everyone? Yes. Will everyone select Pilates as their fitness regimen? No. Not everyone will relate to the Pilates approach, and for certain training goals it may not be the most effective choice. For instance, bodybuilders interested in increasing muscle mass are better served by weight training. Sprinters who wish to gain speed and quickness may prefer plyometrics or another form of resistance training. (Although I believe that even bodybuilders and sprinters would benefit greatly from certain aspects of Pilates, such as the core strength it develops, the heightened awareness it provides, and the flexibility and the control it offers.) Still, the adaptability and wide appeal of Pilates is astounding. It can serve a broad spectrum of the population since its benefits are not limited to the young or the super-fit or super-athletic. I have witnessed positive changes in posture, alignment, weight, and body-mass distribution resulting from Pilates that have startled me in their profundity. I have seen positive changes in self-image, athletic performance, and ability to perform daily activities. My clients have shared heartwarming stories of improvement in their personal and sexual relations. I have witnessed, and experienced myself, rehabilitation programs that use Pilates following surgery and injury that were successful beyond all expectations. It sounds too good to be true. Yet these responses are witnessed time and again throughout the world, and the international community is taking notice. The fact that scientific research now substantiates many of these anecdotal findings adds new (and welcome) credibility to the practice of Pilates.

Of course, Pilates is not a potion that cures all and brings about miraculous changes immediately. Change takes time, commitment, and discipline. If you are dedicated to regular Pilates sessions, three times a week for at least six weeks, some positive changes are inevitable. Although certain changes can and often do occur immediately—for instance, a change in body awareness, muscle activation, or alignment—it takes time for most adaptations to become imprinted in the neuromuscular system, for muscles to transform, and for the transformation to be integrated into a person's life.

I have enjoyed every client I have taught, including many professional dancers, athletes, and celebrities. But one of the most gratifying experiences I have had was working with a woman named Stella who came to me at age 76 with severe scoliosis and an array of muscular and structural imbalances. The medical literature would say that changes could not be made to this woman's alignment, posture, or movement at this point in her life. In fact, it would probably say that without either surgery or bracing during her preteen years, no changes in her physical alignment could have occurred at any point in her life. But Stella worked with a commitment and dedication that I had seldom seen. She inspired all those around her, people of all ages and fitness levels,

including me. After my first session with Stella I realized how unique she was, and she realized that she had found a system that could affect her life greatly. Within the first few sessions her awareness improved and she started recognizing the immense imbalances that had infiltrated her body. After 30 sessions she moved differently, her posture improved, her confidence was elevated—in fact, her whole life changed. She realized early on that these results were only the beginning, that remaining committed for the long haul—not for days, weeks, or months, but for years—was imperative. And remain committed she did! Was it simply the method, the exercises, and the apparatus? I believe not. It was Stella. She has a positive outlook, determination, and a powerful drive. Pilates provided a vehicle and the tools for changes to take place. Did she suddenly have a straight spine?

The Many Benefits of Pilates

Develops every aspect of physical fitness: strength, flexibility, coordination, speed, agility, and endurance

Heightens body awareness

Enhances body control

Teaches correct muscle activation

Corrects posture and alignment

Facilitates optimal function of the internal organs

Improves balance and proprioception

Focuses on breathing and its related physical and psychological benefits (see Breathing on page 7)

Offers a vehicle for concentration and focus

Promotes relaxation and the release of tension

Helps keep musculature and bone structure in an optimal state

Benefits pregnant women by providing a safe, effective, nonimpact exercise activity

Serves as cross-training for athletic pursuits and daily activities

Distributes body mass more aesthetically (people report looking and feeling slimmer)

Provides a path to inner harmony through a finely tuned body

Absolutely not. Such a change to the skeletal structure could not take place at this age. Yet her alignment, muscular control, and efficiency in movement did change. Her level of pain decreased dramatically and she began to enjoy her daily activities, especially her beloved gardening, relatively pain free.

I believe the body is the divine temple of all that lies within. It carries the nucleus of who we are and embodies our true potential. Although I have spent much of my life tuning my body as if it were a fine musical instrument, I knew viscerally from an early age (and later consciously) that physical activity, be it Pilates, yoga, dance, surfing, windsurfing, running, or paragliding, ultimately serves my inner being. The physical benefits are undoubtedly important, but the effects on the inner being carry implications that are infinite. They influence how you function, how you feel, how you relate to yourself and those around you, and how successful you are in every respect. Simplistically, it makes you feel good. And if you feel good, you feel healthy, you function well, you are fulfilled, and life seems more complete. The old adage that proclaims that within a healthy body lies a healthy mind could go one step further: A healthy mind guides a healthy body.

Mind and Body As One

Discussion of the mind–body connection is as old as the ages; it rises up every now and again like a tidal wave. The 1970s and '80s saw trends that focused on the physical being—hard-driving approaches with infamous mottos such as *No pain, no gain* or *Work 'til you drop*. More recently the fitness industry has returned to a mind–body focus—calmer, more introspective, refined, integrated systems of exercise and movement. We've seen resurgence in the popularity of yoga and Pilates, an emphasis on nurturing the body rather than punishing it, and a renewed focus on the power of the mind–body connection. Today this connection is being proven scientifically, not only with surveys but also with research based on brain-scan imaging that reveals changes in the brain that occur as a result of changes in the body, and vice versa.

Joseph Pilates created his system of exercises with the intention that it should positively affect every aspect of a person's life—from movement to interpersonal relationships to heightened performance in daily tasks—leading the way to a state of total well-being. He believed that widespread practice of his system, based as it is on the mind–body connection, would eliminate many diseases and social ills. The Pilates method is more than a series of exercises; it is an approach to life, a philosophy. Time and again Pilates reminds us that his system addresses the whole being. It dictates that we be aware of the changes that occur daily on every level of our being. These changes can be positive (such as rejuvenation and increased energy) or negative (such as rising stress and ailments). To reap the full potency of Pilates, you must make it an integrated part of your life, which will enrich every day. To practice Pilates is to strive to achieve balance and maximize the potential of the body, mind, and spirit.

The key to the positive effects of Pilates lies in its principles, not its exercises and equipment. It is a mind–body system that, unlike many forms of physical fitness, not only addresses the quantifiable aspects of human movement such as strength, range of motion, and endurance but also looks at awareness, balance, control, efficiency, function, and harmony. In so doing stabilization is developed, posture is refined, mechanics of movement are improved, muscle recruitment patterns are reeducated, and function and well-being are reinforced—the ultimate goal of any good conditioning program. Pilates can and will improve every facet of your life.

Three Higher Principles

Return to Life Through Contrology opens with these words: "Physical fitness is the first requisite of happiness." It is a bold statement that could seem judgmental, but on reading further you discover that Joseph Pilates recognized that each person has different capabilities. What his opening statement claims is that the mind and body are intricately linked and that the condition of the body influences the state of the mind, and vice versa. He continuously reinforces this premise in his writing and teachings, reiterating how physical condition relates not only to happiness but also to many other mental states (positive or negative depending on the body's condition), such as relaxation, pleasure, anxiety, and depression. He claimed that by reawakening thousands of dormant muscle cells, we also awaken thousands of dormant brain cells. The body stimulates the functioning of the mind. It is essentially a case of the muscles building the brain.

Despite the size, complexity, and scope of the Pilates method, three themes, which I call the *higher principles,* remain constant. They are guides that help us navigate the lifelong exploration of Pilates. The way in which we define certain elements of the work and describe the movements may change as new research is conducted and modern terminology is created. But these are only words and definitions, the glossary of the system; the philosophy encompassed in these principles never changes. It is the essence of the system itself.

1. **Completely coordinate the body, mind, and spirit.** This goal is the method's driving force—integrating into each exercise the balance of body, mind, and spirit. As Pilates wrote in *Return to Life Through Contrology,* achieving this balance "results in perfect posture." Without recognizing this principle and integrating it into your work, you will feel that your body lacks its life force. Although the body, mind, and spirit share an ever-changing relationship, these components are present throughout our lives. With the practice of Pilates we become aware of their relationship. Finding the balance is a lifelong journey.

2. **Achieve the natural inner rhythm associated with all subconscious activities.** The highest level of motor learning we can attain is when an action is practiced to the point of becoming subconscious. This does not mean that we do it without concentration or awareness; instead, as the movement pattern becomes imprinted in the muscle memory, we can focus on fine-tuning it as opposed being consumed with the action itself. Mastery cannot be achieved in a short time; it is the reward of consistent training over a long period of time, sometimes years. Such training requires discipline and commitment on every level, as well as patience and endurance. But ultimately it is the path to complete health, happiness, and efficiency. As Pilates wrote in *Return to Life Through Contrololology,* "Correctly executed and mastered to the point of subconscious reaction, these exercises will reflect grace and balance in your routine activities" (page 63).

3. **Apply the natural laws of life to everyday living.** Pilates greatly admired nature and the animal kingdom. He often wrote about the graceful and efficient movements of animals, and he considered them far more evolved than humans in terms of movement and muscular development. Many of today's human ills and ailments are a result of people losing touch with the natural laws of living. Sitting at computers for many hours a day, watching television for many more, eating far in excess of our needs (often unhealthy food), and driving and seldom walking are some of the lifestyle changes of the past few decades. Pilates wrote in *Your Health,* "Man has, in the race for material progress and perfection, entirely overlooked the most complex and marvelous of all Creations—Man himself!"

In addition to the *higher principles*, I have identified 10 *movement principles* that are an amalgamation of those cited by Pilates and those that have evolved through my personal experience in this work. Each movement principle applies to every exercise in this book and should be integrated into your practice.

Ten Movement Principles

Pilates practitioners should be mindful of these principles at all times, during both the execution of the exercises and the teaching of the movements. They are the foundation of this mind–body system, serving to guide teachers and students toward understanding, mastery, and well-being. They are what make the Pilates method unique. They evolved from the three higher principles and are closely linked to the underlying philosophy behind them.

If the higher principles are the soul of the system, the movement principles are its personality and character.

Principle 1: Become Aware

The first step into the wonderful world of Pilates, and every step that follows, should be filled with awareness and mindfulness. Be present in the movement with mind and body. In some forms of physical conditioning, everything about the environment seems designed to separate the mind from the body: loud music, television screens, games mounted on exercise equipment, and a myriad of other distractions. Pilates is practiced in an environment that stimulates the mind–body connection, beginning with an awareness of the body.

No one can address the process of realigning the body without an awareness of its structure and how it moves. Often I will say to a client whose leg is not straight, "Please straighten your leg all the way." He will answer, "But it is straight." At other times I will adjust a client's head so that it sits on the centerline of the body, and the response is, "That feels very lopsided." Over time we become accustomed to misalignments, and the less aware a person is, the more severe these misalignments become, until an off-center body part feels centered or a bent limb feels straight. Bringing awareness to the body and the intricacies of movement establishes a foundation for change. Without awareness, little can be achieved.

Principle 2: Achieve Balance

The term *balance* can mean many things. It can relate to components of fitness such as strength and flexibility, to the act of standing on one leg, or to the symmetry of the body. It can also describe a well-designed Pilates program, in which the exercises are proportionately distributed to work different parts of the body in a session (an important consideration in Pilates). Due to the method's focus on the abdominal region, Pilates programs are often excessively weighted toward abdominal work, particularly in forward flexion. This is a mistake. There needs to be a balance in working the various muscle groups as well as the different planes of motion. The word *balance* may also refer to the well-being of the whole individual, a balance of body, mind, and spirit. You should strive to achieve balance, in every sense of the word, and make it an integral part of your Pilates practice.

Joseph Pilates often mentioned the importance of a uniformly developed musculature, stating that only when the muscles are developed in such a way can the body function unhindered, true flexibility be present, and well-being be achieved. This idea touches on several issues, including pure muscular development, ease of function, and the mind–body relationship. Symmetrically and proportionately developed musculature allows the spine to perform its function to support the body and to assist in movement ranging from fine, intravertebral articulation to large powerful actions of the trunk.

Musculoskeletal conditions frequently show patterns of muscular imbalance for multiple reasons. Some patterns are associated with dominance on one side (referred to as *handedness*), some with postural deviations such as scoliosis and kyphosis, and others related to lack of flexibility or excessive flexibility. Imbalances that affect body alignment or result from misalignment are important factors in many painful postural conditions. At times muscles react to protect the body from harm or to reduce pain, with the result that certain muscles become overactive while others are inhibited. Muscle

> The pursuit of awareness is endless—it is what makes Pilates so interesting, intriguing, and rewarding.

imbalance may result as well from occupational or recreational activities that create movement habits in which certain muscles are used persistently while the opposing muscles are inadequately trained. Examples include always holding the phone to the ear on the same side resulting in a chronic tilt of the head, standing with the weight shifted onto one leg resulting in a perpetual tilt of the pelvis, or playing a one-side–dominant sport such as tennis, resulting in asymmetric muscular development.

Each person has different needs in terms of imbalances and how to alleviate them. Identifying and addressing these needs is the first step on the path to achieving balance. As we practice and teach Pilates, we must act as detectives, constantly making observations of our own bodies and those of our students. I provide some basic tools later in the book, such as the roll-down (see page 24), that help assess alignment and identify imbalances.

Principle 3: Breathe Correctly

At the root of the natural laws of life and natural inner rhythm is breathing. Pilates wrote in *Return to Life Through Contrology,* "Breathing is the first act of life, and the last . . . above all, learn how to breathe correctly." Breathing is synonymous with life and with movement. It is all-encompassing; the link between body, mind, and spirit. Breathing is immensely important and powerful, yet it is so often ignored. One deep breath can promote relaxation, release stress, and bring a smile to one's face.

Everything, from the minutest movement to life itself, begins with breath. Breathing is the inner shower that cleanses the body, guides the mind, and rejuvenates the spirit; it promotes natural movement and is the first step to educating the neuromuscular system. Breathing is also a vehicle by which to achieve inner focus, and a path to relaxing the mind and calming the spirit. It is the engine that drives all movement, and it lies at the source of the Pilates method.

Certain muscle groups are recruited during the breath cycle to assist in respiration and therefore must be considered in determining a breathing pattern for a given exercise. For instance, we theorize that exhaling during abdominal work maximizes abdominal muscle recruitment because of the known participation of these muscles in exhalation. Conversely we theorize that since the trunk extensors assist in inhalation, inhaling during trunk extension probably maximizes their recruitment. Clearly both of these muscle groups can be recruited during both inhalation and exhalation, but muscle contraction may be more profound when it corresponds with the breathing. Although scientific proof for these assertions is lacking, my experience as a practitioner and a teacher has convinced me that they are true.

Normal breathing is a complex process that involves many joints and muscles and is responsive to both voluntary and involuntary control. Basic understanding of the breath cycle is important because it offers insight into movement and exercise in general. A crucial muscle to cite when discussing breathing is the diaphragm, a dome-shaped muscle that forms a canopy underlying the rib cage (figure 1.1). The diaphragm plays an important role in breathing and in creating the "muscular corset,"

Breathing

Oxygenates the blood and nourishes the body on a cellular level
Expels toxins from the body
Improves circulation
Improves skin tone
Calms the mind and the body
Encourages concentration
Provides a rhythm for movement
Assists in activating target muscles

the internal cylinder of support that is addressed throughout this book.

During diaphragmatic breathing 75 percent of the respiratory effort comes from the diaphragm. When this muscle contracts, it flattens, increasing the vertical dimension of the thorax. In addition, the external intercostal muscles contract, pulling the lower ribs upward. Because of the orientation of the ribs and their joints (the lower part of the rib cage is wider than the upper part), the lower region of the thorax expands laterally as the diaphragm rises, increasing the lateral dimension of the rib cage. In contrast, as the upper ribs rise they increase the anterior-to-posterior dimension of the thorax, with the sternum moving forward. The overall effect is an increase in thoracic volume, a decrease in intrapulmonary pressure, and air flowing into the lungs—in other words, inhalation.

When the diaphragm relaxes, the organs in the abdominal cavity and abdominal muscles push it upward into its dome shape, thus decreasing the vertical dimension of the thorax. Added to this, the elasticity (recoil) of the lungs and chest wall create decreased thoracic volume and increased intrapulmonary pressure, resulting in air flowing out of the lungs, or exhalation.

In Pilates, we make an effort to emphasize the lateral and posterior expansion of the rib cage during inhalation (called *lateral* or *costal breathing*). Besides drawing air into the lungs, this mode of breathing facilitates the maintenance of abdominal muscle contraction throughout the exercise, which in turn helps stabilize the trunk of the body. During the exhalation phase of Pilates exercises, the abdominal muscles contract further to assist the diaphragm and intercostals in expelling air. (Imagine a process of milking the

Breath is the fuel for what Joseph Pilates called the powerhouse, the engine that drives the movement.

lungs and wringing the air out.) This in turn promotes deeper inhalation on the part of the primary respiratory muscles and the auxiliary muscles (including the back extensors), bringing in a healthy quantity of oxygen-filled air to nourish and rejuvenate the body.

Abdominal muscle contraction typically needs to be maintained throughout the movement, which can be particularly challenging during inhalation. Using lateral breathing with a consistent inward pull of the abdominal wall allows one to maintain abdominal contraction during both inhalation and exhalation; diaphragmatic breathing, by contrast, encourages relaxation of the abdominal muscles during inhalation. This by no means implies that diaphragmatic breathing is undesirable, quite the contrary. However, lateral breathing is the preferred mode of breathing during some forms of physical activity, including Pilates. Many people have commented to me over the years that they have found focusing on breathing, practicing breathing, and learning lateral breathing to be immensely beneficial. Those who have made such remarks include opera singers and rock singers, who typically train using predominantly diaphragmatic breathing—and who need every bit of breath they can get!

Breathing can be practiced anywhere at anytime. I find two exercises particularly helpful in mastering lateral breathing. The first is to wrap a 3-foot length of elastic exercise band around your chest, holding the ends of the band in your hands, and expanding your chest against the resistance of the band. This illustrates and emphasizes how it feels to breathe laterally. The other involves lying supine on a mat in a comfortable neutral spine position, knees bent, legs parallel, and arms by the sides of the body. Visualize that with each breath the chest expands and spreads laterally across the mat in both directions like two waves rising in the ocean and then gently falling

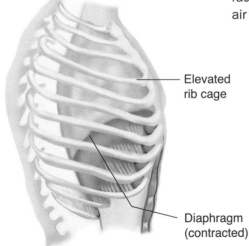

Elevated
rib cage

Diaphragm
(contracted)

FIGURE 1.1 The diaphragm plays a critical role in breathing correctly and maximizing the benefits of Pilates.

Reprinted, by permission, from M.A. Williams, 2000, Cardiovascular and respiratory physiology: Responses to exercise. In *Essentials of strength training and conditioning,* 2nd ed., edited by T.R. Baechle and R.W. Earle (Champaign, IL: Human Kinetics), 121.

back. This is a great form of meditation and good practice for breathing. You can also channel the breath to either side of the chest, if an imbalance is present and one side is not as active as the other. This is often the case when scoliosis is present and one side of the thorax is relatively collapsed. You can channel the breath like a river of energy to the less active side or to any part of the body that needs to be relaxed, released, or activated.

Principle 4: Concentrate Deeply

I view concentration as the bridge between awareness and movement. As you establish the starting position for each movement, I encourage you to go through a checklist of important data: which muscles you need to recruit, how you should align your body, and your chosen breathing pattern. Simply by concentrating on a particular muscle prior to the action, you can motivate it to fire more accurately and intensely than if you do not think about it. Concentrating on your body alignment will help you recruit the correct muscles and avoid unnecessary strain on the body. Concentrating on the breathing pattern will help you maintain a good rhythm for the movement and keep your mind focused. However, keep in mind that concentration can be so intense that it becomes counterproductive. It can morph into tension, which leads to a tightening of the musculature, a restriction in breathing, and halting rather than flowing movement. This is clearly not the intention and should be avoided.

Although awareness and concentration are closely related, I regard awareness as a state of mind—of being mindful and feeling the movement. Concentration is a more cognitive process of understanding the movement. Concentration, combined with awareness, not only promises precise movement but also gives the work a meditative quality. Being meditative does not imply that the work will lack challenge, physical demand, or intensity; it means ensuring a deep focus to the work that allows you to block out unnecessary thoughts and

perform each movement to the maximum of your ability, thus reaping the benefits of Pilates.

Principle 5: Center Yourself

Centering yourself can be defined in purely physical terms—finding where your center of gravity lies. In women the center lies approximately anterior to the first and second sacral segments, floating in the middle of the pelvic bowl. In men it tends to be slightly higher, in the center of the body opposite the navel. Differences in anatomy result in different weight distribution—men tend to be top heavy and women carry their weight in the pelvic region. Discovering and experiencing your body's center of gravity is important because this is the *powerhouse*. The concept of the powerhouse—that all movement emanates from this core—is a common thread in the practice of Pilates and is addressed in more detail in chapter 2 (page 17). In Pilates, centering yourself means more than finding your center of gravity; it means uniting body, mind, and spirit.

The concept of centering is not new. In Eastern practices we learn of *ki* in aikido, *chi* in tai chi, *tan tien* in chi gong, and *chakra* in yoga—all refer, in general terms, to the life force that lies within us like a bottomless well of energy. Interestingly, in all these practices this life force is located in approximately the same area of the body. Martha Graham focused on this area in her modern dance technique and altered the way dancers approached dance and movement; the contraction (a deep flexion of the spine), involving deep abdominal activation, became the foundation of her technique. The feeling of being centered relates not only to the energy emanating from this eternal spring but also to the support provided by the area's strong, intrinsic muscles and a person's ability to tap into this physical and metaphysical support system. It is not uncommon to hear a dancer speak of feeling centered or, conversely, lacking center. As you delve into Pilates and open yourself to finding and moving from your center, you will experience this most gratifying and elevating of sensations.

Principle 6: Gain Control

Gaining control is an amalgamation of all the preceding principles. When you watch people move, particularly during complex movements, it is immediately evident whether they have a high level of control. Few things are as beautiful and inspiring as viewing athletes, dancers, gymnasts, or figure skaters who have immaculate control over their movement. Similarly, watching a lion walk, a cheetah run, or a gazelle leap can evoke a feeling of awe. Kathy Stanford Grant, a student of Joseph Pilates who became a great teacher of his work, periodically sends me phenomenal pictures of animals in balance or in motion. She points out their grace, effortless quality, and unencumbered movement. These characteristics are lofty goals, but something to aspire to.

Initially, achieving control of movement is a conscious process. It occurs through practice, practice, and more practice. Ideally a teacher who has achieved control should guide you in this process. As you continue to train and integrate the work into your body, sometimes for years and many hundreds of repetitions, your own movement control becomes like that of an animal's—a part of your being.

Principle 7: Be Efficient

Who does not want to conserve energy? Waste has become a byproduct of our society in every way. Striving for efficiency teaches us to focus our energy. When performing Pilates we do not grimace during effort, nor grunt as the movements become difficult and demanding. We focus the work where it is needed, exerting the required amount of energy, no more and no less. The remainder of the body is relaxed and calm. I have an internal agreement with myself when performing the work; the more difficult and demanding the movements are, the more consciously relaxed I become. I view efficiency of movement as a laser beam: focused and directed.

Achieving efficiency applies not only to athletic feats but also to everyday movements. An important stage in the process of learning Pilates is transferal, that is, the ability to transfer information learned and practiced in the Pilates session into everyday activities and to integrate it into other aspects of life. A session lasts only about an hour, and this time is often supervised by an instructor. During the remaining 23 hours of the day, we must actively direct our own attention. I recommend creating reminders for yourself to practice transferal. This is like placing notes on a bulletin board, except these notes are mental ones that remind you to keep your head centered, align your spine, use your powerhouse, relax, and ultimately move effortlessly.

When control becomes innate, you have reached the point of mastery.

Principle 8: Create Flow

Like all the principles, flow manifests itself both physically and mentally. It manifests within each movement as well as within the Pilates session as a whole. Flow can be described as the unobstructed channeling and translation of energy into movement. It is also the seamless connecting of movement to movement, creating what appears to be a continuous motion. Despite the fact that teachers offer correction and input to students and may need to stop the class periodically to do so, the overall sense of each individual movement and of the session as a whole should be one of continuum.

If you observe people like inspirational golfer Tiger Woods, dynamic swimmer Ian Thorpe, and brilliant dancer

Mikhail Baryshnikov, you will note a common quality: an effortless flow in their movements. You can experience the same quality through the practice of Pilates.

Flow can be understood physiologically as the immaculate timing of muscle recruitment. In each movement there is an optimal sequence in which the muscles should fire, called a muscle-recruitment or muscle-firing pattern. When muscle recruitment is not only correct but also timed down to the millisecond, the result is flow. Viewing two people who are performing an identical movement can be interesting because often they look quite different from one another. Flow, or lack thereof, is frequently the reason for this difference.

Principle 9: Be Precise

Is precision the domain of perfectionists? I don't think so, although I confess to being one. I certainly would not go so far as to say that someone who is not a perfectionist can't achieve precision. Without precision Pilates work becomes almost meaningless. It is popular in the fitness industry to speak of isolating muscle groups during a particular movement. Isolation depends entirely on precision. Yet often those who claim to isolate muscle groups are doing anything but. Either they lack precision in isolating an area or they rely on external means, such as apparatus, to achieve this goal. For instance, someone who performs a biceps curl using a preacher curl bench is demonstrating nonfunctional isolation, because although he is using the biceps primarily, he is totally reliant on the bench. In life we cannot walk around with this type of support. Isolation is only meaningful when you can stabilize your body and support the isolated movement independently. This is a mindful process that requires returning to the first movement principle, awareness, followed by concentration and control. As you gain more insight into your body, you will be able to achieve increasingly fine muscle isolation. I fantasize that one day I will be able to isolate and control every

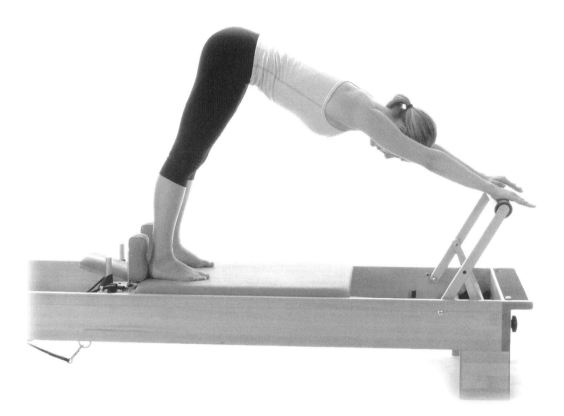

muscle fiber in my body—this is a dream that keeps me grounded and humble!

Precision requires complete muscle integration, which may then be followed by the isolation of certain muscles or muscle groups. You will feel the work more profoundly when you perform every movement with precision down to the finest detail. Precision is the basis of the corrective approach to working the body. Many times when I give students an exercise to perform, they comment on how they feel it more than ever, despite having done it many times. Often it's a matter of adjusting the body one or two degrees this way or that—and suddenly the flame ignites. That is precision. You need a great deal of precision in Pilates, in the execution of each movement and in the activation of each muscle, down to the single muscle fiber.

Principle 10: Seek Harmony

Harmony is the whole, the culmination of all we strive to achieve. It is the ultimate reward for commitment and hard work. Harmony means walking out of a session and feeling completely rejuvenated, being aware of each muscle and sensing the depth of each breath. It means being focused, centered, and in control, moving efficiently coupled with flow and precision. To feel all these things is to be in harmony with oneself and with the environment.

Few forms of conditioning can boast such profound outcomes as Pilates can, as millions are now experiencing. The greatness of human potential is realized when the mind is employed, because the power of the mind is infinite. The principles I've described, individually and united, offer a path to tapping into the resources of the mind. The movements in Pilates, as beautiful and wonderful as they are, are only movements. The principles and philosophy of this system are what make it unique and enable it to transform lives. When correcting alignment and teaching positive movement patterns, you need to do more than address physiological components such as muscle strength and flexibility. You must also consider the principles behind the movements. They will guide you through the internal process of transformation that leads to well-being.

Moving through life in harmony with all around and all within is the achievement of well-being.

The practice of Pilates opens the path to new discovery each day. I can honestly say that I have never done a personal workout and never taught a session where I did not learn something new. Having done thousands of sessions and taught thousands of sessions, that statement itself sings the praises of this system. Of course your body, your mind, and your heart must be open to such learning, but if they are . . . the possibilities are infinite.

CHAPTER 2

Alignment, Posture, and Movement

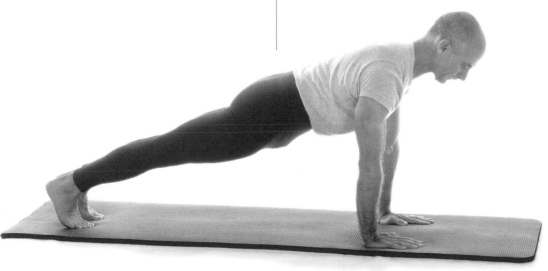

The previous chapter laid the foundation for understanding Pilates—its philosophy, principles, and ability to affect every facet of being, as its creator intended. In the following chapters I discuss concepts that pertain to the science of human movement and their relation to the Pilates method.

The human body is a complex instrument that can be likened, in makeup and function, to a chain with multiple links—the *kinetic chain*. Exploring the kinetic chain is fascinating because it has infinite possibilities. Each body is different, even though they share predictable patterns of movement and muscle development. As a movement occurs, the muscles are activated in a certain order, or pattern. If this pattern is faulty, the movement can still be performed, but it will lack efficiency and could lead to injury. The Pilates method addresses the kinetic chain in its entirety; through a process of refinement it can bring about profound changes and enhance the body's performance.

Musculoskeletal Structure

Let us view the body from the inside out. The skeleton is the body's infrastructure, on which all else is built (figure 2.1a). The skeleton is a well-structured and balanced frame that the muscles are layered on to provide support and movement (figure 2.1b). The bones act as levers and the muscles as cables that move the body part(s) in a desired direction. Because of this ingenious structure, the musculature is able to work effectively. However, if the frame is out of alignment it affects the entire structure, resulting in inefficient muscle action, fatigue, and ailments.

The human body is the most masterful feat of mechanics, engineering, and physics imaginable. For example, consider the patella, the freely moving bone that sits above the knee (the largest sesamoid bone in the body). Besides protecting the knee joint, the patella creates a significant mechanical advantage for the quadriceps. If there were no patella, the quadriceps muscle would need to work approximately 30 percent harder and be much stronger (and larger) to create a force equivalent to that provided with the patella. And if the patella is out of alignment, knee function will be affected dramatically and chronic ailments may result. How often do we

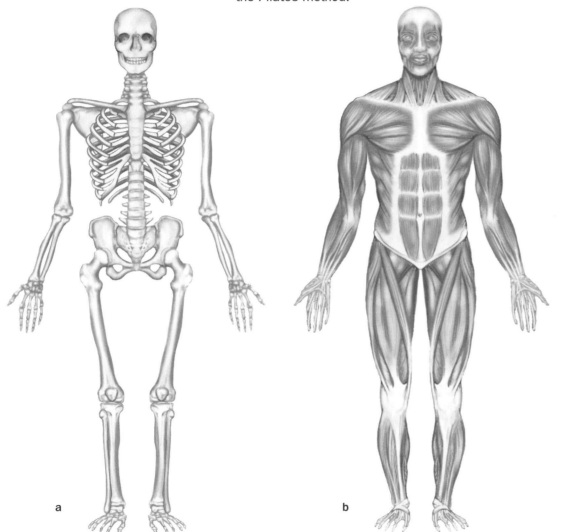

a   b

FIGURE 2.1   **Proper skeletal alignment combines with good muscle mechanics to produce effortless and efficient movement.**

Reprinted, by permission, from P.M. McGinnis, 1999, *Biomechanics of sport and exercise* (Champaign, IL: Human Kinetics), 20 and 22.

give credit to this little bone for offering us such an enormous mechanical advantage in walking, running, and jumping? This is one small example of the body's wondrous mechanics.

Joseph Pilates recognized and respected the marvel that is the structure of the human body. He invented a system that challenges this structure in every conceivable way, offering a path to discovering its full potential. The relationship between the skeletal structure and the muscular system is interesting and unique; it is the basis of all movement analysis. Often when exercising we place so much emphasis on the muscles that we ignore the skeletal structure. To achieve effective and efficient movement, we must consider both the skeletal and muscular systems.

Two well-known first-generation Pilates teachers, Eve Gentry and Bruce King, often described Pilates movements in terms of the *bones* (as opposed to the muscles) moving. Using this imagery facilitates effortless motion, void of tension or excessive force (and the inevitable grimacing and groaning!). It's as if the bones move as a result of an intangible internal force. Focusing on the skeletal structure also draws more attention to alignment. Correct alignment is the first step toward a positive outcome and success in achieving the desired goals.

Spine

One of the most fascinating parts of the skeleton is the spine (figure 2.2). Made up of 24 moving vertebrae and 9 that are fused (this number can vary slightly), the spine can be extremely mobile, allowing multidirectional movement of the trunk. At the same time, it can be very stable, serving as a solid platform to support movement of the limbs. In fact each individual vertebral joint offers very little movement, yet combined they form a highly mobile mechanism. Distributing the work through the spine and maximizing the movement of each vertebral joint is preferable to stressing one or two vertebral joints, which can result in shearing forces and excessive load in that area. The pelvis and lower spine (the pelvic–lumbar region) is of particular interest in Pilates because herein lies the *powerhouse,* the core, from which all movement emanates.

Pelvic Bowl

The pelvic bowl holds the essence of our being, the eternal spring of energy. Here human anatomy meets with the metaphysical, and the musculoskeletal system correlates perfectly with our life force. This concept forms the basis of Eastern and Western practices such as yoga, tai chi, aikido, certain styles of dance, and Pilates. The pelvis is indeed the powerhouse!

Dr. Arnold Kegel, innovator of the much-advocated exercises that bear his name (which involve contracting, holding, and releasing the muscles of the pelvic floor), recognized the importance of the pelvic floor muscles and their development, particularly for women before, during, and after pregnancy. He furthered the premise that training the pelvic floor can help to prevent and cure urinary incontinence and improve sexual function and satisfaction. I am sure he would delight in the attention the pelvic floor muscles are receiving today. A healthy pelvic floor—strong and flexible, able to adapt to changes in internal pressure—is one of the keys to well-being for women and men.

Men are often surprised to learn that they even have a pelvic floor! Both genders need well conditioned pelvic floor muscles (the coccygeus, the iliococcygeus, and the pubococcygeus) for optimal function, and

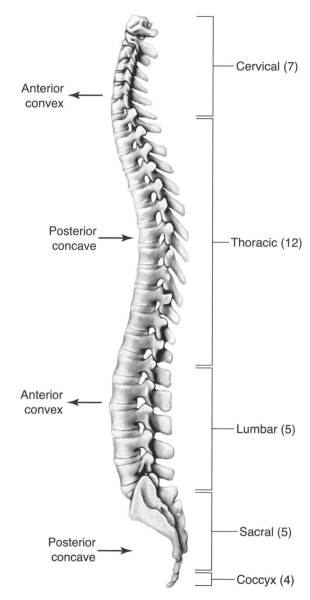

Cervical (7)

Anterior convex

Posterior concave

Thoracic (12)

Anterior convex

Lumbar (5)

Sacral (5)

Posterior concave

Coccyx (4)

FIGURE 2.2 This side view of the spine illustrates natural curves and proper spinal alignment.

recruitment of these muscles should be integrated into a comprehensive exercise program. Fortunately, because of the body's intricate muscle patterning, when the transverse abdominis muscle contracts (as it does throughout the Pilates session), so do the pelvic floor muscles. Also a correlation seems to exist between contraction of the hip adductors and the pelvic floor muscles. In addition, holding in urine activates the pelvic floor muscles. So, by nature's design, they are worked throughout life by default. However, heightening awareness and control of this muscle group will prove extremely beneficial for everyone. A well-conditioned pelvic floor supports the internal organs and viscera and provides added support during pregnancy. In addition it assists in preventing or overcoming urinary incontinence and contributes to heightened sexual function and satisfaction. Actively working the pelvic floor, particularly the coccygeus, influences positioning of the sacrum and may help relieve or prevent lower back pain. Finally, recent literature indicates that the pelvic floor is fundamentally important for core strength and stabilization.

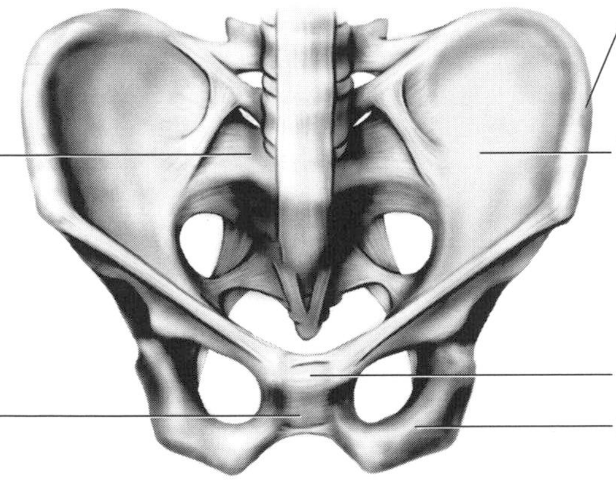

Dr. Noelani Guarderrama, a specialist in urogynecology based in Irvine, California, pointed out to me the uniqueness of the pelvic floor muscles: Like the diaphragm, they sit within a bony structure, in contrast to most of the skeletal muscles, which attach outside the bony structure. (In fact, the pelvic floor is sometimes referred to as the pelvic diaphragm.) The pelvic muscles work synergistically; that is, they work cooperatively in order to adapt to the constant changes of internal abdominal and thoracic pressure. This mechanism of intra-abdominal pressure is thought to unweight the spine and play a significant role in pelvic–lumbar stabilization.

The pelvis is a fascinating structure that serves as a bridge between the upper and lower body. It is made up of three bones—the ischium, ilium, and pubis—bound together by cartilage (figure 2.3). Some people believe that these cartilaginous joints do not move at all; others (myself included) believe they do allow varying degrees of very subtle movement. I must stress that the movement is minute. I often hear people referring to the movement of the sacroiliac joint (SIJ) as if it glides around like the scapulae. This is clearly not the case. At the same time, if these joints become immobile, undue strain is eventually placed on the pelvis and spine. The reasons for either hyper- or hypomobility vary (e.g., genetic, adaptive, or disease related), but for our purposes, simply being aware of the potential imbalances that can occur in the pelvis, and seeking medical advice if a condition prevails, is sufficient.

I like to visualize the pelvis as made up of two rotating discs sitting on their sides facing each other. The rotation of the discs is quite limited in either direction, but the small amount of rotation is significant and essential for healthy function of the pelvis and the body as a whole. The discs work in opposition during many basic activities such as walking and running; as one disc rotates in one direction, the other rotates in the opposite direction.

We need to consider the joints around as well as within the pelvis when discussing its function. The influence of the surrounding joints on the pelvis is profound, and vice versa. In fact, the function of the pelvis can be better understood by viewing the movement of the surrounding joints. If the pelvis is misaligned, it adversely affects the function of body segments up and down the kinetic chain, resulting in inefficient movement, muscular imbalances, and stress on the structure of the body. Detecting the imbalances is the first step toward understanding the body's movement. Remedying them is the next

Anterior superior iliac spine

Sacroiliac joint

Ilium

Pubis

Ischium

Pubic symphysis

FIGURE 2.3 **This front view of the pelvis clearly illustrates its structure and the joints that bind the parts together.**

step, and this is where Pilates can play a crucial role in reeducating the neuromuscular system. Correct pelvic alignment is of paramount importance whether you are performing daily activities, doing Pilates, or sitting at a desk. Balanced development of the muscles around the pelvis is fundamental in achieving a well-aligned pelvis and ideal posture.

One way to view the pelvis is as a suspension bridge with cables (the muscles) holding it from above, below, the sides, and, very importantly, from the inside. As long as all the cables are tensioned correctly and proportionately, little strain is placed on any one cable and the bridge will be stable and level. However, the moment the balance of tension on the cables changes or the bridge is not level, the other cables and the entire bridge will show strain. Although the pelvis will not typically collapse under stress, muscles that encounter excessive tension may become strained or even tear. Simply put, if the pelvis is out of alignment, the body is out of alignment.

We need only look at the list of some of the muscles that act on the pelvic complex—the pelvic floor muscles, spinal flexors and extensors, hip flexors and extensors, hip adductors and abductors, hip external and internal rotators—to understand the impact of the bridge analogy. And this list doesn't include the tendons, ligaments, and joints that also add support and flexibility to this intricate structure. It is no wonder this part of the body is the source of all movement. Pilates provides a path to discovering the powerhouse and unleashing the power of the pelvis. Keep in mind that working with precision when exercising the pelvic–lumbar region is imperative, possibly more so than in any other area of the body.

Muscles of the Powerhouse

In order to achieve good alignment and correct movement mechanics, the body must have the tools to do so; a well-balanced musculoskeletal system is the first step in this quest. Strength is obviously an important aspect of posture, yet other elements, such as habitual muscle activation patterns, genetics, and flexibility, are also key. In many instances a lack of flexibility inhibits ideal alignment and recruitment of the correct muscles. Hypermobility, on the other hand, although not restrictive by nature, demands a great deal of body awareness and muscular control to maintain good alignment. In Pilates we strive to develop strong, flexible muscles that are effective in their function and adaptability.

Certain muscles play a crucial role in providing a stable and pliable core, without which good alignment and efficient function are not possible. These are the deep muscles of the pelvis and trunk (see figure 2.4a). The superficial muscles are sometimes overdeveloped and overemphasized in relation to the deep muscles, often at the expense of a strong, solid core. Being large does not necessarily translate to being functional, and I regard muscle bulk that is not functional as extra baggage to carry around that can ultimately burden the body. As with a tree, the deeper layers, not the bark, provide the support to stand upright and the flexibility to bend with the wind.

The back extensors and abdominal muscles are key in providing the form and function of the trunk. They share a symbiotic relationship, and there should be constant interplay between them. Both the abdominals and back extensors are made up of layers of muscle, and it is the deepest layers that are most prominent in providing stabilization and support to the spine. The abdominal group is made up of the rectus abdominis, the external oblique, the internal oblique, and the transverse abdominis. In addition to having its own layers of muscle, the back serves as the attachment for many dual-purpose muscles such as those connecting to the neck, the upper limbs, the lower limbs, and the pelvis. Within these two major muscle groups, the abdominals and back extensors, two muscles have been identified as

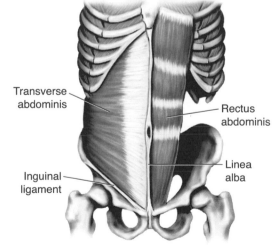

Transverse abdominis

Rectus abdominis

Linea alba

Inguinal ligament

FIGURE 2.4a   A major muscle of the core: the transverse abdominis.

having a particularly profound effect on stabilization and function: the transverse abdominis (TA) and the multifidus (see figure 2.4, *a* and *b*).

The abdominals and back muscles, together with the diaphragm and the pelvic floor, create a cylinder of muscular support in the center of the body. I call this the *internal support system* (ISS). It is congruent with the powerhouse in Pilates, or the core in other forms of training. It is gratifying that scientific research is now substantiating much of what Joseph Pilates advocated so many years ago with regard to the importance of a strong, powerful, and functional core. The muscles of the ISS can be recruited during every exercise, or not at all. Movement is possible without activating the ISS; however, internal support, protection, and efficient function will be absent.

Another component that is important to consider in any discussion relating to the pelvis and the spine is the psoas. There are two psoas muscles, the minor and the major, and the psoas major combines with the iliacus to form the iliopsoas (figure 2.4c). Besides being powerful hip flexors, these muscles are believed to substantially influence spinal stabilization and alignment. Since the psoas is close to the axis of flexion and extension of the lumbar spine, it will compensate for imbalance between the anterior abdominal muscles and posterior spinal

External occipital protuberance

Rectus capitis posterior minor

Obliquus capitis superior

Rectus capitis posterior major

Longissimus capitis

Obliquus capitis inferior

Longissimus cervicis

Semispinalis cervicis

External intercostals

Levatores costarum

Semispinalis dorsi

Quadratus lumborum

Multifidus

Semispinalis capitis

Sternocleidomastoid

Splenius capitis

Iliocostalis cervicis

Splenius cervicis

Iliocostalis dorsi

Longissimus dorsi

Spinalis dorsi

Iliocostalis lumborum

Sacrospinalis

FIGURE 2.4b   Major muscles of the core: the multifidus.

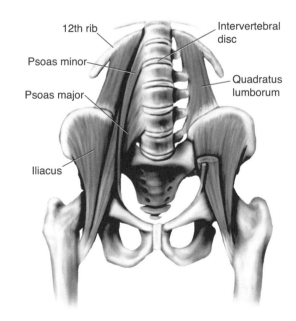

12th rib

Psoas minor

Psoas major

Iliacus

Intervertebral disc

Quadratus lumborum

FIGURE 2.4c   Major muscles of the core: the psoas.

extensor muscles to stabilize the lumbar spine. Some practitioners believe that most defects of the spine and the hip joint structures can and should be related to a disturbance of function of the psoas and iliopsoas. They postulate that tight or weak psoas muscles are associated with pelvic tilt, exaggerated lumbar lordosis, lower back pain, sacroiliac dysfunction, degenerative disc disease, scoliosis, and misaligned posture, among other conditions. With extended sitting, a common by-product of the modern lifestyle, the hip flexors become tight and weak. The psoas and iliopsoas should be addressed in all exercise programs as they affect everyone, from the very active to the sedentary.

The psoas (hip flexor) muscles and the abdominal muscles are agonist and antagonist as well as synergists—they oppose one another's actions and work cooperatively; a dynamic interplay exists between the two muscle groups. The psoas plays an important role in much of the abdominal work in Pilates, particularly in the exercises in which the legs are held up off the ground. Typically, great emphasis is placed on recruiting the abdominals while the role of the hip flexors is minimized or overlooked. I believe that more focus should be placed on controlling and using the hip flexors correctly. They are vital to the successful execution of many Pilates exercises as well as to efficient function and general well-being.

Interestingly, all the muscles of the ISS are what I call *mind muscles;* activating them requires mental focus and a high degree of body awareness and concentration. Controlling the muscles of the ISS requires different skills than those used for controlling superficial skeletal muscles such as the biceps or quadriceps, which are easily accessed and whose activation is readily apparent. Nature intended that the journey toward mastery of movement and control, and the attainment of fitness would demand mind–body exploration and yield a multitude of rewards. As Pilates wrote about the practice of his method in *Return to Life Through Contrology,* "exercises

that produce a harmonious structure we term 'physical fitness,' reflecting itself in a coordinated and balanced tri-part unity of body, mind, and spirit" (pages 32-33).

Principles of Alignment and Posture

People often adopt a simplistic view when assessing posture and alignment; for example, they measure only strength and flexibility and ignore the complexity of the factors involved. Strengthening a certain muscle group or stretching another to improve posture and alignment is not enough. Correcting alignment is a process of neuromuscular reeducation that requires enormous commitment, patience, and the guidance of a scrutinizing eye.

Posture may be observed in terms of the alignment of the joints and bony landmarks and understood in terms of muscle balance and function. It is often described relative to a plumb line—a straight line that runs vertically through the body. Figure 2.5 shows ideal posture viewed from the side. When viewing the body from the side in relation to the plumb line, deviations

Ripple Effect

All movement emanates from the center, both anatomically and energetically. The path of movement is like the ripple effect that occurs when a pebble is dropped into still water. It creates a circular ripple that in turn creates many more ripples moving outward in progressively larger circles. So each movement starts from the inner core (the first circle of energy) and moves outward; the trunk is the second circle of energy, followed by the limbs and finally the periphery, the hands and feet. But don't think of the energy stopping at the fourth circle; it should continue on as if the movement never ends. This is called the follow-through, and it has infinite value in terms of function and aesthetics. It is a concept promoted in all athletic activities from jumping to throwing a ball.

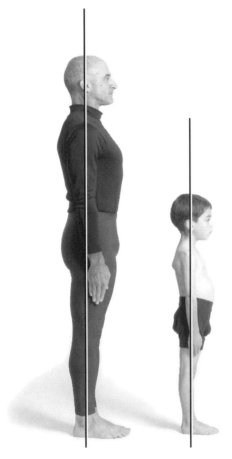

FIGURE 2.5 Posture should also be viewed from the front and back as well, focusing on the symmetry of the body and deviations from the midline in a sideways direction (the coronal plane). Good observation points and landmarks include the ears, shoulders, space between the arms and the trunk, the pelvis, the knees, and the feet. I call these checkpoint areas *windows of opportunity* because they offer so much information regarding alignment.

in an anterior–posterior direction become apparent (in the sagittal plane). The following landmarks of the body should line up vertically on the plumb line: the lobe of the ear, bodies of the cervical vertebrae, shoulder joint, midpoint of the trunk, greater trochanter of the femur, a point slightly anterior to the midline of the knee, and a point slightly anterior to the lateral malleolus (ankle).

Please note that ideal posture is the *ideal,* a goal that one strives for but may never achieve. Each individual is different in body type, center of gravity, habitual movement patterns, mental state, and genes; it is inconceivable to think that one posture will fit all. However, the concept of an ideal posture serves as a guideline and a reference by which we can detect deviations and gauge changes.

Posture affects every movement, exercise, and decision in an exercise program. Consider, for instance, a person who has *fatigue posture,* which is characterized by a rounded thoracic spine and the pelvis being forward of the plumb line in a posterior tilt. Although correction is complex, it generally involves extending the upper back, strengthening the upper back extensors, strengthening the iliopsoas, and stretching the external obliques of the abdomen. Bringing the shoulders into ideal alignment over the pelvis is also often helpful. On the other hand if a person has *lumbar hyperlordosis,* which involves an increased lumbar curve of the spine often accompanied by an anterior tilt of the pelvis, correction generally focuses on strengthening the abdominals and stretching the hip flexors and lower back extensors. Clearly these two people will receive different exercise programs, emphasizing different muscle groups, with the selection of exercises and the cueing appropriate for their particular posture.

Alignment of the Spine

Good alignment translates into less stress on the spine and more economical muscular activity. When the spine is aligned with gravity, the body works in harmony with the laws of nature. The moment the body is not balanced, certain muscles become overworked and others become weak. Maintaining the natural curves of the spine is also important because they act as shock absorbers, protecting the body during impact, whether landing from a jump, running, or carrying a heavy load. We therefore always strive to attain ideal alignment and to develop the musculature to support it.

Although much of our attention focuses on the musculature as it relates to posture and alignment, ideal alignment of the spine also facilitates efficient functioning of the internal organs. Deviations of posture over time can lead to malfunctioning of the inner organs. For instance, I have taught people who have scoliosis and who, with Pilates practice, begin to feel that they can finally breathe into a lung that has seemed dormant for a long time. This is quite typical with scoliosis because the muscles on one side of the thorax become tight, causing the rib cage to compress on that side and limit the function of the corresponding lung. Similarly, with kyphosis (increased thoracic curve of the spine) the rib cage becomes compressed and impairs respiration. Other systems can also be affected; for example, a posture with exaggerated forward flexion places constant pressure on the digestive system, hindering its function.

Placement of the Head

I like to think of the head as a ball balancing on a pin. None of the muscles should be strained; instead they should all act as cables that keep the ball balanced in harmony with the laws of nature. Adjusting the position of the head is one of the most common (and important) corrections I give when I teach. I view the head as simply another vertebra, an integral part of the spine, and as such it should follow the line of the spine. Deviations from this alignment, particularly because of the head's relatively heavy weight, inevitably result in neck tension and strain and are aesthetically unpleasing. It is even more pronounced when a person has a long neck, which essentially acts as an extended lever arm. For instance, if someone has forward head posture (the head is carried anterior to the plumb line), the neck extensors will become tight and overworked and the flexors relatively weak and inactive. The head weighs 12 to 14 pounds (approximately 5 kilograms), so shifting it away from the base of support has a significant effect on the musculature, an effect that grows exponentially as the head moves further away from the plumb line.

During forward-flexion abdominal exercises such as the Mat Work: Chest Lift exercise (page 48), the trunk must lift up and forward and the spine, including the head, must follow a natural curve. When forward flexion is inadequate, the head falls out of the base of support of the upper girdle, and the result is neck strain and tension. This inevitably happens when someone is restricted by weak abdominals or tight lower back muscles and is often exacerbated by attempts to maintain a neutral pelvis when the body does not have the tools to do so (discussed in the next section). To understand proper positioning, visualize the body in forward flexion with the sun shining directly overhead. The shoulder girdle would cast a shadow on the ground below slightly larger than the actual size of the shoulder girdle. This shadow marks the base of support of the upper girdle; the head should be held within this area (figure 2.6a).

The Mat Work: Roll-Up exercise (page 52) offers a good illustration of head alignment and a perfect example of how the art and science of human movement meet. In the sitting phase of this exercise, many people place the head down between the arms. I prefer that the head follow the natural C curve of the spine and be held above the arms, with the arms remaining parallel to the

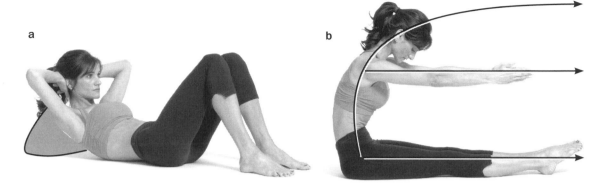

FIGURE 2.6 Best results are achieved when the head follows the natural curve of the spine in forward flexion as in the chest lift (*a*) and the roll-up (*b*).

floor (figure 2.6*b*). Not only does this present a longer, more continuous line, which is visually pleasing, but it also encourages better placement of the shoulders and scapulae, and relaxation of the levator scapulae and upper trapezius.

Neutral Pelvis and Neutral Spine

Neutral pelvis is defined as a position in which the anterior superior iliac spines (ASIS) and the pubic symphysis (PS) are in the same horizontal plane (coronal plane when upright) and the two ASIS are in the same transverse plane. The term *neutral spine* indicates that the natural curves of the spine are present. If the PS is higher than the ASIS, the pelvis is in a posterior tilt; if the ASIS are higher than the PS, the pelvis is in an anterior tilt (see figure 2.7*a, b,* and *c*).

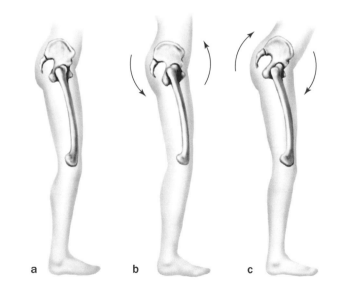

FIGURE 2.7 Neutral pelvis (*a*), posterior tilt (*b*), and anterior tilt (*c*).

The neutral position is a reference point that helps you position your body during Pilates work. This is not to say that you never deviate from it; instead, you can use it to compare and describe all other positions. When the spine is in a neutral position, the pelvis by definition must also be neutral; however, instances do occur in which the pelvis is in neutral and the spine is not, such as during the Mat Work: Single-Leg Stretch (page 56; figure 2.8) and many other abdominal exercises.

Performing exercises in the neutral spine and neutral pelvis position yields several benefits. It encourages balanced muscular development of the pelvic complex and correct muscle recruitment. It teaches and reinforces efficient posture and ideal alignment, which is particularly important when standing. It unloads the pelvis of undue stresses. However, keep in mind that the pelvis is dynamic and constantly adjusts to the body's movements and its ability or inability to perform a movement. At times working with the pelvis in a posterior tilt as opposed to neutral may be advantageous; the neutral position could prove counterproductive and lead to negative results. This is particularly pertinent during abdominal exercises, and appropriate positioning of the spine and

pelvis should be assessed on a case-by-case basis. A neutral pelvis is the ideal, but it may be necessary at first to work with a slight posterior pelvic tilt in order to relax the muscles of the lumbar region and access the abdominals more prominently.

The trend today is to exercise in neutral pelvis and neutral spine positions; however, as stated previously, the two do not always occur simultaneously, and they have different implications. I often encounter students who say they are working in a neutral spine position when they are not (nor should they be). For example, once the head and trunk lift into forward flexion during abdominal exercises, the spine is no longer in a neutral position. In a neutral spine position the natural curves of the spine must be present; in forward flexion the spine has deviated from the natural curves. So to say that you do abdominal work with a neutral *spine* while in forward flexion is a contradiction in terms. However, maintaining a neutral *pelvis* during abdominal work in forward flexion is quite possible and desirable.

I was teaching a mat work class to a large group at a conference recently. I set them up for the chest lift and then instructed them to lift into forward flexion. As I looked around I noticed that they had lifted only their heads, not the entire upper girdle, off the mats. When I inquired why no one was lifting higher, the answer was, "We are trying to maintain a neutral spine position." This revealed a misunderstanding of the neutral spine position; however, even if they had been trying to maintain a neutral pelvis, they were missing the point of the exercise. They were not achieving any significant degree of forward flexion. Neck flexion, yes, but not flexion of the trunk. As a result they were not working the abdominals effectively and probably were achieving more neck tension than abdominal strength.

I have witnessed similar scenarios with oblique abdominal work and rotation of the trunk, such as in the Mat Work: Criss-Cross (page 58). In these cases I have observed a lack of rotation as well as lack of forward

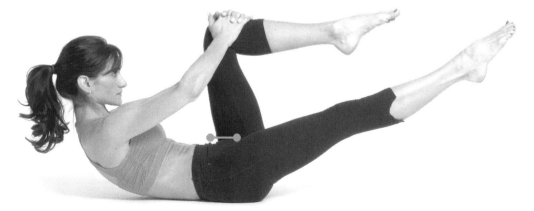

FIGURE 2.8 The single-leg stretch is one of many exercises in which the pelvis is in neutral position while the spine is not.

flexion. Again, I see neck flexion along with flapping elbows and little or no trunk rotation.

I advocate maintaining a neutral pelvic position during many exercises that require pelvic–lumbar stabilization, including abdominal work. But not at all costs. For example, if you have hyperlordosis and a tight lower back, as many people do, performing forward flexion while maintaining a neutral pelvis could result in excessive contraction of the lower back muscles, preventing sufficient forward flexion of the trunk. This translates into ineffective abdominal recruitment, possible excessive hip flexor activation, plus stress on the lower back and probably the neck. In an endeavor to work with a neutral pelvis, people sometimes compromise the outcome of the exercise and reinforce negative movement patterns, coming away with neck pain, back pain, and weak abdominals to boot.

A series of actions allow the lumbar spine to imprint into the mat during forward flexion in a supine position: The abdominal muscles contract, intra-abdominal pressure is increased, the back extensors deactivate sufficiently, and the lumbar vertebrae flatten out. This does not mean that the pelvis should be forcefully thrust into a posterior tilt (commonly called a *tuck*) in order to imprint the back into the mat. Rather the trunk is lifted into forward flexion in a neutral pelvis, and if the pelvis must tilt posteriorly at the end range of the forward flexion in order to achieve maximum abdominal activation,

deactivate the tight lower back extensors, and imprint the lower back into the mat—so be it! Continue modifying the position of the pelvis until you have addressed and overcome the limiting factors. Ultimately you will be able to perform the abdominal exercises with integrity and a positive outcome, void of tension and with a neutral pelvis—the ideal.

Assessing Alignment

Over the years I have found it important to develop convenient methods of assessing posture. Very sophisticated systems of assessment are available yet most are impractical to use at home or during a Pilates session. I recommend the Mat Work: Roll-Down as a simple but useful tool for assessing posture and alignment. It offers valuable information regarding structure, muscular development, and compensations. At the same time it allows one to gently mobilize the spine and coordinate the breathing with the movement. Teachers who are assessing a student's alignment should observe the roll-down from the back, front, and side, since certain postural deviations are more apparent from a coronal (front/back) view and others from a sagittal (side) view. When using this exercise as a self-assessment, you should stand on a firm, level surface in front of a mirror if possible. Self-assessment demands great inner awareness and observation skills that should be honed constantly.

Roll-Down

Muscle Focus

- Abdominals and back extensors

Objectives

- Develop articulation of the spine
- Stretch the back extensors
- Improve control of the abdominals and back extensors
- Align the body and focus the mind

I encourage the use of the roll-down at the beginning and end of a session; however, the exercise is *not* appropriate for everyone and should not be used in certain instances, such as when lower back problems are present. If you have any reservations about yourself or a student doing this movement, substitute a modified roll-down by leaning the back against a wall, placing the feet one to two feet (30 to 60 centimeters) from the wall, and bending the knees. Doing the exercise in this position allows the wall to bear the weight of the body and provides tactile feedback.

During the roll-down, notice deviations from the plumb line and become internally aware of weight shifts within the body. Notice asymmetries and imbalances. Use the roll-down not only as a tool for assessment but also as a vehicle for focusing the mind and tuning the body, just as you would tune a musical instrument before playing it.

Imagery

Imagine your back pressing against a pole that is keeping you upright and aligned. The head fills with water and becomes very heavy. It rolls forward, pulling the body away from the pole one tiny segment at a time. At the bottom the water runs out and lightens the body so that the spine rolls back up the pole, one segment at time.

- ☐ Establish ideal alignment in relation to the plumb line from the outset.
- ☐ Keep the movement relaxed and avoid forcing a stretch of the hamstrings at the end.
- ☐ Relax the hands and hold them with the palms facing the sides of the body.

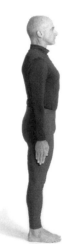

Inhale. Stand upright in ideal alignment with the feet hip-width apart and parallel. Prepare for the movement by going through a mental checklist of ideal alignment.

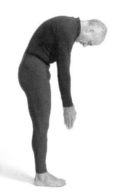

Exhale. Roll down through the spine, beginning with the head and articulating through each vertebra. Allow the knees to bend as you roll down, alleviating any pressure on the lower back.

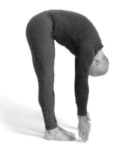

Inhale, holding a relaxed (but not slumped) position at the bottom, feeling the back expand and the vertebrae releasing all tension. Relax the neck and allow the head to follow the line of the spine. Exhale. Roll back up, articulating through the spine and placing each vertebra back on the plumb line establishing ideal alignment and returning to the starting position.

Foot Alignment

The feet are the foundation of the body when upright: standing, walking, running, and jumping. Any misalignment of the feet, in a static position or in motion, results in postural deviations and compensations all the way up the kinetic chain. The foot is made up of many joints and is a complex structure, and citing any one joint or aspect of the foot as particularly vulnerable is difficult. However, I will single out the subtalar joint (often mistaken for the ankle joint) due to its importance to foot alignment. The subtalar joint controls the inward and outward motion (supination and pronation) of the foot and is vital to achieving correct foot alignment. A good guide to achieving neutral alignment of the foot when standing is to observe the Achilles tendon from the back (see figure 2.9). The tendon should be perpendicular to the ground, and fine adjustments of the subtalar joint can be made to achieve this alignment. Becoming acquainted with neutral alignment is particularly helpful during the foot work on the Pilates apparatus.

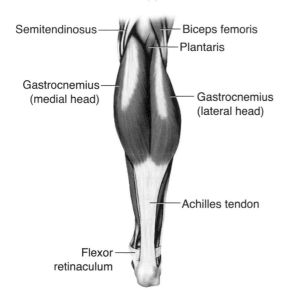

Semitendinosus — — Biceps femoris
— Plantaris
Gastrocnemius — (medial head)
— Gastrocnemius (lateral head)
— Achilles tendon
Flexor — retinaculum

FIGURE 2.9 Alignment of the Achilles tendon.

Effects of Center of Gravity

The body's center of gravity (COG) is important to alignment as well as to understanding the mechanics of exercises. Weight distribution can make exercises easier or more difficult for certain body types. Sometimes difficulty executing an exercise successfully has little to do with lack of strength and much to do with physical build—specifically the weight distribution of the body. For instance, a man with broad shoulders, a well-developed upper body, and short legs may find the roll-up extremely challenging, while a woman with a short, petite torso, substantial hips, and long legs will find the exercise relatively easy. The man is not weaker; in fact he may have far stronger abdominal muscles, but he is top heavy, and the woman's COG is lower. Of course, the man I just described has an advantage in other exercises, such as the Wunda Chair: Full Pike (page 252) and the Reformer: Long Stretch (page 164).

Because each person's COG is slightly different, the way each performs an exercise is also different. Understanding this fact is important in order to make exercises easier or more difficult and, most important, safe. Joseph Pilates had a very muscular build, like a gymnast. Add to this men's naturally strong upper body and the innate inclination to choreograph exercises that feel good (and look good) on oneself, and the result is that it is no surprise that many of the exercises Joseph Pilates created require a strong, well-developed upper girdle. (This in no way implies that women cannot perform the repertoire very beautifully and successfully.) Understanding the mechanics of the body and the exercises will allow you to overcome obstacles for yourself and your students.

Let's take, for example, the Mat Work: Roll-Up (page 52). If a person is struggling with this exercise and it appears to be due to body type rather than weak abdominals or tight lower back and hamstrings, an excellent solution is draping a light (2.2 pounds/1 kilogram) ankle weight over the ankles. This does not allow the person to rely on the ankle weight to pull the body up, as would be the case if the feet were placed under a secure foot strap; it simply changes the weight distribution, adding weight (or, in effect, length) to the legs and lowering the COG toward the pelvis. The individual becomes taller for the sake of the exercise. (If only it were so easy to become tall!) At other times being top heavy or shorter may prove an advantage. Regardless of body type, everyone has challenges to face and obstacles to overcome . . . so enjoy your body and relish the journey!

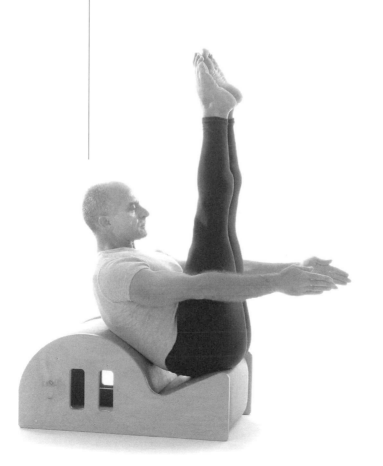

CHAPTER 3

Powerful Pilates Practice

The foundation of the Pilates method, certainly the way I approach it, is working with the *whole* in mind. The body is the most intricate of instruments, and imbalance in one area will inevitably cause imbalances in other areas. Therefore all Pilates programs should be comprehensive, regardless of a person's age, fitness, or ability level. Certainly in some cases you may direct more attention toward a particular area of the body, but you must always keep in mind the intricate patterning of human movement. An injury, compensation, or any other restriction that adversely affects the integrity of the body's ability to function can be regarded as a weak link in a chain. For the chain to function as a complete unit, you must address the weak link without losing sight of the fact that the goal is the efficient function of the chain as a whole.

Structure and creativity seem to be diametrically opposed, yet one cannot exist without the other. Having a structure allows you to be creative and to adapt to personal and specific needs without compromising the concept of the whole. Addressing the body and mind as a whole is what makes this approach so valuable and its effects so profound. If you view Pilates as *only* exercise, and furthermore, exercise for only one part of the body, you risk sacrificing the essence of the system. Adhering to a structure allows one to compile an efficient, comprehensive program. It also allows teachers to keep the flow in a studio when teaching several people at the same time, while offering each person an individualized program and personal attention. I liken it to a conductor leading an orchestra or a chess master who is playing several games of chess at one time—he always knows where he is in each game and what his strategy will be for the next move. This can only be achieved with a clear and well-learned structure.

Over the years I have witnessed Pilates classes that lack structure, direction, and the concept of the *whole*. I have always come away feeling that the session is missing the point; without a logical progression, it lacks the elements that make Pilates so valuable. I sometimes see this happening in medical environments, where Pilates is used as a treatment modality. A therapist might take a patient through a few exercises on the reformer, and then move on to another treatment. Using a Pilates exercise here and there is not Pilates. The exercise happens to be done on Pilates equipment and it might or might not be a Pilates movement, but what is being practiced is not Pilates because it does not embody the system's philosophy and approach. I cannot say this is wrong; I can only say it is not the system that Joseph Pilates created. Therefore it cannot achieve the outcome that Joseph Pilates described in *Return to Life Through Contrology* as "the highest accomplishments within the scope of our capabilities." (Of course many therapists have studied Pilates in depth and have integrated it very successfully into their practices as a complete system.) The method's creator was explicit in his belief that you must address both the mind and body, concurrently and comprehensively. This belief has been proven to be a powerful approach to wellness and is now receiving the widespread recognition it deserves.

Structuring Your Practice: The Block System

With the aim of finding a useful structure for Pilates practice, I have developed a system for organizing a comprehensive program. The block system is the nucleus of my approach to Pilates. It is the result of many years of practicing and teaching the method and directing Pilates programs around the world. It is solidly grounded in the Pilates method and, at the same time, it adheres to the principles of exercise physiology. Its structure ensures that practitioners address the whole body, simultaneously providing a framework for individual development and creativity, and offering clear guidelines and flexibility. This filing system organizes the vast Pilates repertoire in a way that each exercise has a home, a block it belongs to. It can be likened to a family tree; all the exercises are related to each other, some more closely than others, all emanating from the same roots. Familiarity with the intricacies of the whole tree is essential in order to implement the block system successfully; this familiarity can then be used to compile programs that are individualized according to level, personal needs, restrictions, and goals.

Without such a system, the hundreds of Pilates exercises become just that—exercises, like words with no story. They are valuable in and of themselves, but they convey a message only when put together in sentences. The more finely crafted the sentences, the more profound the message. So it is with Pilates. The teacher compiles the session with the blocks, which are like chapters in a book; together, they create the whole story. Each movement takes on more meaning when it is placed within a well-thought-out structure and sequence of movements—like poetry in motion. This is where the art and the science of human movement unite. At this level, mind and body work as one and all the principles of Pilates are in effect; the work becomes deeper and yet more effortless. This is the level we strive for, where the greatest and most productive changes take place.

Fully grasping the many levels of the block system can take years. However, even in its simplest form the system provides a way to categorize the vast repertoire, to maximize the work time and use the session to its full potential. Because it is a standardized system it allows practitioners who are trained in it to communicate and collaborate in a seamless and meaningful fashion, wherever they may be in the world. As I visit studios in the many countries this system has spread to, I am filled with pride when I see how successfully the block system has been implemented in different cultures.

In this book all the exercises on the apparatus are laid out according to the block system, which enables you to learn each exercise and its place in the overall structure concurrently. For example, the exercises on the reformer that focus on the upper girdle fall into the arm work block, which offers you a pool of upper body exercises of varying levels of difficulty to choose from. Each block comprises individual exercises or series of exercises. A series is a compilation of several exercises that complement each other to create a complete, integrated *exercise unit* for a particular area of the body.

The blocks that make up this system are as follows:

Warm-up. Prepares the body for the work, both physically and mentally. Typically a selection of mat work exercises.

Foot work. Devoted to the lower limbs, foot work is performed on the reformer, cadillac, and wunda chair. The focus is the entire leg: foot, ankle, knee, and hip. This block is regarded as part warm-up and part specific training for the lower limbs.

Abdominal work. A selection of exercises focused on developing the abdominal muscles. Although the abdominals work throughout the Pilates session, these exercises are specifically aimed at this region and address all the abdominal muscles.

Hip work. This section demands work and control of the hip joint and is typically performed with the feet in the straps on the reformer or using the leg springs on the cadillac. Focus on control of the pelvic–lumbar region is key because of the close relationship of the pelvis to the hip joint.

Spinal articulation. This block is devoted to spinal mobility and developing control of the trunk muscles. Spinal articulation exercises can be found on almost all the apparatus, including the mat. These exercises integrate the muscles of the core.

Stretches. Selections from this block can be performed on or off the apparatus and typically include one or two stretches for the hip flexors and hamstrings. The selection of exercises depends on the needs and ability of each person.

Full body integration (FBI) I and II. Although all Pilates exercises work the entire body, these exercises defy categorization by muscle group or area of the body and are specifically geared to full-body motion. The exercises in FBI I are fundamental and intermediate, and those in FBI II are advanced and master level.

Arm work. This block is devoted to the upper girdle of the body. I have compiled several series consisting of exercises that work the various muscle groups of the arms. Typically a complete series is practiced to ensure comprehensive training of the upper body.

Leg work. These are exercises for the lower body to supplement the foot work. They typically emphasize the hip abductors and the hip adductors. However, the block system allows flexibility, so that this section may be utilized for specific skill training for dancers, skiers, and runners, for example, or for corrective work and rehabilitation of the lower limbs.

Lateral flexion and rotation. This block refers to exercises that work the lateral flexors and rotators of the trunk, with an emphasis on the oblique abdominal muscles. These muscles are vital to healthy functional movement and support of the spine. Often imbalances exist between the muscles on either side of the body. The reasons for these vary from scoliosis to one-side–dominance (handedness) to the practice of certain athletic activities. I recommend always working toward balance and symmetry.

Back extension. This block is devoted to exercises for the trunk extensors. These muscles lie along the spine and span the back in layers. The superficial muscles are long, large muscles that are responsible for gross movement. The deeper intrinsic muscles are intervertebral muscles that control fine intricate movement of the spine. As with the abdominals it is the deeper layers that are largely responsible for stabilization. This section should *not* be compromised.

I sometimes hear an unjustified criticism of Pilates: that the rotation and extension exercises are inadequate. My standard answer is simple: "Sorry, but either you or your teacher does not know Pilates." There are myriad options in the Pilates repertoire for both spinal rotation and extension, which are important components of any comprehensive exercise program.

As we age, spinal extension becomes all the more important in an exercise program. Over time gravity tends to pull us forward into flexion. Add to this our modern lifestyle, with hours spent in front of computers, driving cars, and taking part in recreational pursuits that also demand forward flexion, and the result is a bleak picture that includes a high incidence of round-shoulder syndrome and other shoulder problems, nonspecific lower back pain, and neck tension. If one then studies Pilates with a teacher who is obsessed with working the abdominals, the majority of exercises will be performed in trunk flexion, and the picture gets even worse. Effective abdominal work is important but must be in proportion with correct and sufficient work of the back extensors, a key component in achieving good alignment, balance, peak performance, and general well-being.

I often look to babies and young children for guidance. Seldom do you see toddlers with bad alignment; they have strong backs and straight spines. I recall a wonderful incident when Lolita San Miguel, one of the Pilates "elders" and a first-generation teacher, was visiting me. My son Elan, who was about 2 years of age, was taking a bath and Lolita and I were standing in the bathroom looking on. Together we marveled at the amazing musculature and posture of this little rambunctious ball of energy as he stood, sat, jumped, splashed, and showed off his athletic skills to his guest. This is the type of spine nature intended us to have, not only as infants, but throughout our lives. Yes, little ones also have little potbellies, and as they reach their early teens emphasis on developing the abdominals is important. However, we should not lose sight of the importance of keeping the back muscles conditioned and of working to prevent the deterioration that can occur over time.

Exercise Descriptions

In order to fully understand an exercise or movement, you must analyze it. You will then be able to apply the movement at the right moment and in the most appropriate manner to achieve the desired outcome. I have formulated a clear and succinct form of analyzing each movement. This analysis opens the door to understanding as well as learning and teaching the movement. It is also invaluable in compiling exercise programs. In the following section I explain the categories used in chapters 4 through 11, which describe and analyze each movement on the various pieces of apparatus.

Each exercise is presented by name, apparatus, block, level of difficulty, and the amount of resistance to use (if applicable). This information is followed by a discussion about the exercise, its muscle focus, its objectives, and the imagery that I suggest using to achieve the desired results. Imagery is a very personal teaching tool, so what I offer might work for you or it might spark your imagination to create your own imagery. I also include a checklist of key points you should observe to ensure a successful outcome for each exercise. Finally, photographs illustrate the movement and are accompanied by the breathing pattern.

Classifying the Movement

The blocks are used to classify the exercises, but each one is also defined by its level of difficulty—fundamental, intermediate, advanced, and master level. (Master-level exercises, as the name implies, take years to master. I offer only a few in this text, as more would be beyond its

scope. I do plan to make available more of this level of the work in an upcoming book.) Classifying movements by level is a subjective process since what is difficult for one person may be relatively easy for another. Thus I allocate levels according to the complexity of the movement—the more complex the movement, the higher the level of difficulty.

I must emphasize that this system is not one in which, once you have learned an advanced movement, you no longer practice the fundamental or intermediate movements that prepared you for that advanced move. Each exercise is an additional tool in a large toolbox or another dance step to use and enjoy. When I construct programs for advanced students, I select exercises from all levels, not only from the advanced repertoire. Including a range of exercises in a program is important both physically and mentally. The level should not be a goal in and of itself, but a milestone in the lifelong process of learning.

I have spent much of my career mastering the most difficult moves in this method, and I certainly enjoy the exhilaration of performing the master-level work, which I do in its entirety. Yet it is only part of the picture. With commitment, people can reap the same benefits at any level of practice. The benefits depend not only on the movements performed but also on their quality and the integration of the principles into one's work and life. Too often I see the master-level repertoire becoming the sole focus, at times being performed by people who have little experience in this work. Talented gymnasts or dancers could probably perform all the master-level work almost immediately. Does this mean they know Pilates? No. It means that they can learn choreography and perform it. Pilates is not the performance of choreography; it is the never-ending process of learning about the body, controlling movement, and striving for well-being.

I see as much value in the Mat Work: Pelvic Curl (page 45), one of the most fundamental exercises, as I do in the single-leg high bridge (not included in this book), one of the most advanced movements in the repertoire. In this example, the two exercises are actually closely related. The relationship between fundamental and advanced work should be established early on in the practice of Pilates. These relationships allow you to prepare methodically for the next level and grow in the system. The process of working through the levels and understanding each building block, not the performance of an advanced exercise, is the path to reaping rewards. You can do an exercise thousands of times and always find new meaning in it. I do not believe that any movements are *simple*. Besides the enormous complexity in terms of neuromuscular and biomechanical activity, each movement embodies an entire philosophy. The work manifests itself on so many different levels. Fundamental? Possibly. Simple? Never.

Some people try to learn the repertoire as quickly as possible, steering away from the fundamental exercises, preferring to move on to the more difficult work. But every movement has infinite complexity, regardless of the level. I encourage you to delight in the process of becoming intimately familiar with each exercise rather than rushing. The development of familiarity and understanding, not whether or not you can perform an advanced exercise, reflects true learning.

Resistance

Pilates is recognized for its ingenious use of both gravity and springs for resistance. In exercises utilizing gravity for resistance, the degree of resistance has not been stated, as it will always be consistent. However, in exercises using springs for resistance (the majority of exercises on the apparatus), the appropriate amount of resistance is noted. In some instances there is an effect from both the springs and gravity, and an understanding of the mechanics of the apparatus is essential. Springs provide *progressive resistance,* meaning that the resistance increases as tension on the spring increases. This differs from *constant resistance,* in which the resistance does not change. Take into account that when working with resistance, whether constant or progressive, the effect on the muscle varies because of the mechanical advantage or disadvantage at certain angles of the joint.

Much debate surrounds the question of which type of resistance is preferable. This cannot be resolved simply, and I think the points made in favor of each are valid. Ultimately, it comes down to personal preference. I personally favor working with springs because they can be easily adapted to simulate other activities and can be more functional in their effect. They also feel alive with energy, a sensation that I enjoy.

The spring settings on the equipment are a complex issue. Settings vary from one piece of equipment to another, and even the same piece of equipment varies with the manufacturer. Unfortunately no universal standard exists. Adding to the complexity is the fact that the spring setting for an exercise will also differ based on a person's fitness level, experience, and restrictions. In addition, you can dramatically change the goal and intensity of an exercise by increasing or decreasing the tension. Even the age of the springs can be a factor to consider when choosing a setting.

Let me also distinguish between absolute and relative resistance. *Absolute resistance* means, for instance, that two springs are always two springs. *Relative resistance*, on the other hand, refers to how heavy or light the tension feels for a particular exercise. For example, two springs are typically regarded as light for foot work but heavy for arm work.

The Pilates professional must become familiar with the resistance settings on each piece of apparatus, as they are unique to each one. As an example, when doing foot work on the reformer, heavy might mean four springs, on the cadillac the equivalent might be two springs, and on the wunda chair two springs on the top setting. The only way to learn about spring settings and their effect on an exercise is through practice—doing each movement many times, experimenting with different spring settings. There will always be a logical range within which to execute an exercise. Determining your place within that range requires patience, practice, and experience.

Because of the variables mentioned previously, I have not included an actual spring setting for each exercise. Instead I offer a scale featuring an absolute weight range, which translates to a limited number of spring setting options. You must then make microadjustments according to your individual needs.

The following are Body Arts and Science International guidelines for resistance and spring settings on the reformer. The same concept can be applied to the other apparatus, although the number of springs will change. Through experience you can establish the setting for each resistance category on the respective piece of apparatus.

Extra-light	→	0.5 spring (25 to 50 percent spring)
Light	→	1 to 1.5 springs
Medium	→	2 to 3 springs
Heavy	→	3.5 to 4 springs
Extra-heavy	→	4.5 to 5 springs

Muscle Focus

The muscle focus identifies which muscle or group of muscles the exercise targets. Although it is usually one muscle or muscle group, because of the complexity of the movement and the changing positions, there may be more. Identifying the muscle focus assists you in achieving the desired goal of the exercise. Note that in many instances, increasing or decreasing the resistance or adjusting the body position even slightly will change the muscle focus.

You are encouraged to recruit the internal support system (ISS)—the transverse abdominis, pelvic floor, diaphragm, and, in most instances, the multifidus—throughout the session, therefore these muscles are not mentioned in each exercise as target muscles. The muscle focus refers to muscles other than the ISS unless the exercise is specifically for one or more of these core muscles.

Objectives

Whereas the muscle focus is very specific, the objectives relate to an exercise or an action in a broader context, often describing the action of that muscle and other muscles involved. Although an exercise may have one muscle focus, it can have several objectives that do not necessarily relate only to the area of the muscle focus. For example, in the Mat Work: Hundred (page 50), a signature Pilates abdominal exercise, the muscle focus is the abdominals and the objectives are to strengthen the abdominal muscles, develop trunk and scapular stabilization, and stimulate the cardiovascular system.

Control

I use the word *control* in a specific context that requires explanation. Often the term *strengthen* is thrown around too liberally in Pilates. In order to strengthen a muscle, certain criteria need to be in place, one being *overload.* If insufficient overload is placed on a muscle, it will not increase significantly in strength. There may be muscle activation, which in itself has value in terms of neuromuscular patterning and body awareness. However, the muscle is not being strengthened significantly. So I use the term *control* when a muscle is being recruited but not overloaded sufficiently for significant strengthening to occur. Several other terms used frequently in the objectives warrant discussion.

Stabilization

A frequent objective is to develop stabilization in a particular area of the body. Each exercise can be broken down into muscles that stabilize movement (stabilizers) and muscles that produce movement (movers). Both are important in maintaining the integrity of the exercise. A subcategory is the synergists, which are recruited to neutralize undesired muscle actions and assist in achieving the correct movement. For instance, in the Reformer: Seated Chest Expansion (page 172), a shoulder extensor exercise, the following sequence of events should occur. First the stabilizers are recruited, initially the stabilizers of the trunk (local stabilizers), then those of the scapulae and the elbow (global stabilizers). The movers—the shoulder extensors—come next, of which the latissimus dorsi is prominent. The latissimus dorsi is a shoulder extensor, shoulder adductor, and shoulder internal rotator. In this exercise we encourage the first two actions but do not want shoulder internal rotation. Therefore, we must engage the shoulder *external* rotators to neutralize the *internal* rotation component of the latissimus dorsi and prevent the shoulder from internally rotating. The shoulder external rotators function as synergists to keep the shoulder in the desired neutral position and assist the prime mover in maintaining the integrity of the exercise.

In any exercise, I encourage first focusing on the stabilizers because without correct stabilization efficient movement cannot occur. Once you have achieved correct stabilization, focus on the initiators and then the movers. I call this the *SIM (stabilize-initiate-move) formula*. The initiator may be described as the initial cue or prime focus of the movement; it functions as a crucial link in the movement. After this process has been learned and practiced many times it becomes second nature, an instinctive response to the movement.

Most traditional forms of movement analysis address the stabilizers and movers but not the initiator. This is understandable because the initiator is in fact either a stabilizer or a mover, and therefore falls into one of these categories. However, using the concept of the initiator encourages mental focus, body awareness, and control, which in turn promise maximum effect from the exercise.

Besides highlighting the importance of stabilization, Pilates incorporates full ranges of motion of the joints as well as different types of muscle contraction. The stabilizers, which are fundamental to this system and are now also recognized as fundamental in most exercise and rehabilitation regimens, work isometrically, meaning that the muscles contract with no change in their length or in the angle of the joint(s) they are acting on. The movers work isotonically, both concentrically (the muscles decrease in length, and the angle of the joints they are acting on decreases) and eccentrically (the muscles increase in length, and the angle of the joints they are acting on increases). Pilates also encourages a symbiotic relationship between agonist and antagonist muscle groups: typically, as one contracts concentrically the other contracts eccentrically. In certain instances they act as stabilizers, both contracting isometrically to stabilize an area. It is important to strive for a good balance between opposing muscle groups in terms of strength, flexibility, and control.

Stabilizing the Trunk The term *trunk stabilization* describes a stable position of the spine and is synonymous with *spinal stabilization, core stabilization,* and *torso stabilization.* I typically use the term *trunk stabilization* when the trunk is stable and the upper girdle is being mobilized because of the close relationship the two regions share. The movement of the arms has a direct influence on the thoracic spine and, conversely, certain muscles of the thoracic region play an important role in correct mechanics of the shoulder girdle. Furthermore, achieving good head alignment or shoulder function is impossible without correct alignment of the trunk.

Holding a stable position of the trunk is fundamental to the success of many Pilates exercises. In order to achieve trunk stabilization the ISS must be recruited. However, depending on the position of the trunk, certain muscles may be activated more than others. For instance in the Mat Work: Front Support (page 83), the abdominals play a vital role in stabilizing the trunk and avoiding collapse through the center (see figure 2.4a, page 17). However, in the Mat Work: Back Support (page 88), although the abdominals are recruited to add support to the structure, it is primarily the back extensors, together with the hip extensors and shoulder extensors, that hold the structure up (see figure 2.4, *b* and *c*, page 18).

Similarly, in the Mat Work: Rolling Like a Ball (page 55), stability of the trunk needs to be sustained in forward flexion. In this case the abdominals play a far greater role than the back extensors; in fact, disengagement of the back extensors may be necessary to achieve the smooth, rolling motion. The Mat Work: Swan Dive (page 104), however, demands a great deal of back extensor work to achieve the desired position. Yet, the abdominals are crucial in maintaining stability, distributing the load through the spine, and protecting the lower back from excessive pressure.

In a standing position, the gravitational pull is equal in the front and back of the body (ideally). In this case the abdominals and back extensors work in a state of co-contraction to stabilize the trunk. The back extensors hold the body upright and prevent it from folding forward. At the same time, the abdominals play an important role in creating a girdle of support around the midsection and functioning as a second spine, preventing excessive stress on the spine.

Note that the abdominals tend to decondition more quickly than the back extensors, and the back extensors tend to respond to conditioning more readily than do the abdominals. Add to this the fact that the back extensors are being used most of the time in order to keep us upright, and the result is that they are typically better conditioned than the abdominals. However, the fact that the back extensors are in use almost constantly can in itself create a problem, especially for the superficial layers; they may become hypertonic (overused) and feel very tight. "Switching them off" to allow the abdominals (plus the intrinsic extensors such as the multifidus) to fully engage is a first crucial step in creating balance in the trunk and healthy trunk stabilization. Other extensors that appear to play a profound role in trunk stabilization are the quadratus lumborum, longissimus, and iliocostalis.

The muscles of the trunk must be well conditioned to support a variety of activities, and the trunk should be worked in all ranges of motion: flexion, extension, lateral flexion, and rotation. A safe guideline in exercising the muscles of the trunk is equal balance between the flexors and extensors, with the lateral flexors receiving 50 to 75 percent of the time allotted for the spinal extensors. In addition, consider that exercises geared toward endurance as opposed to strength appear to have a more positive effect on enhancing spinal stability. The block system ensures that each of these factors is addressed in a well-rounded Pilates session.

Stabilizing the Pelvic–Lumbar Region Another important area to consider when discussing stabilization is the pelvis and lumbar spine. With pelvic–lumbar stabilization, as with trunk stabilization, the position of the spine and the direction of the pull of gravity determine which muscles are recruited and to what extent, yet the ISS is fundamental to achieving stabilization and is recruited at all times. I use the term *pelvic–lumbar stabilization* when the lower extremity is being mobilized because such action has a direct impact on the pelvis and lumbar spine.

Stabilizing the Scapulae The terms *shoulder stabilization* and *scapular stabilization* are synonymous. We tend to think of the shoulder as only the glenohumeral joint, the ball-and-socket joint that allows arm movement in every direction, but it is an intricate structure that involves precise interplay between various bones, joints, and muscles. The humerus, scapula, and clavicle form the shoulder complex, which is connected to the axial skeleton only at the tiny sternoclavicular joint. Because of the lack of bony and ligamentous support, the shoulder is *muscle dependent*—it relies heavily on the musculature for its function and stability. *Scapular stabilization* is a more precise term than *shoulder stabilization* because the stabilization mechanism always emanates from the scapulae. Scapular stabilization does not necessarily mean keeping the scapulae still, but preventing them from moving excessively in an undesired direction. For instance, in many exercises the scapulae tend to elevate and adduct, requiring that they be depressed and abducted to maintain the integrity of the movement.

In this book I use *scapular* or *shoulder stabilization* interchangeably to refer to keeping the scapulae in the correct position.

The shoulder complex is of great personal interest to me because I inherited a hooked acromion process. Throughout my life I have participated in activities with a high level of shoulder activity (swimming, dancing, yoga, gymnastics, and Pilates) and my supraspinatus eventually tore and retracted on both sides. This resulted in extensive open rotator cuff surgery on both shoulders to

shave the acromion process and reattach the muscles. This was followed by recuperation and rehabilitation, after which began a personal journey of exploration to find solutions within Pilates that would bring me back to 100 percent function. I learned a tremendous amount, including how difficult and painful rehabilitation can be. I recognized anew the power of Pilates and its limitless possibilities. But probably the most important lessons I learned are how intricate the mechanics of the shoulder are, how few people use their shoulders correctly, and the far-reaching implications of incorrect use. One of the most common corrections in Pilates studios worldwide is "Relax your shoulders."

The back extensors, particularly those of the mid-back, play an important role in correct shoulder mechanics, not only because of their direct participation in those mechanics but also because of their importance in alignment and posture of the body (figure 3.1). As mentioned earlier, our modern lifestyle lends itself to certain postural deviations, such as round-shoulder syndrome, which is caused by the fact that so much of what we do is in a forward-oriented direction. We work on computers, drive for hours, eat, and sit for much of the day—and then when we go out for recreation we ride bikes, play golf, or go to the gym and do 500 push-ups, crunches, and bench presses! The pattern is clear; all these activities involve forward motion and typically lead to weak back extensors and shoulder external rotators; tight pectorals, hip flexors, hamstrings, and shoulder internal rotators; and an overactive levator scapulae and upper trapezius. Throw in some psychological tension, and you have a recipe for the neck, shoulder, and lower back problems that are so prevalent in our society.

So where do we start? We start with the muscles that hold us up, the back extensors, supported by the ISS. As long as the body is in good alignment, as close to the plumb line as possible, achieving good shoulder mechanics is possible. Conversely, without good alignment of the trunk, good shoulder mechanics are impos-

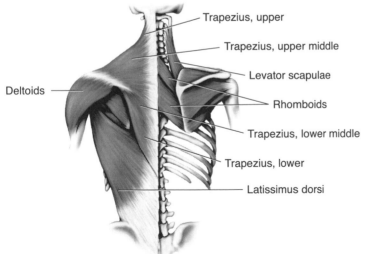

Deltoids —

— Trapezius, upper

— Trapezius, upper middle

— Levator scapulae

— Rhomboids

— Trapezius, lower middle

— Trapezius, lower

— Latissimus dorsi

FIGURE 3.1 The muscles of the mid-back help with scapular stabilization, an important objective in many Pilates exercises.

sible—and faulty shoulder mechanics will probably result in shoulder problems. Rounded shoulders can lead to impingement, impingement can lead to rotator cuff inflammation, inflammation to tearing and potentially to incapacitation and surgery. This downward spiral starts with innocent habitual movement patterns that cause incorrect posture and muscular imbalance.

Disassociation

Disassociation is a wonderful concept because it depicts so well two of the pillars of human motion: stabilization and movement. Stabilization plus mobilization equals disassociation. One area of the body remains motionless while a connecting part moves as freely as possible. Ineffective stabilization translates to an unstable base of support. Ineffective movement lacks efficiency, fluidity, strength, and range of motion, and typically relies on muscle-substitution patterns (compensations) to perform the motion. The more solid the foundation is, the more precise and efficient the movement can be. This is the basis of correct mechanics of movement. The formula is as follows: *Better stabilization equals better movement, and better movement equals safer movement.*

Muscle Isolation

The process of achieving muscle isolation involves heightened body awareness and control. Muscle isolation and muscle integration seem to be diametrically opposed functions; however, achieving true muscle isolation means incorporating all the principles of Pilates and achieving muscle integration. Much of the conventional equipment found in gyms can be used to facilitate isolation of a muscle group, without requiring integration. I do not consider this functional isolation because the support is provided by extrinsic rather than intrinsic means; the equipment provides the stabilization not the body. *Better integration equals better isolation*, and Pilates offers the tools to master both sides of this equation.

Imagery

One of the tools commonly used when doing or teaching Pilates is imagery. An image can convey a large amount of information instantaneously, whereas explanations involving large amounts of technical information and in-depth description can at times be confusing and counterproductive. In fact, describing a directive anatomically is often almost impossible. For example, if you want the movement to flow, how could your instruction be described in concrete and anatomical terms? Yet simply saying, "Flow," accompanied by an illustrative gesture or calming tone, will most likely produce the desired effect.

Imagery should be used with insight to avoid misunderstandings and breakdowns in communication. The image should be suited to the client's *image* vocabulary so that he or she can relate to the image and infer meaning. If not, the image may seem meaningless or even ludicrous. Common expressions such as "navel to spine," "scooping the belly," and "hollowing the center" are examples of imagery. These phrases refer to the action of engaging the ISS, specifically the transverse abdominis. Teaching the recruitment of the ISS (and use of the powerhouse) is challenging because of the high level of awareness, concentration, and control required. Imagery is often the key.

Effectively cueing an exercise (for yourself or others) by using imagery requires good understanding of the movement. Cueing is an art that comes in different forms—tactile, verbal, and visual—and you can deliver each type in different ways. Through cueing, information can be conveyed, received, and integrated instantaneously. Succinct cueing is equivalent to good communication between teacher and client, and good communication leads to better understanding. Good understanding is the basis of quality practice; *consistent, high-quality practice is the path to mastery and success.*

A key component in improving cueing skills is experience in practicing and teaching the method. This process takes time. Just as a student cannot learn all the nuances of an exercise in one session, so a teacher cannot learn all the cues in one page of a book. Cues for an exercise may also change from person to person and day to day. Knowledge, practice, experience, intuition, compassion, and understanding are all ingredients that make for good cueing.

Following is a brief discussion of some of the terms I often use in my imagery, both in a studio setting and in this book.

Lengthening

The term *lengthen* is frequently used in Pilates. This is a complex directive that can mean different things to different people. Working full ranges of motion can encourage lengthening. It is also helpful to think of the co-contraction of the muscles along a kinetic chain (such as a limb) and the joints being in full extension. This can give the appearance and feeling that the whole kinetic chain is functioning as one long segment (reaching out in space) rather than as short individual links.

When using imagery, stressing the difference between concept and physiological fact, and not confusing the two, is important. For example, commands such as "Lift the leg from the back [the hamstrings], lengthening out of the hip joint" and "Reach up from under the arm" both utilize imagery to aim for a physically apparent result but are anatomically imprecise. This is not to say these images cannot and should not be used. Absolutely they can, and often very effectively. But one should always be aware of the distinction between fact and poetic license.

A related point of discussion is the question of how straight is straight? Because of the often-heard instruction not to lock the knees or elbows, many people no longer straighten their limbs completely. This results in inefficient movement, incomplete use of the joint, an unstable joint, inadequate muscle recruitment, and even the onset of problems such as patella femoral syndrome (caused by misaligned tracking of the patella). *Locking*

refers to hyperextension of the joint, which should be avoided when doing Pilates. However, this note of caution does not mean that you should never completely extend the joint; it means that you should reach the straightest line possible without going beyond true extension (a straight line). This is achieved by becoming aware of what *straight* is. First, create an imaginary straight line across the joint. Then activate both the agonist and antagonist muscles groups (co-contraction). In the case of the knee, the hamstrings and quadriceps should be in a state of co-contraction with the knee joint fully extended. In this position the joint is well supported, the correct muscles are activated fully, and a long line has been achieved.

Remember, a straight limb is longer than a hyperextended or slightly bent one. This is easy to feel on the reformer when doing the foot work (pages 112 to 121). As long as the carriage is traveling away from the foot bar, the leg is still straightening. Once the leg is completely straight, the carriage will no longer move in that direction and it is time to bend the knee and return. If the knee continues extending past the straight line into hyperextension, the carriage will actually start returning toward the foot bar. It is a slight but distinct movement, illustrating that hyperextension is shorter than full extension.

Ultimately, creating length is both an anatomical and an inner quality and is conveyed better through relaxed, rather than tension-filled, movement. A wonderful dance teacher once showed me how a straight arm can look short or, by contrast, appear infinite in length. It was difficult to identify exactly what the difference was, but it was clearly apparent and I have never forgotten that lesson. I try to re-create that quality in every move I do.

Relaxing the Ribs

In discussing imagery we need to pay particular attention to the lower rib cage, which tends to thrust forward in an upright position or lift off the mat in a supine position. This can lead to a tightening of the lower spinal extensors and hyperlordosis. I think of the lower ribs being connected to the pubic symphysis with a rubber band that allows the ribs to move, sliding up and down the front of the body, but remain controlled. This image encourages the muscles of the lower back to relax, which increases the chance of improved abdominal activation. You will often hear Pilates teachers say, "Drop your ribs" or "Relax your ribs." What is being implied in physiological terms is to engage the abdominal muscles and decrease contraction of the lower spinal extensors (without going into spinal flexion), resulting in ideal alignment with appropriate muscle activation. Breathing can play a valuable role in this process. Often one deep exhalation achieves the desired result. Try it right now—inhale and exhale fully!

Imprinting

Credit for the concept of *imprinting* must be given to Eve Gentry, one of the great first-generation Pilates teachers. It was a central motif of her teaching and of the powerful imagery she used with great success. I had the pleasure of experiencing Eve's teaching firsthand, and a true pleasure it was.

Lying on a mat, visualize the body sinking into soft sand, making an imprint. The bones are then moved out of and back into the imprint. In this form of work the focus on the individual muscles may be minimized while attention is shifted to the motion of the body part. Ideally, this results in movement that is fluid and void of tension. For example, when performing the pelvic curl you may imagine an imprint of the spine in the sand. Each vertebra is first lifted out of its imprint and then returned. The result is sequential articulation of the spine without excess muscle activity (or at least without the tension associated with trying too hard). You can apply this concept to any part of the body in any position. It allows the body to move with graceful correctness without being bogged down with information.

In conclusion, effective learning and teaching strategies may vary with the type of movement patterns. Furthermore, different people may prefer different learning modes. Some people learn better when presented with a picture or a model of the movement, which they then emulate and practice. Others learn better by breaking the motion down into small movements. Still others prefer an explanation or the use of touch. In most cases a combination of approaches is best, using every angle to improve performance and increase understanding.

The following general guidelines will prove helpful in achieving a positive outcome:

- Precede the movement with the breath.
- Set up the exercise before moving (engage the ISS).
- Concentrate on the muscle focus.
- Keep the head aligned with the spine.
- Direct the eyes forward, in line with the head.
- Breathe throughout the exercise (even if it is not the set breathing pattern).
- Keep the shoulders and neck relaxed.
- Create long lines in the movements.
- Move with flow.

Movement Description

Each exercise in the following chapters includes a description of the movement, with step-by-step instructions for correct execution. Although the words *exercise* and *movement* can and are used interchangeably, I often use the word *movement* rather than *exercise* in an endeavor to differentiate the Pilates approach from the notion that an exercise is merely a physical action. The physical motion of an exercise is only one of many layers (and the most superficial one at that). Even the most basic exercise has many layers of information. This is not meant to devalue the physicality of an exercise but to bring attention to this approach, in which the movements are a means to an end and vehicles for a higher purpose.

Preparation—setting up the body to perform the movement correctly—is important before starting an exercise. I often say to students that the setup is 90 percent of the exercise and the movement is 10 percent. Without a good, precise setup the movement has little chance of being correct and producing the desired results. The setup allows the mind and body to work together to achieve optimal alignment and muscle recruitment.

The setup may take 5 seconds or 30 seconds—take the time you need to engage the ISS and establish a connection with the muscle focus of the exercise. Review the breathing pattern, and do a body scan to make sure that every body part is aligned and in place. Go through a checklist of the nuances of the movement. If you are working alone, cue yourself and make corrections to the movement before the mistakes or deviations ever occur.

The better you know your body and recognize your own compensations, the more refined this process becomes. In essence the exercise begins long before movement is apparent.

Achieving Symmetry

Is symmetry attainable? Is it desirable? My wife, Adelle, likes to remind me that in nature there is no absolute symmetry—close, but not absolute. So should we strive for symmetry in our bodies? This question leads to the interesting issue of symmetrical versus asymmetrical training. I have worked with athletes involved in such activities as tennis and volleyball who have questioned whether to tamper with the asymmetries their sport has resulted in. One of them might argue, "I am one of the top tennis players in the world. I want to refine my muscular development and enhance my performance. I want more core strength but I don't want to tamper with the balance (or imbalance) in my body because it is serving me well." And it often is. Personally I like to promote symmetry as an ideal, a reference point to strive for that can measure improvement as well as serve as a guideline for cueing. I believe that training toward symmetry ultimately enhances performance and function, in both everyday and skill-specific activities—and it prevents undue stresses on the body and eventual breakdown.

Furthermore, when practicing movement on one side of the body, a transferal of information to the other side occurs. That means that if one side is injured, exercising the noninjured side has a positive effect on the injured side, as information is transferred. This transferal applies not only to injuries but to all motor skills, including athletic activities.

Training toward symmetry is complex, therefore a conservative approach is the most prudent one. Do not rush to make drastic changes. I use the following steps when dealing with imbalances. Note that I use the first and second steps in a well-rounded session for several

Repetitions in Pilates

Joseph Pilates spoke of *mindless repetition;* I like that term because I believe that high repetition invariably becomes mindless, with diminished return. You can spend hours on an exercise routine that is based on a high number of repetitions with no real focus or control, and it becomes mindless as opposed to mindful. Being mindful in each exercise and each repetition is the goal. In order to achieve this, both physically and mentally, I recommend a limited number of repetitions, usually 5 to 10, depending on the intensity and complexity of the movement. The more complex the movement is, the fewer repetitions are required. Use the low end of the scale for the very difficult and complex repertoire, and the high end, 10 repetitions (still relatively low compared to a typical gym workout) for the fundamental work.

The main reason that such pronounced effects are achieved from so few repetitions is because of the high degree of precision, which recruits the desired muscles to the maximum. If many repetitions are done, compensations often creep in—other muscles (usually the larger, superficial ones) take over, and the work and effect on the desired muscles is minimal at best. Other negative effects of doing excessive repetitions are fatigue, wear and tear on the joints, boredom, and in some instances, injury. Pilates encapsulates the concept of *Less is more* (quality versus quantity), which holds the key to deeper work and enhanced performance.

months before proceeding (only if necessary) to steps 3 and 4.

1. Work bilaterally, raising awareness of asymmetrical muscular activity and development.
2. Work unilaterally, using the same number of repetitions and resistance on both sides.
3. Work unilaterally, loading the weaker, less-dominant side more than the other.
4. Work unilaterally, working only the weaker, less-dominant side.

Moving With the Energy Lines

As a dancer I was taught to think of movement in terms of energy lines or paths; this is a concept that adapts well to Pilates. Energy paths can be straight, circular, or spiral shaped. Fundamental movements such as the Mat Work: Pelvic Curl (page 45) or Mat Work: Chest Lift (page 48) are comprised of only one or two energy lines (see figure 3.2a). More complex movements have more energy lines, since various parts of the body reach in different and often opposing directions. For example, the Mat Work: Spine Twist (page 72) has longitudinal, horizontal, and circular energy lines (see figure 3.2b). The longitudinal line, which travels up and down the spine and continues into space, keeps the trunk upright. The horizontal line, running across the shoulders and traveling outward in both directions, keeps the arms, shoulders and back as broad as possible and on one plane. We add to this a spiral, which travels up the trunk, illustrating the rotation that occurs. The energy moves in all these directions at the same time, making this movement relatively complex.

Think of the energy lines as a form of notating the energy of the exercises. Understanding these lines will bring clarity and simplicity to the exercises and result in precise movement. You can utilize this principle in every exercise. Once you understand the energy lines

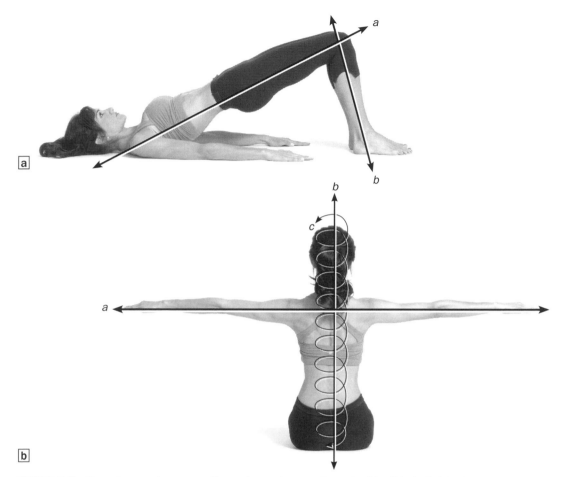

FIGURE 3.2 Focusing on the energy lines of exercises such as the Mat Work: Pelvic Curl (a) and the Mat Work: Spine Twist (b) will direct you to the correct movement path.

of an exercise, the choreography becomes clear and the correct muscles will be activated in the most effective manner.

Adapting Exercises

There is no need to reinvent the wheel. I've seen people create variations of Pilates exercises simply to be different or to avoid boredom. Others choreograph variations because they are unfamiliar with the original exercises. I do not support changing an exercise for any of these reasons. I believe the essence of the exercise is often lost in a mass of choreography, at times ceasing to have any resemblance to the original exercise or its intention. Yes, we must evolve. But evolution does not mean throwing out this vast, ingenious body of work. It means refining it according to gains in scientific knowledge and building on the foundation of the original work. This promotes growth, keeps the system alive and up to date, and allows us to adapt the work to individual goals and the needs of modern society.

The original body of work must be seen in the context of the time and place it was created, the early part of the 20th century in Europe and New York. That world was very different from the 21st century in terms of people's habits, occupations, and lifestyles. Computers were nonexistent, cars were scarce, air travel was a dream, the Internet was decades away, recreational activities were different—surely evolution is justified. But in the process, we must not lose sight of the value of Joseph Pilates' work.

Modifying exercises or adding props (assists) to them is necessary at times in order to avoid negative movement patterns, compensations, and contraindications and to achieve the desired objectives. When I say *modification,* I mean changing the choreography of an exercise to meet certain goals. However, maintaining the essence of the exercise is critical, which means that one must understand the intention and mechanics of the exercise and its possible contraindications. Discovering modifications is an integral part of being a creative, interactive teacher.

This approach to modifications applies also to *assists*. Assists are external aids such as springs, rubber bands, cushions, balls, or adjustments to the apparatus that help achieve the goal. Again, complete understanding of the exercise and the exerciser is essential. Also important is being well informed about the many choices of apparatus and which would be best suited for each scenario. In short, intimate familiarity with the Pilates repertoire, the human body and its movements, and the myriad choreographic directions and apparatus available make this work an evolutionary process.

I have intentionally abstained from offering many modifications and assists in this book. My reasons are twofold; first, I think that initially gaining knowledge, understanding, and experience in the original repertoire is important. Too much information and too many variations can lead to confusion. Second, I like to encourage individual creativity. Once you have learned the original exercises—their form, function, and intent—and gained knowledge of the equipment, human science, and the body you are working with, the possibilities for developing variations become infinite.

CHAPTER 4

Mat Work

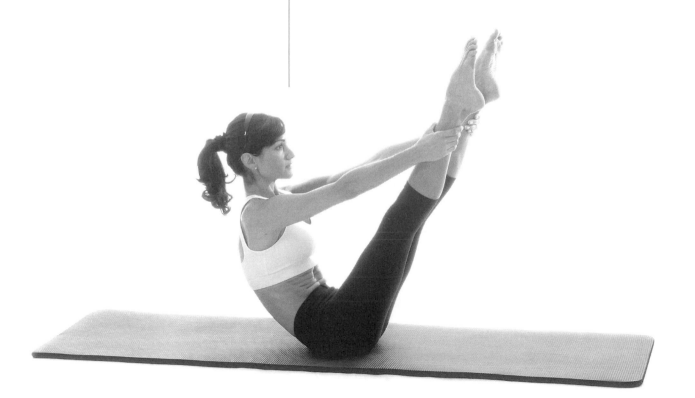

Pilates mat work is the foundation of the system, the spring from which the water flows. It is the source of all that follows, the root of every other exercise in the repertoire, and it never ceases to challenge. Without an intricate familiarity with the mat work, you will lack a fundamental component in your practice.

Mat work can be practiced anywhere and everywhere, with no special apparatus other than a mat. You can practice it any time of day, at any level of difficulty, from fundamental to advanced. You also can structure it to meet different goals: as a warm-up for a Pilates class on the apparatus or other athletic activities, as part of a daily conditioning program, for general body awareness and neuromuscular reeducation, or as a pre- and postnatal activity.

Note that the exercises are presented with both progression and a block system in mind. Therefore not all fundamental exercises appear at the beginning of the chapter, and there is some shifting back and forth in terms of the level of challenge associated with the exercises.

Mat work embodies flow as no other apparatus does. It lends itself to the integration of transitions and movement without pause, and because of this fact, it also promotes cardiovascular endurance more than any other aspect of the Pilates method. I have created several mat work sequences based on level and dura-tion—I call them *flow sequences*—that offer a unique way to practice traditional mat work. They incorporate the original movements yet place them in a sequence that flows seamlessly from one exercise to the next. The flow sequences, which are invigorating and challenging for all levels, embody the principle of flow and organize the exercises in a way that works the entire body. The idea is to view the mat work as one continuous movement, starting with the first breath and ending with the final movement.

I typically conclude a mat work session with some relaxation and focusing, which lasts anywhere from 1 to 5 minutes. It sometimes involves moving through slow, guided movements that are simple and enjoyable to perform, or it may involve sitting in one position, still and comfortable, listening to calming words or music or going through a short, guided meditation.

This relaxation period serves as a cool-down for the body and a time to mentally and spiritually integrate the work that you have just done. I find this possibly the most valuable part of the session because it creates an inner feeling that you can preserve for the rest of the day. This is the moment when the transformation occurs, when body, mind, and spirit unite. Don't view the mat work as the underdog in this system; it is the crown jewel. Enjoy!

Pelvic Curl

The pelvic curl is a foundation exercise that has a myriad of benefits. Not only does it mobilize the spine and prepare it for exercise, but it also teaches correct recruitment of the internal support system (ISS; page 17). The pelvic curl develops body awareness and brings focus to the *powerhouse*. This exercise promotes mobility in the pelvic region, releasing both physical and mental tension in the process.

Imagery

The image I like to use is that of a banana peel being peeled off the fruit slowly and deliberately. Allow the feeling of gentle resistance and fine movement to prevail throughout.

☐ Begin and complete the movement in a neutral spine position.

☐ Tilt the pelvis slightly posteriorly and stretch the hip flexors in the up phase.

☐ Keep the shoulders and neck relaxed and uninvolved.

Muscle Focus

- Abdominal muscles
- Hamstrings

Objectives

- To improve spinal articulation
- To establish pelvic–lumbar stabilization
- To develop abdominal and hamstring control

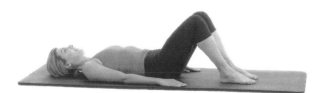

Inhale. Lie supine with the spine in a neutral position, keeping the entire body relaxed. Bend the knees and place the feet hip-width apart. Sense the elongation through the spine while gliding the scapulae down the back, placing the arms straight by the sides with the fingers reaching toward the feet. Make sure the neck is relaxed with the chin tilted slightly to the chest.

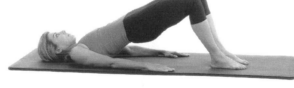

Exhale. Draw in the abdominal muscles. Begin to curl the pelvis, lifting the lower back vertebra by vertebra off the floor. Midway through the motion, recruit the hamstrings to lift the pelvis and trunk higher off the mat. Then as you inhale, keep the body still, with the legs parallel. Engage the shoulder extensors to accentuate the extension of the upper back.

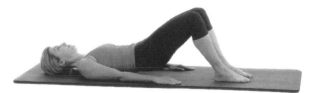

Exhale. Articulate the spine in reverse order from the top of the spine, vertebra by vertebra, accentuating the flexion through the lumbar region. Return to the starting position.

Leg Changes—Single and Double

Muscle Focus

- Abdominal muscles

Objectives

- To develop pelvic–lumbar stabilization
- To develop hip-joint disassociation
- To improve abdominal and hip flexor control

This exercise uses the abdominal muscles as stabilizers rather than as movers. It is particularly useful when pelvic stability is lacking or abdominal strength is insufficient to lift into forward flexion. By keeping the entire body still, particularly the pelvic–lumbar region, and moving only one leg up and down, you learn to bring awareness to the powerhouse and how to stabilize the pelvis. To raise the level of difficulty and challenge, unload both legs and alternate the leg lifts, with the leg change occurring simultaneously.

Imagery

The pelvis should be as stable as a rock and the legs as light as feathers, floating up and down without affecting the pelvis. These opposing images help create the sensation that occurs in the body.

- ☐ Avoid tension in the lower back and possible hyperlordosis when lifting the legs.
- ☐ Move the leg(s) as one unit, maintaining a right angle at the knee.
- ☐ Minimize the weight shift onto the supporting leg when lifting the opposite side.

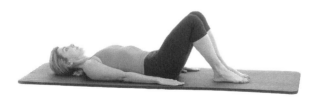

Inhale. Prepare as you would for the initial position of the pelvic curl (page 45), emphasizing pelvic–lumbar stability and distributing the weight evenly on the feet.

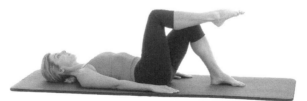

Exhale. Lift one leg, focusing movement in the hip joint only, maintaining a perfect right angle in the knee throughout the full range of motion. Continue the movement until your hip reaches a right angle with the floor (tabletop position).

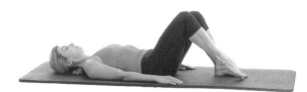

Inhale. Keep the knee at a right angle and lower the leg gently, touching the floor with the tip of the toes without placing any pressure on the foot. Repeat several times before changing to the other side.

Supine Spine Twist

This exercise prepares the body (specifically the spine) for rotational movements. It also activates and brings awareness to the oblique abdominal muscles. The degree of the rotation should be dictated by your flexibility and abdominal control. Maintain strong pelvic–lumbar support, avoiding hyperlordosis throughout the movement. This is particularly pertinent when in rotation because the tendency to exceed the controllable range of motion often results in the back arching excessively.

Imagery

Imagine the pelvis turning like a doorknob, with the pelvis, knees, and feet as one unit rotating fluidly from side to side.

☐ Keep the shoulder girdle and neck relaxed and still.

☐ Focus the movement in the waist area, initiating it with the transverse abdominis, followed by the oblique abdominal muscles.

☐ Keep the knees and feet together, avoiding any gliding back and forth.

☐ Maintain a long line across the chest from the fingertips of one hand to the fingertips of the other.

Muscle Focus

▪ Oblique abdominal muscles

Objectives

▪ To improve flexibility for spinal rotation

▪ To increase abdominal control

▪ To encourage pelvic–lumbar stabilization

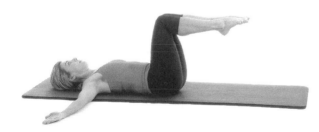

Exhale. Lie supine with the arms in the T position, palms facing upward. The hips and knees are at right angles; the ankles are in line with the knees. Draw the lumbar spine into the mat, maintaining a slight posterior pelvic tilt.

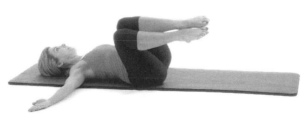

Inhale. Rotate the spine; moving the pelvis and the legs as one unit to one side, keeping the knees together. The movement is in the transverse plane, with the shoulder girdle providing a stable base around which the movement occurs.

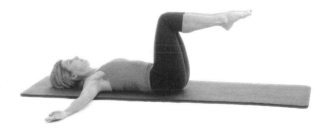

Exhale. Draw the pelvis and legs as one unit back to the center. Repeat the steps on the opposite side

Chest Lift

This exercise strengthens the abdominal muscles, teaches correct recruitment of the internal support system, and lays the foundation for much of the abdominal work that follows. Although it resembles the infamous *crunch,* it is a completely different exercise. Most notably the pace is much slower, to eliminate momentum and let the movement be driven by the strength of the abdominal muscles as well as the positioning of the spine and pelvis. The chest lift should be challenging regardless of your fitness level. Remember: *Exercises do not get easier (as we get stronger); they get better (more intense)!*

Muscle Focus

▪ Abdominal muscles

Objectives

▪ To strengthen the abdominal muscles
▪ To develop pelvic stability and control

Imagery

Imagine creating a hollow-bowl shape in the area of the navel as the abdominal muscles sink down to the spine and the lower spine imprints into the mat. The pelvic floor and the upper spine gently rise on either side, forming the walls of the bowl.

☐ Avoid pulling on the neck.
☐ Lift the head, shoulders, and upper trunk as one unit.
☐ Maintain a neutral pelvis, keeping the hip flexors as relaxed as possible.

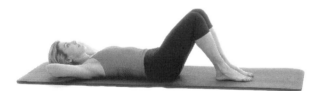

Inhale. Lie supine with the pelvis and spine in a neutral position and the knees bent with the feet hip-width apart. Feel a sense of elongation through the spine. Interlace the fingers and cradle the head in the hands. Make sure the neck is relaxed with the chin slightly tilted to the chest. Engage the internal support system, highlighting awareness of the abdominal region.

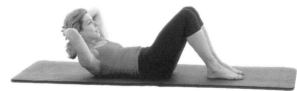

Exhale. While drawing in the abdominal muscles, allow the lumbar spine to sink into the mat and begin lifting the upper spine from the top of the head. Sense a hinging action just under the sternum, and maintain absolute stability of the body below this point. Continue lifting the upper spine vertebra by vertebra until the bases of the scapulae have risen off the mat. Inhaling, maintain the maximum height you can achieve with the upper trunk. Draw in the abdominals further.

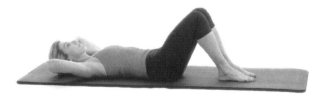

Exhale. Lower the spine without releasing the abdominal muscles. Return to the starting position.

Chest Lift With Rotation

This exercise is an extension of the Mat Work: Chest Lift (page 48), adding the element of rotation, which challenges the abdominal muscles further by loading the oblique muscles in a bilateral pattern. This lays the foundation for much of the rotational abdominal work, such as the Mat Work: Criss-Cross (page 58), and prepares the body for the many rotational activities that everyday life and athletic activities demand.

Imagery

A good image for this exercise is a combination of a doorknob turning described in the supine spine twist (page 47) and the hollow-bowl image described in the chest lift (page 48). These images together demonstrate the type of movement used in this exercise.

☐ Move the head, arms, and upper trunk as one unit.

☐ Avoid pulling on the neck and moving the elbows forward.

☐ Maintain forward flexion as you transition from side to side.

Muscle Focus

▪ Oblique abdominal muscles

Objectives

▪ To strengthen the abdominals, emphasizing the obliques
▪ To develop pelvic stability while performing spinal rotation

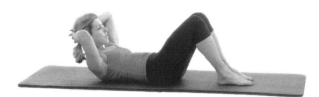

Inhale. The preparation position for this exercise is the up phase of the chest lift (page 48).

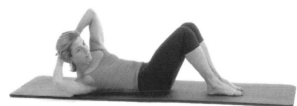

Exhale. Rotate the upper girdle to one side. Focus on drawing in the abdominal muscles and moving from the waist area without any lateral flexion of the trunk. Maintain stability of the pelvis throughout.

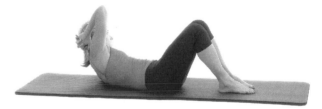

Inhale. Rotate the upper girdle through the center to the opposite side without lowering the trunk. Continue moving from side to side. On the final repetition rotate back to the center, hollowing the abdominal cavity further before returning to a supine position.

Hundred

Muscle Focus

- Abdominal muscles

Objectives

- To strengthen the abdominal muscles
- To develop trunk stabilization
- To stimulate circulation and warm up the body

This exercise is one of the signature abdominal exercises of the Pilates method, highlighting the powerhouse. The name of the exercise is derived from the breathing pattern—each breath cycle should last for 10 counts (5 counts for the inhalation and 5 counts for the exhalation) and this pattern is repeated 10 times, totaling 100 counts. This does not mean taking 100 breaths! I often use active breathing, or what Ron Fletcher coined as *percussive breathing,* during this exercise, but not if it induces tension. The percussive quality does make the breath more active and dynamic—a good thing if done well.

The hundred can be counterproductive if certain elements are not in place, including strong abdominals and the ability to lift the trunk into adequate spinal flexion. I encourage you to practice preparation exercises to build up to the hundred. For example, you can start by keeping the feet on the floor or performing the exercise with legs bent in a tabletop position,

thereby eliminating or decreasing the load on the hip flexors and making the exercise less demanding for the abdominals. If you have tight hamstrings, I recommend bending the knees for this exercise, again reducing the load on the hip flexors. When doing the full version with the legs straight, keep them at a height that you have the abdominal strength and control to support; holding the legs perpendicular to the floor is less challenging than bringing them closer to the floor.

Imagery

Visualize the movement of the arms generating energy like a turbine, which then helps keep the body stabilized, the abdominal bowl hollow and active, and the legs supported.

- ☐ Draw in the abdominal muscles throughout the exercise, imprinting the lower back into the mat.
- ☐ Relax the neck and shoulders throughout.
- ☐ Keep the pumping motion smooth, small, and free of tension.

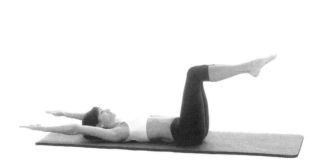

Inhale. Lie supine with the knees and hips bent at 90 degrees (tabletop position). Hold the arms straight and directly above the head.

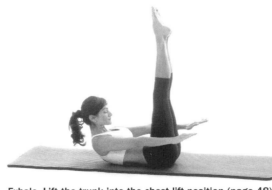

Exhale. Lift the trunk into the chest lift position (page 48), straightening the legs to the appropriate height for you. Lower the arms to the sides of the body, parallel to the floor. Inhale. Prepare for the movement by drawing in the abdominal muscles more deeply.

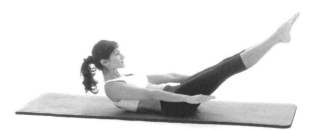

Exhale for the duration of five counts as the arms pump up and down with a small pulsing movement. Inhale for the duration of five counts, continuing to pump the arms. Keep the arms close to the sides of the body throughout. Repeat this cycle 10 times. Return to the starting position.

Leg Circles

This exercise is an excellent example of coordinated stabilization and mobilization resulting in the disassociation of the hip joint. While the pelvis remains anchored and the lumbar spine still, the hip joint fluidly rotates and the leg circles effortlessly. Hip mobilization and disassociation, a pattern often found in Pilates exercises, is required for many activities such as cycling, running, and certain dance and gymnastic movements. When executed correctly it may help release lower back tension and remedy sacroiliac dysfunction.

Leg circles can be performed with a rubber exercise band draped over the foot and held in the hands. This allows the hip flexors to relax and assists in achieving the desired fluidity of the joint as the leg rotates—a very helpful option when tight hamstrings are present.

Imagery

Imagine the leg as a big spoon that is stirring thick syrup in a big pot. The motion should be gentle and smooth, with a continuous flow. Thinking of a fall-and-retrieve action, like a yo-yo rolling down and then up, may also be helpful.

☐ Maintain a neutral pelvis and spine throughout the exercise.

☐ Keep the movement in the hip joint unrestricted and fluid.

☐ Keep the neck, shoulders, and chest relaxed.

Muscle Focus

- Abdominal muscles
- Hip flexors

Objectives

- To develop pelvic–lumbar stabilization
- To improve hip disassociation
- To develop control of the hip flexors
- To relax the muscles around the hip joint

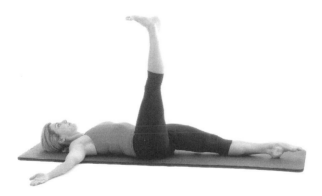

Exhale. Lie supine and place the arms by the sides of the body or in a T position. Keep the legs straight and together with the feet gently pointed. Bend one leg to the chest and then straighten it upward, perpendicular to the floor; dorsiflex the foot. Keep the other leg straight and actively engaged, with the foot plantarflexed.

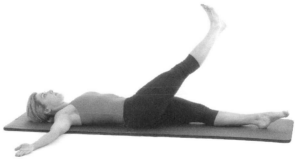

Inhale. Circle the raised leg inward, bringing it slightly across the centerline of the body, then down and around. Make the circle only as big as you can make it while maintaining a stable pelvis. Exhale, alternating the breathing on each circle, pausing slightly each time the leg is perpendicular to the floor, and repeat 5 to 10 times.

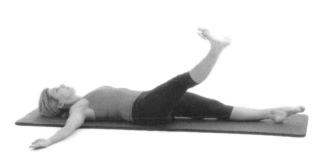

Inhale. Reverse the circle and repeat the breath pattern. Emphasize pelvic–lumbar stability and the free-flowing movement of the hip joint. Repeat 5 to 10 times, returning to the perpendicular leg position after the final repetition. Then bend the leg to the chest and return to the starting position.

Roll-Up

Muscle Focus

■ Abdominal muscles

Objectives

■ To strengthen the abdominal muscles
■ To develop spinal mobility and stability
■ To stretch the muscles of the back

The roll-up activates the abdominal muscles both as movers and as stabilizers. In the initial phase, the abdominals are recruited to move the body into spinal flexion. Next the hip flexors are introduced to lift the trunk and pelvis off the mat, flexing at the hip joint as the abdominals stabilize the trunk, maintaining the C curve of the spine. In the top position, with the shoulders directly above the hip joints, concentrate on further engaging the abdominals, remaining in the C curve and stretching the muscles of the back.

I have made several choreographic changes to this exercise from the classic form. The first is that I advocate pausing in the position described above, with the shoulders above the hips rather than reaching all the way forward with the trunk over the legs. The reason for this change is to avoid stretching the hamstrings early in the session. My objective is to warm up the abdominal muscles by activating them and to warm up the back muscles by stretching them.

The second change is the positioning of the head, which I discuss in chapter 2 (page 21). In the classic form, the head is taken to a point between the arms. I prefer that the head follow the natural line of the spine, in which case it is held higher up so that the neck and face can be clearly observed from the side.

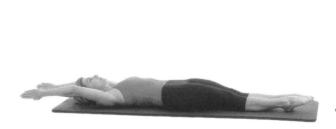
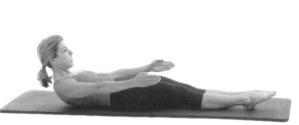
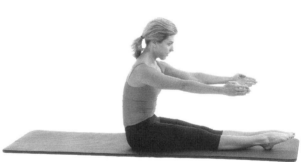

Exhale. Lie in a supine position with the arms overhead, palms facing each other, legs straight and together, and feet softly plantarflexed. Draw the ribs down and together while accentuating the overhead reach of the arms. Keep the arms shoulder-width apart.

Inhale. Engage the abdominal muscles and begin the movement with the arms, following with the head and upper spine. Pause in this position, deepening the hollow in the abdominal area and imprint the lower back deep into the mat. Prepare to lift forward off the mat to a sitting position by activating the hip flexors.

Exhale. Draw the abdominal muscles in as you lift and peel the spine off the mat vertebra by vertebra, maintaining the C curve of the trunk. Pause when the shoulders are above the hips. The curve should extend from the fingertips through the spine to the tips of the toes—hollow and deep.

Finally, in the classic form the feet are dorsiflexed. I like the feet to be in a relaxed plantar flexion position, with the knees soft. When the feet are dorsiflexed, there is a strong tendency to overuse the quadriceps and extend the knees fully. This wastes energy and needlessly activates the rectus femoris. I encourage downplaying the activity of the hip flexors in this exercise, particularly the rectus femoris. The "cherry on the top" of my version of this exercise is that it has longer lines and is aesthetically much more appealing (in my personal opinion).

Imagery

As you roll up, visualize holding the reins of a horse and being gently raised off the mat and then lowered back down. The movement should appear effortless and the gentle curve of the body should remain constant.

☐ When supine, do not allow the ribs to thrust upward as the arms reach overhead.

☐ Maintain a C curve of the trunk when lifting off the mat and in the sitting position.

☐ Keep the head aligned with the spine through the full cycle of this exercise.

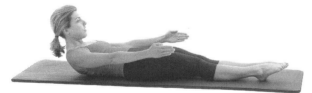

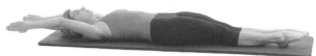

Inhale. Deepen the hollowing of the abdominal region and accentuate the curve of the spine. Do not bury the head between the arms. Hold the arms at shoulder height or lower to help create the long neck position, keeping the neck and shoulders relaxed. Exhale. Roll down vertebra by vertebra through the spine, establishing a stable core with the abdominal muscles.

Lower the head and take the arms back overhead to return to the starting position.

Muscle Focus

- Abdominal muscles

Objectives

- To improve trunk stabilization
- To learn to use energy efficiently
- To release the lower back muscles and deepen the abdominal work

Rolling Like a Ball

This exercise embodies the concepts of stabilization and internal energy flow. The more still and stable the position is, the smoother the movement will be. It illustrates well the controlled release of the back muscles (in particular those of the lower back), the deep engagement of the abdominals, and the gentle and consistent rounding of the spine, which is so necessary for the success of much of the abdominal work in Pilates. It also introduces balancing on the sit bones, a position that repeats itself in several increasingly challenging exercises. The key to the success of the exercise is keeping the ball shape of the body as contained and stable as possible.

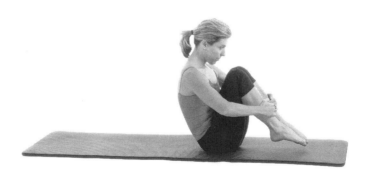

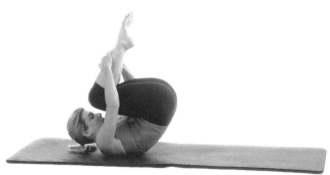

Exhale. Sit on the mat, holding each leg at the ankle. Draw the spine into an elongated C curve and lift the feet slightly off the mat. Balancing on your sit bones, keep the head aligned with the natural curve of spine. (Do not bury the head between the knees.) Deepen the C curve and solidify the position.

Inhale. Allow the weight to shift within the body and roll back, visualizing a further hollowing and rounding of the lower back region. Roll only as far as the shoulder girdle, avoiding pressure on the cervical spine.

Imagery

Visualize an inflated wheel that rolls effortlessly and without obstruction. The more inflated it is, the more smoothly it rolls. When it is deflated, its movement is staggering and halting, just as this exercise appears when a consistent, smooth spinal curve is not maintained, usually because of a tight lower back or a lack of abdominal control.

☐ Keep the trunk as still and stable as possible throughout the movement.

☐ Maintain a consistent curve in the spine from the head to the tailbone.

☐ Pause momentarily on the sit bones and on the shoulders.

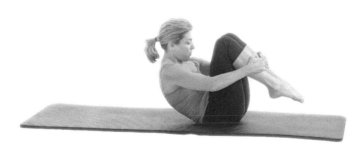

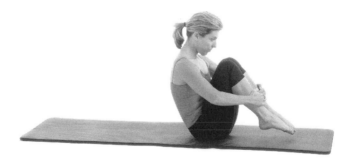

Exhale. Pausing (but not stopping), reverse the internal energy and the direction of the roll. Continue holding the trunk in a strong C-curve position, placing moderate pressure on the legs with the hands. Roll forward through the thoracic and lumbar vertebrae, returning to the initial position.

Inhale. Focus on the internal work occurring in the body to maintain this dynamic, balanced position, and keep the internal energy flowing as you prepare to repeat the movement.

Double-Leg Stretch

Muscle Focus

▪ Abdominal muscles

Objectives

▪ To strengthen the abdominal muscles
▪ To develop trunk stabilization

The double-leg stretch is a challenging abdominal exercise that emphasizes trunk stabilization. The lower back remains firmly anchored on the mat as the arms and legs simultaneously stretch away from the center of the body and are then drawn back toward the center. Keep the eyes focused forward, head stable, and the neck and shoulders relaxed. The abdominal muscles provide support for the structure; imagine them, not the hip flexors, drawing the knees toward the forehead. As the hips reach approximately 80 degrees of hip flexion and the shins are parallel to the floor, place the hands firmly on the knees, pause the movement, and deepen the abdominal contraction.

Imagery

I use the image of a rubber band being stretched from both sides and then rebounding, just like the arms and legs are stretched out in each direction and are then pulled back to center. This recoiling quality provides the dynamic essence of the exercise.

☐ Maintain a stable spine from the tip of the head to the tailbone.

☐ Reach the arms as far overhead as possible without lowering the trunk or elevating the shoulders.

☐ Keep the feet slightly above eye level throughout (if abdominal strength allows).

☐ Imprint the lower back into the mat throughout the movement.

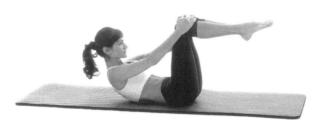

Exhale. Lie supine with the knees bent toward the chest and one hand on each knee. Lift into forward flexion, establishing the chest lift (page 48) position with the trunk.

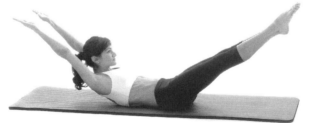

Inhale. Move the arms overhead and simultaneously straighten the legs in the opposite direction, keeping the trunk stable and the feet slightly above eye level. Imprinting the back into the mat is vital at this point in order to focus on recruiting the abdominal muscles.

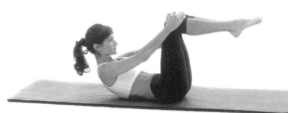

Exhale. Circle the arms around from overhead out to the sides, simultaneously drawing the knees in toward the forehead to return to the starting position. Keep the trunk stable, the shins parallel to the floor, and firmly place the hands on the knees.

Single-Leg Stretch

This exercise develops abdominal strength in a stabilizing mode (isometric contraction), holding the trunk and the pelvis absolutely still as the legs perform the movement. It is important to pay attention to the positioning of the head, which should be aligned with the spine, supported, and absolutely still. The pumping action of the legs should accelerate the abdominal work, which occurs independently of the pelvis. With each repetition, press down firmly into the knee as if driving the hip into the mat, bearing down on the bent knee with the hands to accentuate the abdominal contraction. The third photo illustrates an alternative arm position in which the outside hand reaches toward the heel.

Imagery

The combination of the legs moving in and out simultaneously conjures up the image of the pistons of a machine as they fire in and out with absolute precision. The powerhouse of the body serves as the engine that drives the pistons.

☐ Keep the trunk still throughout the movement.

☐ Keep both feet at approximately eye level as they alternate in and out.

☐ Make sure the shin of the bent leg is parallel to the floor and do not bring the knee in too close to the chest (the angle of the thigh should be at approximately 80 degrees).

Muscle Focus

▪ Abdominal muscles

Objectives

▪ To strengthen the abdominal muscles

▪ To develop stability of the pelvic–lumbar region

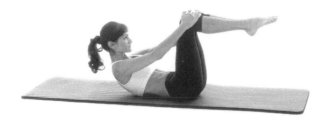

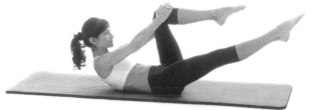

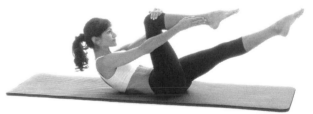

Inhale. Lie supine and draw the knees to the chest. Lift the trunk into forward flexion as in the chest lift (page 48), with the scapulae off the mat, the thighs at approximately 80 degrees of hip flexion, and the shins in a tabletop position, parallel to the floor. Place the hands on the knees.

Exhale. Straighten one leg and place the hands firmly on the shin of the opposite leg just below the knee. The bent knee is slightly closer to the chest than in a typical tabletop position; however, the shin remains parallel to the floor (as in the tabletop position).

Inhale. Simultaneously change legs, keeping the feet on the same horizontal plane and the legs close to the centerline of the body. Exhale as you straighten the opposite leg, transferring the hands to the bent knee. Return to the starting position after the final repetition.

Muscle Focus

- Oblique abdominal muscles

Objectives

- To strengthen the abdominal muscles, especially the obliques
- To develop pelvic stabilization and trunk rotation

Criss-Cross

The action of the lower body is identical to that of the Mat Work: Single-Leg Stretch (page 57): a pumping motion, keeping the feet at the same level and creating a sense of resistance as you draw the knee of the straight leg toward the chest.

The rotation of the trunk is key because it emphasizes the work of the oblique abdominal muscles. There is a tendency to laterally flex the spine and flare the ribs as the trunk faces the bent knee; this results in a swivel-type motion as opposed to a true rotation. You can prevent this by contracting the muscles on the flaring side, drawing the lower ribs toward the pelvic crest. In addition, because of the intensity of the exercise and the load on the abdominal muscles, sometimes the height of the trunk in forward flexion

decreases and the lower back starts to lift off the mat into hyperlordosis. If this occurs, immediately pause and reestablish the proper position before continuing. If muscle fatigue has set in or if you are unable to achieve the correct position, stop rather than compromise good form. Practicing incorrect form, even with the best of intentions, is counterproductive and can lead to negative habitual movement patterns and possible physical ailments.

One other common mistake is flapping the elbows in and out with minimal or no rotation of the trunk. The upper body, including the head and arms, must move as one unit as in Mat Work: Chest Lift With Rotation (page 49), an excellent preparation for the criss-cross.

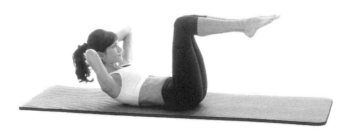

Inhale. Lie supine and draw the knees to the chest. Lift the trunk into forward flexion (as in the single-leg stretch, page 56) with the scapulae off the mat, the thighs at approximately 80 degrees of hip flexion, and the shins in a tabletop position, parallel to the floor. Interlace the fingers behind the head and hold the elbows wide.

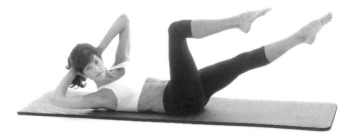

Exhale. Straighten one leg, rotating the trunk toward the bent knee.

Imagery

Use the same imagery as for the Mat Work: Single-Leg Stretch (page 57). The feeling in the waist should be like a rotating disk with the lower section (the pelvis) held absolutely stable and the top section (the trunk) rotating on an axis. Or imagine a chicken turning on a skewer that runs longitudinally through its body.

☐ Keep the elbows wide and stable.
☐ Rotate from the waist, avoiding lateral flexion.

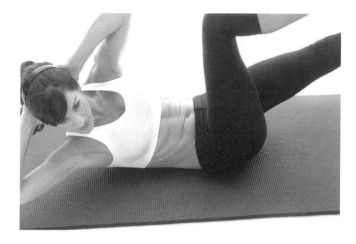

Note in this closeup the pure rotation of the trunk and the stability of the pelvis resulting in strong abdominal oblique activation.

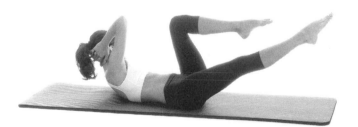

Inhale. Change the legs simultaneously as the trunk passes through the center. Then exhale as you complete the straightening of the leg and the rotation of the trunk to the other side.

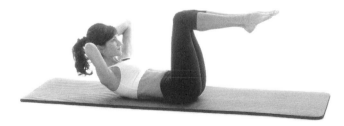

Inhale. Return to the starting position.

Hamstring Pull

Muscle Focus

- Abdominal muscles

Objectives

- To strengthen the abdominal muscles
- To develop pelvic–lumbar region stabilization
- To increase hamstring and hip flexor flexibility

The hamstring pull prepares you for the high level of pelvic–lumbar stabilization and abdominal challenge needed for other intermediate, advanced, and master-level exercises. With each leg pulse, you should focus on deepening the abdominal contraction rather than pulling the hamstrings as the name implies. The support for the position emanates from the abdominal muscles rather than the act of holding onto the leg.

Anchoring the lower leg creates a stable foundation both for stretching the hamstrings of the upper leg and for elongating the hip flexors of the lower leg, as well as facilitating deeper abdominal work. Keep a neutral and stable pelvic position, lifting the leg only as high as your flexibility and pelvic control allow. The leg movement should be viewed as independent of the pelvis.

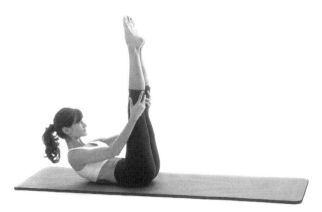

Inhale. Lie supine and lift the head and chest forward into the chest lift position (page 48). Bend the knees toward the chest, and then straighten the legs toward the ceiling, perpendicular to the floor.

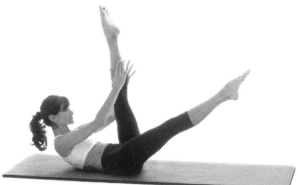

Still inhaling, place the hands behind the calf of one leg and lower the other leg to the mat and anchor it.

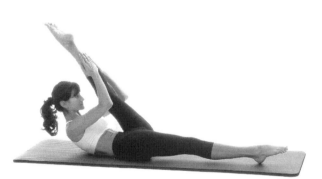

Exhale. Draw the leg slightly closer to the face, deepening the abdominal contraction, and do two small pulses with the leg. Use percussive breathing, which means exhaling with two puffs of air, one with each pulse.

This exercise offers many options to accommodate individual needs. People with tight hamstrings or hip flexors can bend the knees slightly, which allows better alignment and positioning of the pelvis. Those with weak abdominal muscles can switch the legs one at a time; then, as they gain more strength, perform the switch with both legs simultaneously.

Imagery

A wonderful image for this movement is a handheld fan opening and swishing closed, then opening in the other direction. The legs move so swiftly that they create a blur of movement.

☐ Maintain pelvic–lumbar and trunk stability as you change legs.

☐ Cradle the leg with the hands behind the calf (if flexibility allows).

☐ Keep the shoulders and neck relaxed.

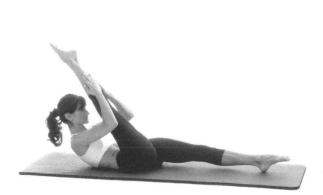

Inhale. Change the legs simultaneously—one going to the mat, the other lifting to the 90-degree angle. The switch should be swift, with absolute stillness in the torso. Continue alternating the legs.

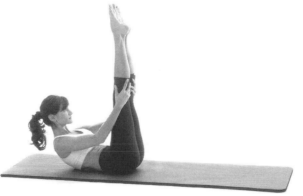

Finish the exercise in the beginning position, with both legs perpendicular to the floor.

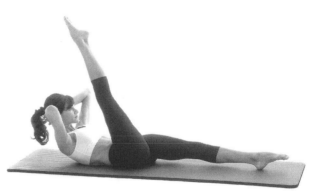

For an additional challenge, place the hands behind the head with the fingers interlaced, keeping the trunk in the same position as for the regular hamstring pull or rotating it as in the criss-cross (page 58). The leg action is the same as for the regular hamstring pull.

Shoulder Bridge Prep

Muscle Focus

- Abdominal muscles
- Hamstrings

Objectives

- To strengthen the hamstrings
- To stabilize the pelvic–lumbar region
- To develop hip disassociation
- To improve back extensor control

This exercise combines pelvic–lumbar stabilization with hip disassociation. It places the body in a challenging suspended position, starting from the top phase of the Mat Work: Pelvic Curl (page 45) and then lifting one leg and supporting the body with the other. The single-leg support of this exercise demonstrates a *forced couple* muscle pattern of the hamstrings and the abdominal muscles, both pulling the pelvis toward a posterior tilt. You may sense an energy line running through the body that creates opposing forces, one pulling diagonally outward and upward through the knees and the other diagonally downward from the knees through the shoulders. This sense of opposition helps you keep the body aligned from the shoulders to the knees and balances the work of the flexors and extensors of the trunk, which are co-contracting.

Imagery

Visualize a suspension bridge on which a mechanical arm goes up and down without affecting the stability and strength of the bridge. Also visualize a straight line that runs from the shoulders through the hips to the knees. This energy line provides the foundation for the exercise.

- ☐ Keep a consistent 90-degree angle in the knee of the moving leg.
- ☐ Initiate the movement from the hip joint.
- ☐ Maintain hip extension in the supporting leg.
- ☐ Avoid lowering or tilting the pelvis.

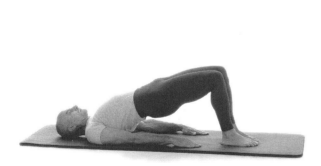

Inhale. Perform a pelvic curl (page 45) and hold the top position. Distribute the weight evenly on the feet, keeping the legs parallel. Maintain the stretch of the hip flexors while engaging the shoulder extensors to support and accentuate the upper and mid-back work.

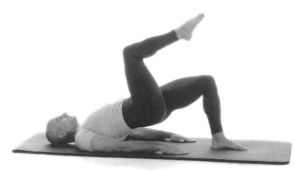

Exhale. Lift one leg from the hip joint, maintaining a 90-degree angle in the knee. Keep the pelvis stable and level throughout the leg lift, with a minimal weight shift to the supporting leg.

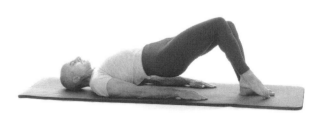

Inhale. Lower the leg and touch the mat lightly with the foot. Lift the leg again with an exhale. After several repetitions switch legs, again with a minimal weight shift, and repeat the sequence with the other leg. Complete the exercise by placing both feet on the mat rolling down as in the pelvic curl (page 45).

Spine Stretch

As with the Mat Work: Pelvic Curl (page 45), this exercise teaches articulation of the spine, but in a sitting rather than supine position. It also resembles the roll-down discussed in chapter 2 (page 21). Emphasize rolling or peeling the spine vertebra by vertebra as the trunk moves into forward flexion and then extension, returning to the upright position along the plumb line. There is a prominent interplay between the spinal flexors and extensors in this exercise, which aids spinal mobility and stability, and enhances core strength. This exercise can improve seated posture enormously.

As the upper body rolls forward and then back to the seated position, focus on keeping the legs shoulder-width apart, the pelvis stable, and the feet dorsiflexed.

Keep the toes facing the ceiling; this will ensure that the legs remain in a neutral position rather than succumbing to the tendency to externally rotate.

Imagery

Visualize the motion of a young tree being pulled over by its top branches and then slowly being released to find its stable, upright position.

☐ Maximize articulation of the spine when moving from spinal extension to spinal flexion and vice versa.

☐ Keep the feet dorsiflexed, with the toes toward the ceiling.

☐ Keep the shoulders relaxed and the neck elongated.

Muscle Focus

▪ Abdominal muscles
▪ Back extensors

Objectives

▪ To develop spinal articulation
▪ To develop core control and trunk stabilization
▪ To improve hamstring flexibility

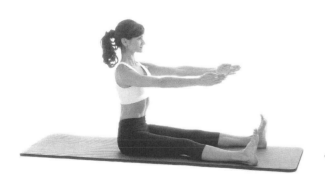

Inhale. Sit with the trunk upright, the legs straight and shoulder-width apart. Dorsiflex the feet and reach the arms forward, shoulder-width apart and parallel to the floor with palms facing each other.

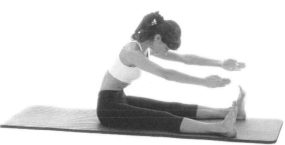

Exhale. Roll down and forward through the spine, starting from the head.

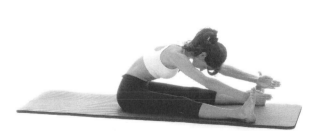

Inhale. Deepen the abdominal work, drawing the spine further into forward flexion and stretching the back muscles. (Alternatively, once you have accomplished the illustrated version, you can extend the spine on a diagonal, beginning from the lower back and completing the movement with the arms in line with the ears.) Exhale. Restack the spine back to the starting position. Or, for the option with back extension, return to forward flexion and then restack the spine.

Roll-Over

Muscle Focus

- Abdominal muscles

Objectives

- To develop spinal articulation
- To stretch the lower back and hamstrings
- To improve control of the abdominal muscles

You must follow certain guidelines to make this exercise effective and meet its objectives. Flexion of the back, particularly the lower back, achieved by employing deep abdominal contraction, should facilitate the roll-over. Avoid the tendency to take advantage of the momentum and lever action of the legs to roll over; instead maintain a constant angle of 90 degrees in the hip joint during the roll-over phase, which will force you to maximize the abdominal work. On the return, you can enhance the stretch in the hamstrings and the lower back by drawing the thighs close to the chest, creating a tight pike position.

People who have neck problems should be extremely cautious when approaching this exercise; some individuals may need to avoid it completely (as with all other Pilates exercises that place weight on the cervical spine), even though most of the weight should be borne on the shoulder girdle rather than the neck.

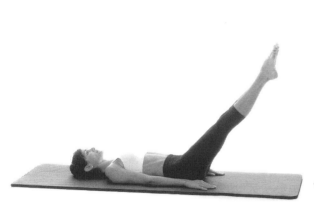

Exhale. Lie supine with the arms by the sides and the legs straight and together at a 60-degree angle to the mat.

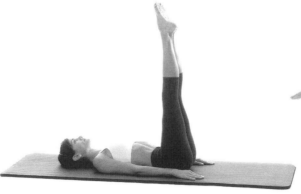

Inhale. Lift the legs to a 90-degree angle in the hip joint.

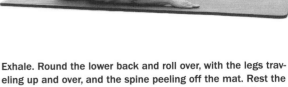

Exhale. Round the lower back and roll over, with the legs traveling up and over, and the spine peeling off the mat. Rest the weight on the shoulder girdle, keeping the legs parallel to the mat.

Imagery

In the roll-over phase, visualize creating a ball out of the lower back (see also Mat Work: Rolling Like a Ball, page 55). The feeling should be like a metal spring being bent in half and then opening out to the beginning position.

☐ Do not use momentum to roll over.

☐ Keep the hip joint at a constant 90-degree angle during the roll-over phase.

☐ Deepen the abdominal contraction to achieve maximum lumbar flexion.

☐ Keep the thighs close to the chest in the roll-back phase.

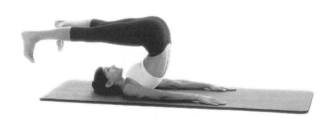

Inhale. Dorsiflex the feet and separate the legs to shoulder-width.

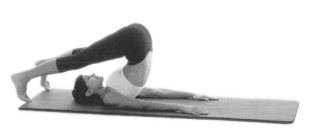

Continue inhaling as you lower the feet toward the floor (touch the floor if flexibility allows).

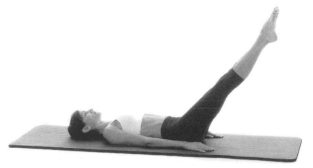

Exhale. Lower the legs toward the chest, articulating each vertebra of the spine down to the mat. Anchor the pelvis on the mat, and circle and lower the legs, joining them together. Return to the starting position.

Neck Pull

Muscle Focus

- Abdominal muscles

Objectives

- To strengthen the abdominal muscles
- To improve spinal mobility
- To increase hamstring flexibility
- To develop back extensor control

Ironically, contrary to what the name implies, pulling on the neck is the one thing to avoid in this exercise. Tackle this exercise only after having achieved proficiency in the Mat Work: Roll-Up (page 52). Placing the hands behind the head (as opposed to the arm movement in the roll-up) alters the center of gravity and the levers of the movement, making it more difficult than its cousin the roll-up. In addition, reaching forward over the legs with the trunk requires more flexibility than the roll-up. Extending the spine in a sitting position and establishing an upright alignment of the trunk demands core strength and well-conditioned trunk stabilizers, particularly back extensors, as well as adequate hamstring flexibility.

In the learning stages of this exercise, allow the spine to roll down one vertebra at a time from the sitting upright position. Once proficiency has been achieved, attempt to hinge the trunk backward as one unit prior to articulating the spine down during the descent to the starting position. Due to the demands of this exercise, it should be performed later in a session and not as part of a warm-up.

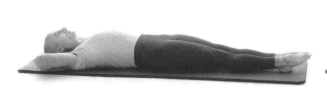

Exhale. Lie supine with the legs straight and together, feet gently plantarflexed. Interlace the fingers behind the head and keep the elbows wide.

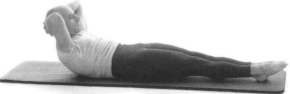

Inhale. Lift the head and shoulder girdle, sinking the lower back into the mat.

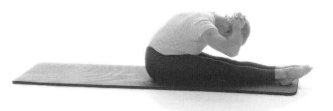

Exhale. Roll up, continuing the movement forward until the trunk is over the legs.

Imagery

The smooth, rolling motion that is desired in this exercise is similar to that of a carpet rolling up and unrolling. The second phase, the move from forward flexion into the upright sitting position, can be likened to pulling over a young tree and then allowing it to spring back up.

☐ Avoid pulling on the neck and thrusting the head forward during the roll-up phase.

☐ Keep the elbows wide throughout the exercise.

☐ Hinge back with a straight trunk before rolling down through the spine.

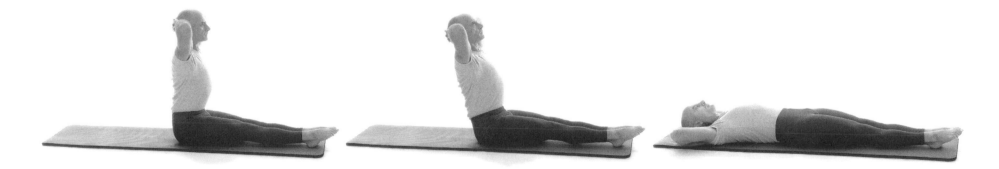

Inhale. Roll the spine up to a sitting position, articulating each vertebra on the longitudinal axis.

Exhale. Lean back slightly, keeping the trunk straight.

Roll down to the starting position, articulating each vertebra.

Control Balance

Muscle Focus

- Hip extensors

Objectives

- To strengthen the hip extensors
- To improve hip flexor flexibility
- To strengthen the core

In addition to requiring a great deal of core strength, this exercise relies greatly on hip flexor flexibility and hip extensor strength. The extensors, primarily those of the hip and back, facilitate the leg lifting perpendicularly to the floor, essentially creating a straight line through the trunk and up through the leg.

This exercise serves as an excellent preparation for the Mat Work: Jackknife (page 94) in that it is a one-legged version of that exercise. Both this exercise and the jackknife place greater pressure on the cervical spine than does the Mat Work: Roll-Over (page 64), so I advise erring on the side of caution when performing them. They are absolutely contraindicated for anyone with neck problems, particularly those related to disc dysfunction.

Imagery

I like to visualize two energy lines in this exercise: one that runs from the shoulders through the trunk and the upright leg to the ceiling, and the other creating a stabilizing force by stretching from the hip joint down through the leg into the ground.

- ☐ Keep the focal point of your weight on the shoulder girdle.
- ☐ Keep the pelvis and trunk still as the legs change.
- ☐ Minimize bearing weight on the cervical spine.

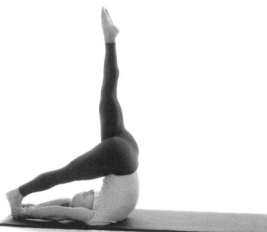
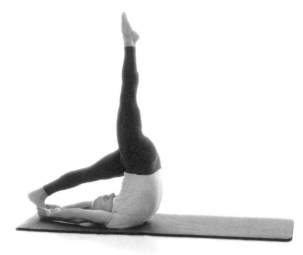

Inhale. Perform a roll-over (page 64) and remain in the position with the legs overhead. Circle the arms around and overhead to hold onto the feet.

Exhale. Extend one leg upward toward the ceiling. Perform two pulses, as in the hamstring pull (page 60), with the leg at maximum height (aiming to increase the hip extension). Use percussive breathing that corresponds to the two pulses.

Inhale. Switch the legs simultaneously, keeping the pelvis and trunk as still as possible. After the final repetition, place both feet on the floor overhead and roll back down.

This exercise demonstrates the fundamental principles of Pilates clearly and profoundly. Not only does it integrate awareness, balance, breath, and control, but it also epitomizes concentration, center, efficient use of energy, precision, and flow of movement and harmony. It demonstrates coordinated activation of the abdominal muscles and the trunk extensors. The open-leg rocker is an exceptional preparation for more advanced full-body exercises such as the Mat Work: Teaser series (pages 100 to 101) as well as the teaser on other apparatus (see pages 215 and 284).

People who have tight hamstrings or who lack strength in the back extensors should modify the position by bending the knees and holding the legs behind the thighs.

Imagery

The image of an inflated tire rolling smoothly (see Mat Work: Rolling Like a Ball, page 54, and Mat Work: Seal Puppy, page 105) applies here too. The point of balance, when you are sitting on the sit bones in the V shape, should feel effortless. This pinnacle is where body, mind, and spirit unite and is the culmination of every Pilates principle—the *point of harmony*.

☐ Use the back extensors to complete the movement.

☐ Keep the arms straight throughout the exercise.

☐ Hold the legs firmly without pulling on them.

Muscle Focus

- Abdominal muscles
- Back extensors

Objectives

- To develop trunk stabilization
- To improve balance
- To increase spinal mobility

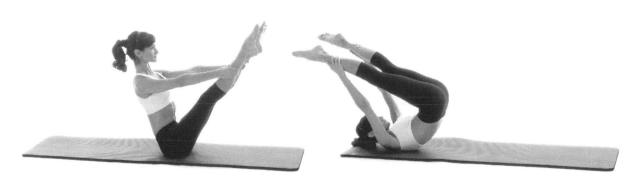

Exhale. Sit balanced on the sit bones in a V position with the back and legs straight. Hold the ankles firmly with the hands, keep the legs shoulder-width apart, and focus the eyes straight ahead.

Inhale. Round the back, initiating the movement from the lumbar spine, and roll back to the shoulders. (The head should barely touch the mat, if at all.)

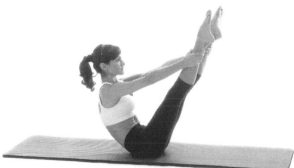

Exhale. Roll back up, first keeping the spine round and then extending it as you return to the starting position. Balance momentarily before rolling back again.

Saw

Muscle Focus

- Hamstrings
- Adductors
- Back extensors

Objectives

- To improve flexibility of the hamstrings and adductors
- To develop strength of the back extensors
- To develop control of the oblique abdominals

This exercise is an intricate interplay of extending and rotating the trunk and stretching the hamstrings and adductors. Maintain an extended back, rather than a rounded back, as the trunk and arm reach forward over the leg during the stretch phase. This maximizes the hamstring stretch and offers the added benefit of strengthening the back extensors. When reaching forward over the leg, keep the spine aligned over the leg and the head aligned with the spine. Some instructors recommend rotating the trunk in this position and looking toward the back arm. People have enough problems achieving straight alignment of the trunk; adding rotation to this difficult position often results in severe compensations and bad alignment. Additional rotation should be added only after the version presented here has been mastered.

Note that the saw requires that the trunk move as one unit rather than through segmental articulation of the spine. Also, remain true to the longitudinal axis when rotating the trunk in the initial phase, and return to this exact position on the longitudinal axis in the final stage of the exercise before returning to face center. In the sitting upright positions, whether facing front or rotated, keep the spine elongated over the stable base of the pelvis.

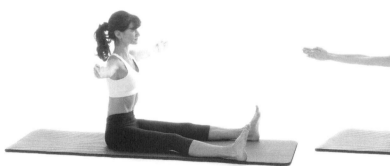
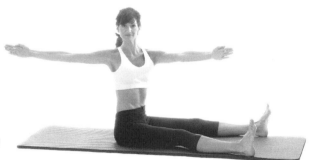
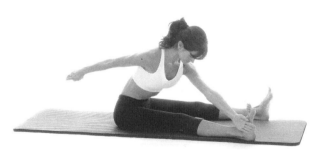

Exhale. Sit upright with the legs straight and open slightly beyond shoulder-width and with the feet flexed. Hold the arms in a T position, reaching them as far out to the sides as possible.

Inhale. Rotate the torso around the longitudinal axis. Keep the pelvis anchored, and move the arms and head with the trunk.

Exhale. Reach forward over the leg with the trunk. The front hand extends past the small toe, and the back hand reaches back with the palm facing the body. Feel the oppositional pull of the arms.

Imagery

Visualize a pole strapped to the back, which you rotate around in the upright position before folding over the leg. When folding the trunk over the leg for the stretch, maintain the feeling of the pole strapped to the back to accentuate spinal extension and alignment.

☐ Keep the back extensors engaged when reaching forward.

☐ Keep the feet dorsiflexed with the toes toward the ceiling.

☐ Anchor the pelvis and distribute your weight evenly on the sit bones throughout the exercise.

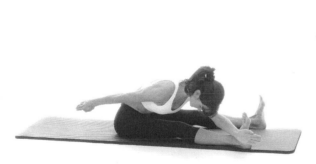

Inhale. Extend the spine further to accentuate the hamstring stretch. Then exhale and reach forward and down again to deepen the stretch of the hamstrings and the lower back, keeping the abdominal muscles engaged.

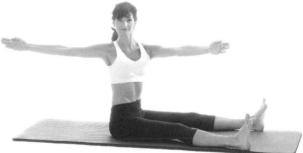

Inhale. Extend the back further before lifting to the longitudinal axis while facing the side.

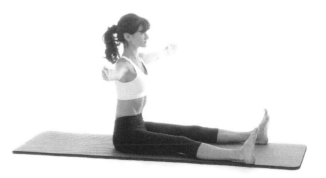

Rotate back to the center starting position. Repeat the movement to the other side.

Spine Twist

Muscle Focus

- Oblique abdominals
- Back extensors

Objectives

- To strengthen the oblique abdominal muscles and back extensors
- To improve trunk mobility

This exercise emphasizes organized rotation of the spine around the longitudinal axis. Proper engagement of the oblique abdominal muscles allows correct rotation of the spine. Daily activities, such as cleaning and gardening, and recreational sports, such as golf, volleyball, and tennis, are activities in which incorrect rotation can lead to backaches or more severe injuries. People tend to use the shoulders and arms when they rotate to compensate for lack of mobility in the trunk, rather than using the powerful trunk muscles and focusing on spinal rotation. Tremendous improvement in performance can be gained when trunk rotation is maximized and the powerhouse is employed.

Imagery

Imagine two poles or energy lines, one longitudinal, running up and down the back, and the other in the transverse plane reaching across the shoulders from the fingertips of one hand to the fingertips of the other.

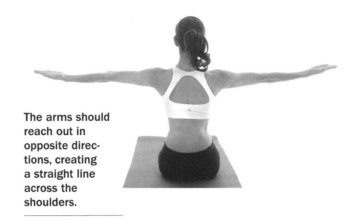

The arms should reach out in opposite directions, creating a straight line across the shoulders.

The transverse pole rotates around the longitudinal one, while both poles remain in their respective planes of motion.

- ☐ Keep the pelvis and legs still.
- ☐ Initiate the movement from the waist, not from the shoulders, keeping the arms aligned.
- ☐ Move the head with the trunk.

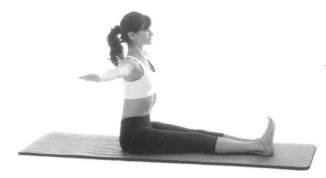

Inhale. Sit upright with the legs straight and together and the feet dorsiflexed. Hold the arms in a T position with the palms facing upward (shoulders in external rotation).

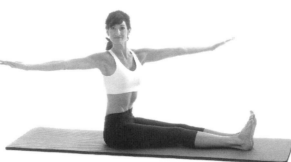

Exhale. Rotate the trunk to one side using two pulses, mobilizing from the region of the waist. (The pulses assist in achieving maximum range.) Keep the arms aligned with the shoulders.

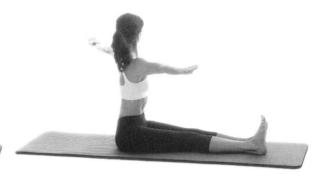

Inhale. Pass through the center and repeat the movement to the other side. Complete the exercise by facing forward in the starting position.

Corkscrew

This exercise builds on the principles of the Mat Work: Supine Spine Twist (page 47) but incorporates a longer lever arm (the legs), intensifying the hip flexor work and the abdominal work, particularly that of the oblique abdominals. The pendulum motion and circling of the legs demand intricate control of the spine and coordination of the abdominal muscles and hip flexors, which act alternately as movers and stabilizers at various points in the exercise. Note that the pelvis rocks from side to side with the movement of the legs, with one side lifting off the floor briefly as the legs move to the opposite side; however, it anchors soon afterward as the legs move through the center of the arc to the other side. The lower back should imprint into the mat as the legs pass through the center and should only momentarily leave the mat as the legs go out to the sides before returning to the imprint. Use the starting point (12 o'clock) as the reference position that you always return to.

Imagery

Visualize drawing a big circle on the ceiling as the legs arc around in one direction and then the other.

☐ Keep the legs and feet together and aligned throughout the exercise.

☐ Keep the shoulder girdle, neck, and head still and relaxed.

☐ Focus the movement in the waist region.

☐ Bend the knees if necessary to reduce strain on the hip flexors and lower back.

Muscle Focus

▪ Abdominal muscles

Objectives

▪ To strengthen the abdominal muscles

▪ To develop pelvic–lumbar stabilization

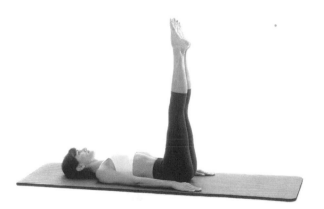

Exhale. Lie supine with the arms in a T position or at the sides of the body and the legs at 90 degrees to the floor. Imprint the lower back into the mat.

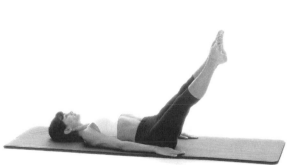

Inhale. Shift the pelvis and both legs to one side, keeping the shoulders stable and relaxed. The upper leg must reach out further to stay aligned with the lower leg.

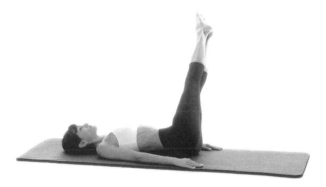

Exhale. Circle the legs downward in an arc through the center and around to the opposite side. As the legs pass through the center, again imprint the lower back into the mat. Once the legs reach the opposite side of the arc, bring them back to the starting position. Alternate the direction.

Muscle Focus

- Oblique abdominals

Objectives

- To strengthen the lateral flexors
- To stabilize the pelvic–lumbar region
- To develop hip adductor control

Side Leg Lift

Every good, well-balanced exercise program should include lateral flexion of the trunk. The side leg lift is relatively simple to execute and teach yet profound in its effect. In addition to strengthening the lateral flexors of the trunk, this exercise develops pelvic and lumbar stabilization, in which the oblique abdominals play a vital role.

The ideal alignment of the body is a straight line with the spine in a neutral position, with the trunk flexors and extensors co-contracting as well as the lateral flexors on both sides. The lower back extensors frequently overpower the abdominals and take over, which in extreme cases can result in hyperextension of the back. To avoid this, keep the legs slightly forward of the centerline, creating a banana shape.

Imagery

The body creates an elongated bow shape as the legs lift. Imagine a long energy line reaching out and then up. Another helpful image is that of a fish on its side with its tails swooping upward.

☐ Recruit the oblique abdominals on both sides.

☐ Keep the adductors engaged throughout.

☐ Maintain a sense of lengthening in the lower leg, keeping it alongside the top leg.

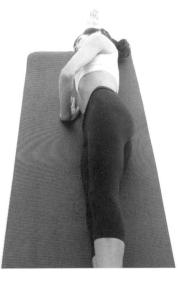

The ideal alignment is a plumb line on its side.

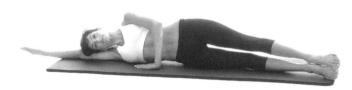

Inhale. Lie on one side with the bottom arm straight in line with the body and the head resting on it. The pelvis is "stacked" perpendicular to the mat and the legs are pressing together. The top arm is bent, with the hand placed on the mat, or straight and resting on the side of the body (more challenging).

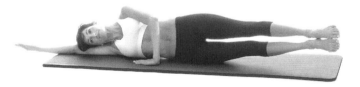

Exhale. Lift both legs by flexing the trunk laterally (without sinking into the mat), keeping the legs together and the body aligned. Inhale. Lower the legs without allowing the feet to touch the mat. Following the final repetition, lower the legs to the starting position and repeat on the other side.

Side Kick

This exercise reinforces the concept of trunk and pelvic stabilization with hip disassociation. In a side-lying position you rely on a much smaller and narrower base of support than you do in exercises in which you are supine or prone. Consequently the level of difficulty is increased and the lateral stabilizers of the body are recruited more strongly. By focusing on scapular and trunk stabilization, you minimize the pressure on the elbow and maximize stability. While the leg swings back and forth, spinal flexors and extensors are in a state of balanced co-contraction as they hold the trunk stable. When the leg swings forward, there is a need to use the extensors more (to avoid spinal flexion); when it swings back, there is a need to use the abdominal muscles more (to avoid spinal extension). These are subtle internal adjustments that produce a stable spine.

This exercise is an excellent example of how the body adapts to changes in the center of gravity. In this instance as the leg swings back and forth, the pelvis adapts by shifting slightly in the direction opposite the leg. This small anterior–posterior motion of the pelvis assists greatly in maintaining a balanced, stable position, both in this exercise and in everyday movements.

Imagery

Imagine the swinging motion of a pendulum. Now place the pendulum on its side without affecting its movement. The motion of the leg should feel like that of a pendulum, free and effortless.

☐ Minimize rocking the trunk backward and forward.

☐ Maximize the range of motion of the leg.

☐ Did not sink into the supporting shoulder or allow the underside of the rib cage to drop.

☐ Avoid thrusting the ribs forward as the leg swings back.

Muscle Focus

- Abdominal muscles and back extensors
- Hamstrings
- Hip flexors

Objectives

- To develop pelvic–lumbar stabilization
- To increase hip flexor and hip extensor control and flexibility
- To develop hip disassociation

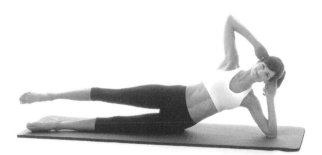 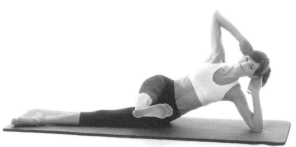 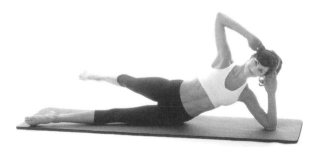

Inhale. Lie on one side, leaning on the elbow of the lower arm with the hands behind the head. Engage the underside oblique abdominal muscles and shoulder stabilizers to support the trunk. Stabilize the bottom leg on the floor and hold the top leg at hip height.

Exhale. Swing the top leg as far forward as possible, dorsiflexing the foot and pulsing twice when reaching the maximum range. Avoid tucking (posteriorly tilting) the pelvis; keep it in a neutral position.

Inhale. Swing the leg back as far as possible, plantarflexing the foot and elongating the leg, pulsing twice when reaching the maximum range. Again, maintain a neutral position of the pelvis. Repeat the forward-and-back leg swing several times, finishing in the backward swing position.

Basic Back Extension

Muscle Focus

- Back extensors

Objectives

- To strengthen the back extensors
- To develop abdominal and scapular control

This exercise provides a foundation for subsequent back extension mat exercises, such as swimming (page 77), double-leg kick (page 79), rocking (page 80), and swan dive (page 104). Proper abdominal recruitment plays a crucial role in supporting the back and achieving correct alignment during this exercise. Developing movement through the entire vertebral column, activating each intravertebral joint, helps to prevent shearing forces on the lower lumbar vertebrae, which often occur when extension is isolated to the lower back rather than distributed through the spine. Again, abdominal recruitment assists in achieving this goal.

With the pelvis serving as an anchor, relax the lower body and focus on working above the pelvis. Another area of stabilization that deserves special mention (besides the abdominal region) is the group of muscles that depress the scapulae. These muscles, particularly the lower trapezius, serve as both scapular stabilizers and mid-back extensors. Take advantage of this unique and beneficial relationship in all back extension exercises and establish good alignment and movement mechanics of the back and shoulders in general.

Imagery

The image of an airplane hovering just above the ground helps you achieve an elongated position and a feeling of flight as opposed to arching into an extreme arc.

- ☐ Maintain abdominal support throughout the exercise.
- ☐ Keep the head aligned with the spine.
- ☐ Use the scapular stabilizers, pressing the arms against the sides of the legs, with the fingers reaching toward the feet.

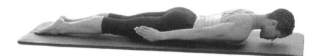

Inhale. Lie prone with the forehead on the floor. Keep the arms by the sides with the palms pressing against the legs. Keep the legs together with the feet gently plantarflexed.

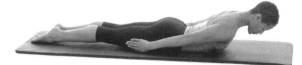

Exhale. Lift the upper trunk, head, and chest slightly off the mat. Keep the legs, including the gluteal muscles, relaxed and together. Press the pubic symphysis gently into the mat while engaging the abdominal muscles.

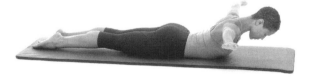

Inhale. Reach the arms out and up into a T position, then exhale and return the arms to the sides of the body, keeping the trunk stable throughout. Lower the upper body, keeping all the muscles mentioned activated. After the final repetition, lower the body to the starting position.

Swimming

I love this exercise! It is so valuable in terms of strength development and cross-pattern coordination of the back extensors and hip extensors. When the right side of the back is working, the left hip extensors are activated, and vice versa. We use this type of cross pattern frequently in everyday movements and recreational activities, the most common being the normal gait cycle (walking). As we stride forward with the right leg, the left leg goes backward while the trunk rotates to the right, resulting in the exact pattern of the swimming exercise—the back extensors of the right side working with the left hip extensors. Beginners can make this exercise easier by allowing the arm and leg that are not being lifted to remain on the mat. This provides some leverage and recuperation time for the limbs that have been working.

Imagery

Imagine doing little flutter kicks with the arms and legs as if both were doing the leg movement of the front crawl swimming stroke in opposite directions. The trunk, from head to tailbone, is like a plank, with the arms and legs hinging around small independent axes and having no effect on the stability of the plank.

☐ Maintain trunk and pelvic stability throughout the movement.

☐ Avoid elevating the shoulders.

☐ Keep the movements of the arms and legs small.

Muscle Focus

▪ Back extensors

Objectives

▪ To strengthen the back extensors
▪ To develop trunk stabilization
▪ To build coordination and cross-patterning
▪ To improve shoulder flexor and hip extensor control

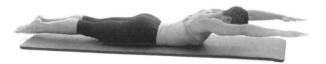

Exhale. Lie prone with the arms reaching forward and the legs together. Lift the chest, arms, and legs slightly off the mat.

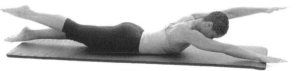

Inhale. Alternate lifting the left arm and right leg higher, then the right arm and left leg. Start slowly and then speed up the movement. Repeat four cycles each of the right arm–left leg movement and the left arm–right leg movement while inhaling.

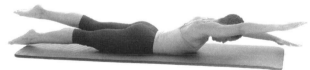

Exhale while repeating four cycles on each side. Continue this pattern for 10 inhalations and exhalations. Complete the exercise by suspending the body in back and hip extension for a moment before lowering it.

Single-Leg Kick

Muscle Focus

- Hamstrings

Objectives

- To develop knee flexor and hip extensor control
- To strengthen the mid- and upper back extensors
- To improve trunk stabilization

The setup in this exercise is important because the positioning of the body can place excessive pressure on the lower back if good abdominal support is not employed. The back extensor work should focus on supporting the mid- and upper back. The arms of course also add support, and good scapular stabilization is imperative. Position the lower arms either in a triangle shape with the fingers interlaced or parallel to each other. In either case, place the elbows directly under the shoulders and stabilize the scapulae.

In the case of discomfort or excessive pressure in the lower back, I recommend performing this exercise in a prone position with the hands together and the forehead resting on the hands.

Imagery

The body position for the single-leg kick should be like a sphinx. The leg movement should be disassociated from the rest of the body's stable position, with the lower legs opening and closing like handheld fans (when viewed from the side).

- ☐ Maintain scapular depression throughout the movement.
- ☐ Keep the pubic symphysis lifting up toward the sternum.
- ☐ Keep the legs lifted off the mat throughout.

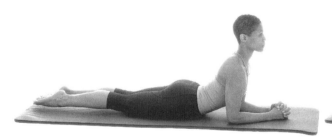 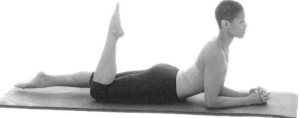 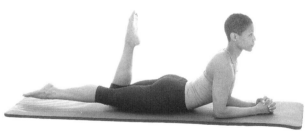

Inhale. Lie prone and, while engaging the abdominal muscles, lift the chest and extend the back. Place the elbows under the shoulders, positioning the forearms in a triangular shape with the fingers interlaced. Straighten the legs and lift them slightly off the mat.

Exhale. Bend the right leg and pulse it twice (exhaling on each pulse) then straighten it, simultaneously bending the left leg.

Repeat the pulses with the left leg (continuing to exhale on each pulse). Repeat the same pattern of right and left leg bends, this time inhaling on each pulse, without changing the body position.

Double-Leg Kick

This is an exceptional back extension exercise with several important benefits besides strengthening the back extensors. First, the arms add support to the back extension, monitoring the load on the back. Second, holding the arms together provides an excellent thoracic and shoulder stretch. This exercise also provides good hamstring work and prepares you for Mat Work: Rocking (page 80). An elongated body position is important, emphasizing the activation of the mid- and upper back as opposed to a high arched position, which would focus the work in the lower back.

Imagery

This is one of several exercises in which I like to visualize an archer's bow and arrow. The body is the bow and the arms form the twine. This powerful image also reinforces the elongation desired in this exercise.

☐ Keep the legs lifted slightly off the mat throughout.

☐ Relax the elbows to the floor during the down phase, placing the hands high up on the back.

☐ Keep the head aligned with the spine when lifting into back extension.

Muscle Focus

▪ Back extensors

Objectives

▪ To strengthen the back extensors
▪ To develop hamstring control
▪ To stretch the thoracic region

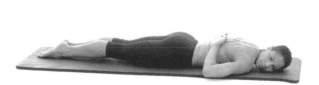

Inhale. Lie prone with the fingers interlaced behind the back. Allow the elbows to fall to the floor, and turn the head to one side, resting it on the cheek. Straighten the legs, keeping them together, and lift them slightly off the mat.

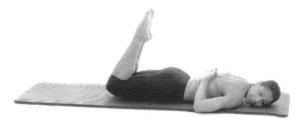

Exhale. Bend both legs together and pulse them three times (exhaling on each pulse).

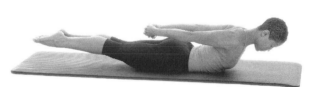

Inhale. Extend the back to lift the chest off the mat. Simultaneously straighten the arms and the legs, and bring the head to the center. Then lower the body to the starting position, resting the head on the opposite cheek.

Muscle Focus

- Back extensors
- Hip extensors

Objectives

- To strengthen the back and hip extensors
- To improve hip flexor flexibility
- To stretch the chest

Rocking

Rocking relies on the stable shape of the body and an inner energy to "get the ball rolling." It is difficult to articulate verbally how this happens; once you establish the shape, you shift the center of gravity slightly forward and away you go! A good preparation for this exercise is to lift into the rocking position and then lower down to the floor, repeating this action several times without the rocking.

I cannot overemphasize the importance of the hip extension. Reach the feet to the ceiling and the body will tip forward. Once it has tipped forward, momentum will keep you going. Like the Mat Work: Swan Dive (page 104), this exercise relies more on stability and intricate muscle coordination than on flexibility.

Imagery

The body is the shape of an archer's bow: The body is the bow; the arms the twine. This is similar to the image in the Mat Work: Double-Leg Kick (page 79), however in this case the bow is taut in preparation for shooting the arrow. The position is much more arched. Another good image is that of a boat rocking forward and backward as it sails through the waves.

☐ Keep the head still and aligned with the spine.
☐ Maintain scapular depression with the arms straight.
☐ Keep the legs adducting, only opening as much as is needed to avoid stress in the pelvis or the back.

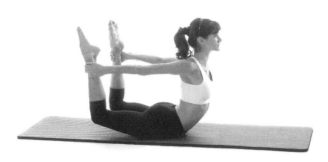

Inhale. Lie prone. Bend the knees and reach back with the arms, taking hold of the ankles and lifting the trunk and legs into an arch.

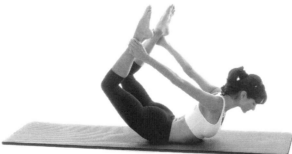

Exhale. Rock forward.

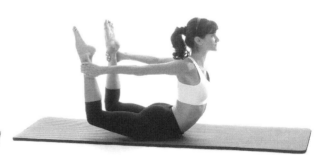

Inhale. Rock backward.

Rest Position

This exercise is usually done after back extension work. The rest position serves as a necessary pause as well as a good transition into the exercises that follow in the mat work sequence. In a kneeling position with the upper body on the mat, allow the pelvis to sink toward the heels, releasing the neck, shoulders, and lower back muscles. This position is like the child's pose in yoga.

If you have a preexisting knee condition, place a large triangular cushion under the pelvis between the lower and upper leg so that the flexion of the knees is not as extreme. If you have back problems or other discomforts, you can drape yourself, prone, over a large ball that offers support to the trunk.

Imagery

Imagine the back spreading or melting over the legs. The back, pelvis, and shoulders drape themselves over the thighs. With each breath the back expands laterally and the relaxation deepens.

- ☐ Breathe naturally and deeply throughout.
- ☐ Allow the pelvis to sink toward the heels.
- ☐ Allow the eyes to close if it feels comfortable.

Muscle Focus

- ▪ Lower back extensors

Objectives

- ▪ To relax the back and shoulders
- ▪ To rest the body
- ▪ To stretch the muscles of the back, particularly those of the lower back

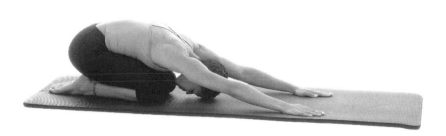

Kneel with the chest on the thighs and the pelvis resting on the heels. Place your forehead on the ground, with the arms reaching forward or at the sides of the body, whichever feels more comfortable. Comfort is key.

Cat Stretch

This exceptional exercise achieves two important goals: spinal flexion (focusing on the abdominals) and spinal extension (focusing on the back extensors). It has the added benefit of stretching and releasing the muscles of the lower back during the flexion phase and improving pelvic–lumbar stabilization during extension. It can prove particularly valuable for low-load abdominal and back work, like that required during pregnancy, rehabilitation, and for the older population.

Imagery

Spinal flexion invokes an image of a ball of energy, or a whirlpool that stirs up in the abdominal region, creating a firm, round shape. Spinal extension evokes a feeling of elevating the sternum to create the distinctive look of the sphinx, proud and determined. Also, as the name implies, the image of a cat awakening and taking a lengthy stretch is essential to the dynamic of this exercise. Visualize the cat's spine rounding and arching, displaying its phenomenal mobility.

☐ Keep the hips above the knees and the shoulders above the hands throughout the exercise.

☐ The movement occurs in the trunk, between the hip joints and shoulder joints.

☐ Maximize flexion of the lower back during the first phase and extension in the mid- to upper back during the second phase.

Muscle Focus

- Abdominal muscles
- Back extensors

Objectives

- To develop abdominal control
- To increase flexibility of the lower back
- To improve shoulder stabilization and control
- To strengthen the mid- and upper back extensors

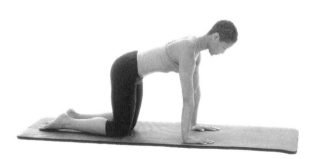

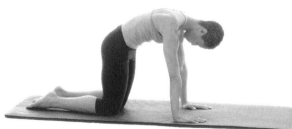

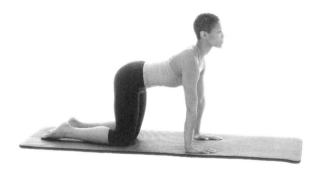

Inhale. Kneel on the hands and knees with the knees hip-width apart and the hands shoulder-width apart. The spine should be in a neutral position, with the weight evenly distributed on the legs and the arms. Sense the elongation of the spine from the tailbone to the top of the head while drawing awareness to the ISS.

Exhale. Engage the abdominal muscles and draw the spine into flexion while accentuating the curve in the lower back and allowing the head and pelvis to follow the natural line of the spine. Avoid rounding the upper back excessively, letting the head go too far between the arms, or tucking the pelvis under. Inhale. Return to the neutral elongated spinal position while still co-contracting the abdominal and back muscles.

Exhale. Extend the thoracic spine by arching the back while maintaining stability of the pelvic–lumbar region. Externally rotating the shoulder joints slightly helps to facilitate and accentuate the upper back extension. Follow the extension by returning the starting (neutral spine) position.

Front Support

Also known as the *plank* or *push-up* position, the front support exercise utilizes two critical areas of stabilization: the pelvic–lumbar region (core) and the shoulder girdle. Strengthening these two regions and establishing good muscle mechanics provides efficient stabilization for subsequent weight-bearing exercises in a similar position on all the equipment. When good alignment and solid stabilization are not present, the trunk and the shoulder region "collapse," resulting in inefficient and sometimes harmful positions. This may take some relearning, since many people are accustomed to doing hundreds of push-ups—incorrectly.

Imagery

Imagine the body as a strong, solid bridge or ramp that will not budge under immense weight.

☐ Keep the body in a straight line from head to toe.

☐ Maintain scapular abduction and depression throughout the exercise.

☐ Keep the hands directly under the shoulders.

Muscle Focus

▪ Abdominal muscles

▪ Scapular stabilizers

Objectives

▪ To develop trunk and shoulder stabilization

▪ To strengthen the upper body

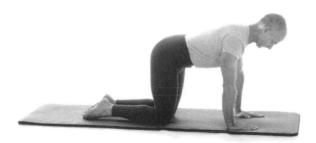

Exhale. Starting in the setup position of the cat stretch (page 82), establish a solid neutral spine position. Stabilize the shoulders, feeling an even distribution of the weight between the upper and lower body.

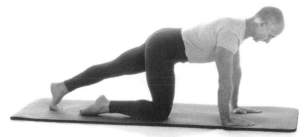

Inhale. Reach one leg back with a minimal weight shift. Further stabilize the shoulder region.

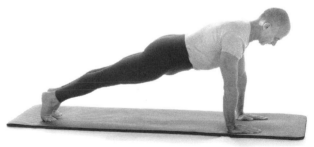

Exhale. Extend the other leg back into the front support position, with the arms and legs firm and straight. Hold this position while deepening the use of the internal support system, maintaining stability throughout the body.

Shoulder Bridge

Muscle Focus

- Abdominal muscles
- Hamstrings

Objectives

- To strengthen the hip extensors
- To develop pelvic–lumbar stabilization
- To develop hip flexor control and flexibility
- To improve hamstring flexibility

This challenging exercise builds on the Mat Work: Shoulder Bridge Prep (page 62) and the Mat Work: Pelvic Curl (page 45). The key to the exercise is maintaining a stable pelvis that is not affected by the leg swinging up and down. You should feel the front of the moving leg elongating on the way down (stretching the hip flexors) and the back of the leg stretching on the way up (stretching the hamstrings). This stretching is enhanced by the dorsiflexion of the foot.

Orient the pelvis toward a posterior tilt when in the bridge position. This is to prevent the pelvis from tilting anteriorly, which could cause hyperlordosis, particularly when the leg is lowered. The tendency to anteriorly tilt the pelvis is exacerbated when the hip flexors are tight.

Imagery

Visualize a ride at an amusement park featuring a carriage on the end of a girder that swings like a pendulum. The leg is the girder that swings in an arc shape.

- ☐ Maintain consistent height of the pelvis from the mat.
- ☐ Avoid tipping the pelvis to one side.
- ☐ Position the pelvis toward a posterior tilt.

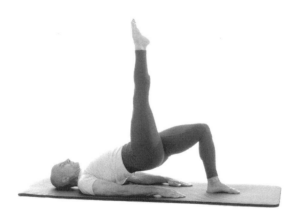

Inhale. Lie supine with the knees bent and the feet firmly placed on the ground. Perform a pelvic curl (page 45), pausing in the top position. Lift one foot off the ground, bending the knee toward the chest, and then straighten the leg directly toward the ceiling.

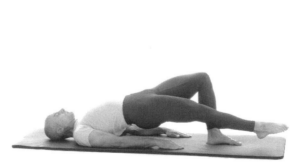

Exhale. Lower the straight leg toward the floor with the foot plantarflexed.

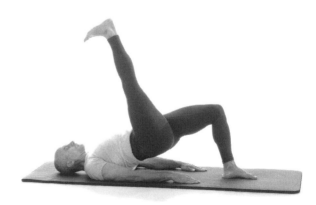

Inhale. Kick the straight leg upward, dorsiflexing the foot. On the final repetition, pause with the leg straight up and plantarflex the foot. Bend the knee and place the foot on the floor to return to the starting position. Switch legs and repeat the sequence with the other leg. Complete the exercise by placing both feet on the mat and rolling down.

Leg Pull Front

Mastering the Mat Work: Front Support (page 83) before learning this exercise is imperative because it is the foundation on which the leg pull front exercise is built.

The key to the exercise is maintaining stillness in the body except for the leg that lifts and lowers. The leg movement makes this difficult position less stable and therefore more challenging. Note that when the leg lifts to the back, the pelvis remains stable, which means that the leg may move back no more than a few degrees (depending on hip flexor flexibility) before the pelvis starts tilting anteriorly. Dancers may be tempted to do a full arabesque, but I urge them to keep the pelvis neutral and maximize height without tilting it. Then when the pelvis is allowed to tilt and open to maximize turnout and height, the leg will be higher and stronger than ever before.

Imagery

First create the bridge described in the Mat Work: Front Support (page 83). Now add to that bridge a swinging gate to allow tall ships to pass under it. The bridge does not move, only the gate.

☐ Maintain the plank position of the body throughout the exercise.

☐ Keep the pelvis neutral with a bias toward a slight posterior tilt.

☐ Maintain scapular abduction and depression.

Muscle Focus

■ Hip extensors
■ Abdominal muscles

Objectives

■ To strengthen the hip extensors and shoulder girdle
■ To develop trunk stabilization

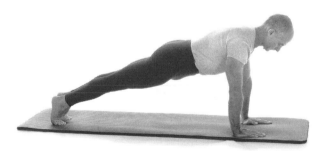

Inhale. Start with a front support (page 83, third photo). Lift one leg off the ground only slightly; plantarflex the foot.

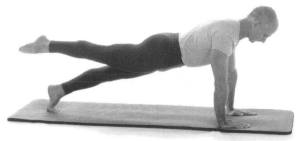

Exhale. Extend the hip to lift the leg higher.

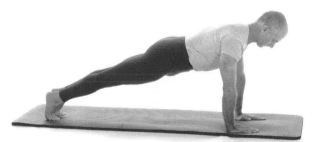

Inhale. Lower the leg so the toes just touch the ground, maintaining the plantarflexion. On the final repetition dorsiflex the foot and place it on the ground, returning to the front support position. Repeat on the other side.

Muscle Focus

▪ Triceps

Objectives

▪ To strengthen the elbow extensors and pectoral muscles
▪ To develop trunk stabilization

Push-Up

Unlike a typical push-up, the Pilates push-up is a sequence of movements that involve the entire body, shifting from the front support position to standing upright and back again. Within this sequence is the standard push-up, which, with the elbows kept close to the sides of the body, emphasizes the triceps. Of primary importance is keeping the scapulae still as the elbows bend and the body is lowered and then lifted back up. The scapular stabilization determines the depth of the elbow flexion—as soon as the scapulae start to move, lift the body back up and regroup.

Few people are initially able to keep the scapulae stable in a neutral position. Many a "muscle man" has crumbled trying to do push-ups while keeping the scapulae still. During a presentation at a large forum in China in 2003, I asked for a volunteer to do no more than 10 push-ups correctly. (I defined *correctly* as holding the trunk and scapulae absolutely stable and moving only the arms.) A hulk of a man with muscles bulging everywhere came up. I must admit I thought that I'd met my match and my experiment would fail. As he proceeded with the utmost confidence, I stopped him each time his scapulae began to move. He did not get very far, and when I feared that the pool of sweat that had built up under him was about to drown us both, he collapsed and, with a slight smile, conceded

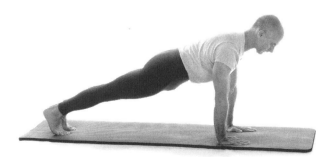

Exhale. Start in the front support position (page 83).

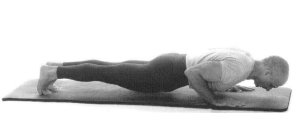

Inhale. Bend the elbows (as in a standard push-up).

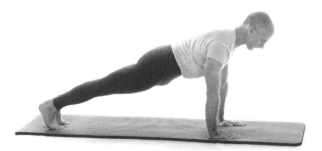

Exhale. Extend the elbows (as in a standard push-up). Repeat the push-up twice. After the second repetition, extend the arms and pause momentarily.

that he needed to learn how to do push-ups again (after 20 years of doing 500 a day). We gave each other a hug, and no words were necessary to express the understanding, camaraderie, and respect we both felt for each other . . . and the work.

Once you have mastered moving from the front support position to standing and back again, I advise gradually decreasing the number of arm walks until you can do the movement with no "walking"—just one swoop up and then a dive back to the front support position. This demands pushing off from the arms to transfer the weight to the feet, lifting the pelvis high,

and then rolling up through the spine. Reverse this sequence to return to the front support position.

Imagery

See Mat Work: Front Support (page 83) and Reformer: Up Stretch (page 163).

☐ Engage the abdominal muscles throughout the exercise.
☐ Keep the elbows close to the sides of the body.
☐ Do not allow the scapulae to adduct or elevate.

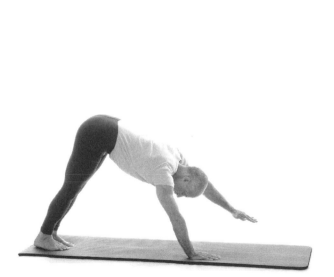

Lift the pelvis upward and walk the hands toward the feet, transferring the weight to the feet.

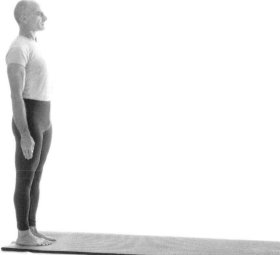

Roll up to a standing position. Inhale in this position, establishing good upright alignment.

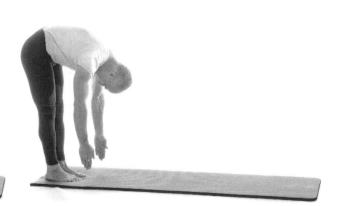

Exhale. Roll down and walk the hands forward to the front support position. Repeat the sequence three to five times.

Back Support

Muscle Focus

- Shoulder extensors
- Hip extensors
- Back extensors

Objectives

- To develop trunk stabilization
- To strengthen the shoulder and hip extensors
- To improve back extensor control

This exercise emphasizes the co-contraction of the trunk flexors and extensors. Although it directly strengthens the back, shoulders, and hip extensors, it indirectly addresses the need for flexibility of the opposing flexors, particularly the shoulder and hip. Strong back, hip, and shoulder extensor muscles and sufficiently flexible hip and shoulder flexors, which tend to tighten over time, are vital for correct alignment.

The first movement, once the setup position has been achieved, is hip extension supported by shoulder and back extension. The hamstrings must engage *before* the gluteal muscles do during the hip extension. Deviating from this sequence of muscle recruitment may lead to incorrect positioning of the pelvis and lack of hamstring activation. The gluteals are strong and tend to overpower the hamstrings during hip extension.

Tight pectorals, abdominal muscles, and hip flexors will limit one's ability to do this exercise, which is why many men find it challenging or seemingly impossible. This limitation, of course, is no reason to eliminate the exercise; instead, the flexibility of these muscles must be addressed.

Finally, although vertebra-by-vertebra articulation of the spine is often used in Pilates, in this case you must strive to keep the spine in a stable position and hinge from the hip joint, lifting the trunk as one solid unit.

Imagery

Two visuals enhance this exercise. The first is to imagine the hips as the hinge of a door, opening (as the pelvis lifts) and closing (as the pelvis lowers). The second is to visualize two poles (or energy lines): one running from the head through the trunk to the hip joint, the other running from the ankles through the knee to the hip joint. As the pelvis lifts, the two poles connect and become one. As the pelvis lowers, they again split to become two poles.

- ☐ Avoid flaring the ribs.
- ☐ Lift the pelvis from the hip joint in a hinging action, keeping the back and legs straight.
- ☐ Allow the head to follow the line of the spine.

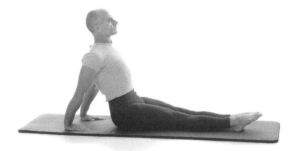
Inhale. Sit with the arms extended about a foot behind the pelvis with fingers facing the pelvis. Straighten the legs out in front and softly plantarflex the feet. Engage the back extensors and scapular stabilizers.

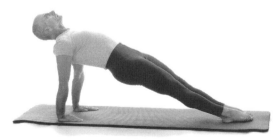
Exhale. Lift the pelvis off the floor, hinging at the hip joint until the body establishes a straight line.

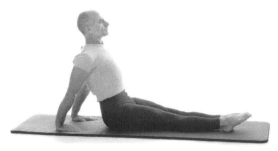
Inhale. Lower the body down to the starting position, again hinging at the hip joint.

Leg Pull Back

The Mat Work: Back Support (page 88) is a necessary prerequisite to learning and mastering this exercise. As with the leg pull front, the key to the exercise is maintaining stillness in the body except for the one leg that lifts and lowers.

Flexibility is a major factor in the success of this exercise. Without it, your ability to perform the exercise will be limited. The flexibility of the shoulders and trunk is already challenged by the back support position. Now, as the leg lifts forward and up, hamstring flexibility plays a vital role.

Imagery

Using the concept of the poles or energy lines discussed in Mat Work: Back Support (page 88) , keep the central pole stable and straight and visualize the leg as yet another pole attached to the side of the pelvis. The leg swings up and down without affecting the central pole.

☐ Isolate the movement of the leg as you lift and lower it.

☐ Keep the hip (supporting leg) and back extensors engaged.

☐ Align the head with the spine.

Muscle Focus

- Hip, back, and shoulder extensors
- Hip flexors

Objectives

- To strengthen the hip and shoulder extensors
- To develop trunk stabilization
- To improve hip flexor control

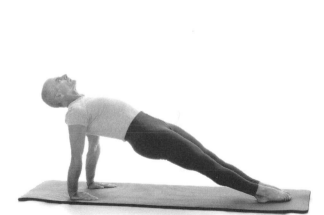

Inhale. Assume the back support position (page 88).

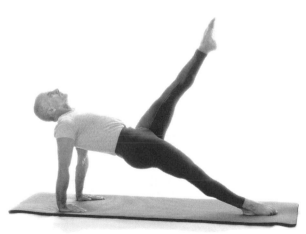

Exhale. Flex the hip, lifting one leg up toward the ceiling.

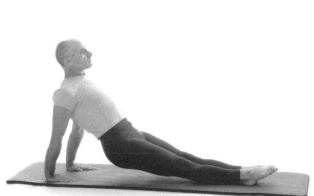

Inhale. Lower the leg to the starting position. Repeat several times before changing to the other leg.

Muscle Focus

- Hip extensors
- Hip flexors

Objectives

- To develop hip extensor and flexor control
- To improve hip extensor and flexor flexibility
- To develop shoulder and pelvic–lumbar stabilization

Scissors

The scissors is a challenging exercise in large part because of the hyperextended position of the lower back. This position feels precarious and demands a high level of pelvic–lumbar stabilization in order to do the exercise correctly. Because it is the same as the Step Barrel: Scissors (page 275), picturing the spine being supported on a rounded barrel is helpful. (In this case the arms take the place of the barrel.) The pelvis should be stable and anchored as the legs perform a scissors action, alternating as they pass through the centerline (the starting point) perpendicular to the floor.

Note that the elbows should be directly under the pelvis (no splaying); without their support, the pelvis sinks and the whole structure starts to collapse. Keeping an equal angle of split between the legs creates the desired wide V position and an equal stretch of the hip flexors and hamstrings.

Imagery

I recommend an image that seems to help create the desired movement and dynamic. Imagine the legs opening wide like a handheld fan, then closing and opening to the other side.

- ☐ Maintain an arc shape of the spine.
- ☐ Keep the elbows parallel to each other (or as close to it as possible).
- ☐ Cradle the pelvis with the hands.

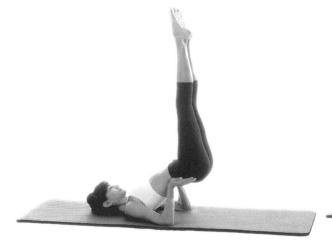

Inhale. Lie in a supine position and draw the knees toward the chest. Create a ball shape with the body and roll over onto the shoulder girdle. Place the hands under the pelvis, as if holding a bowl, and create a bridge shape with the trunk. Now straighten the legs up toward the ceiling.

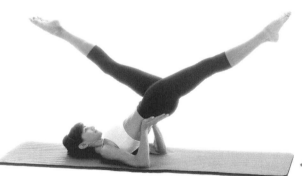

Exhale. Open the legs equidistant from the centerline in a wide V position. Pulse the legs twice in the open scissors position, exhaling on each pulse.

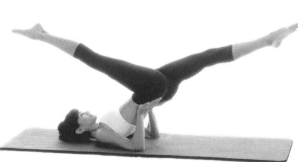

Inhale. Switch legs, passing through the starting position, and repeat the pulses in the open V position, again exhaling on each pulse.

Bicycle

The bicycle is an extension of the Mat Work: Scissors (page 90), so proficiency in doing the scissors is required. Although both legs perform a cycling action (one bending and the other straightening simultaneously), at one point in each cycle they are in the scissors position, which becomes a reference point. Flexibility, awareness, and strength developed from previous exercises enable you to tap the foot of the back leg on the floor as the knee bends—a position that demands spinal hyperextension and flexible hip flexors—without compromising pelvic–lumbar stabilization and creating excessive pressure on the low back. Both legs should function symmetrically, and emphasis should be placed on the abdominal muscles to achieve the support needed for this exercise and to protect the lower back. The feeling can be likened to having a barrel under the back that supports the trunk in this challenging position.

Imagery

The large, fluid, circular motion of the legs conjures up an image of cycling a penny-farthing bicycle (an old-fashioned bike with one large wheel in front and a small one in back).

☐ Maintain an arc shape of the spine.

☐ Perform elongated movements with maximum fluidity.

☐ Keep the legs parallel, avoiding external rotation of the hips, particularly when bending the knee of the leg that is in hip extension.

☐ Keep the elbows parallel with each other (or as close to it as possible).

Muscle Focus

▪ Hip extensors
▪ Hip flexors

Objectives

▪ To develop hip flexor control
▪ To improve flexibility of the hip extensors and flexors
▪ To develop shoulder and pelvic–lumbar stabilization

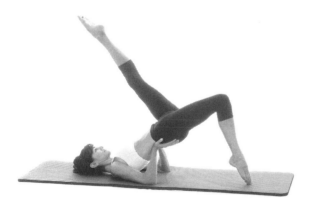

Inhale. Start in the same position as the scissors (page 90), splitting the legs into the wide V position. Exhale. Extend the back leg (furthest from the face) toward the floor. Bend the knee and tap the floor with the toes.

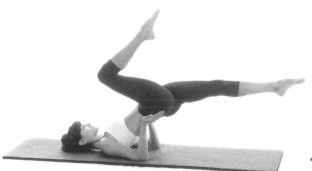

Inhale. Flex the hip and bring the leg up to the chest. At the same time take the straight leg over to replace the "old" back leg.

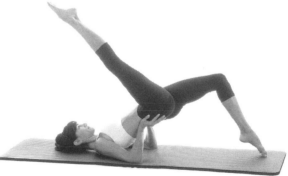

Begin straightening the bent leg in front of the face as the straight one starts bending to tap the floor with the toes. Continue this large cycling action. After several repetitions, reverse the direction of the cycling (a challenging exercise in coordination).

Hip Circles Prep

Muscle Focus

- Abdominal muscles

Objectives

- To strengthen the abdominal muscles
- To promote pelvic–lumbar and shoulder stabilization
- To develop trunk rotation

The hip circles prep is an offshoot of the Mat Work: Corkscrew (page 73), which is done in the supine position. Certain elements of the corkscrew apply to this exercise; however, the sitting V position of the body requires a higher level of stabilization, strength, and control. The shoulder girdle needs to remain stable, and the focus of the movement is in the region of the waist as the pelvis rotates from side to side. The legs reach out to one side and then circle down and around to the other side and back to center. It is crucial to maintain abdominal support in order to avoid stress on the lumbar spine.

Perform five circles in one direction and then five in the other, rather than alternating as in the corkscrew. In the advanced version of this exercise, arm support is eliminated, and the upper body (including the arms) moves as one unit in one direction, while the legs and pelvis move as one unit in the opposite direction. Repeating the movement several times before changing direction allows a greater sense of flow. The trunk rotation and the power it requires enhance athletic pursuits as well as deepening the understanding of activation of the powerhouse.

Imagery

The visual of tracing a cone from the pelvis out through the feet offers a clear picture of the movement, with the feet describing the large part of the cone. The bigger the cone, the more support and stabilization you need. If you are performing the advanced version, the arms describe one cone and the legs another; one clockwise and the other counterclockwise.

☐ Avoid hyperextending the lumbar spine as the legs circle.

☐ Prevent the top leg from sliding backward.

☐ Keep the shoulder girdle still, the scapulae depressed, and the mid- and upper back extensors engaged.

☐ Move the pelvis from side to side as the legs draw a large circle.

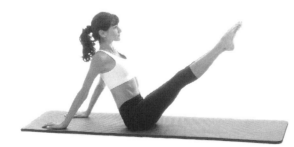

Exhale. Sit in a V position with the arms extended behind the body and the hands resting on the floor. Face the fingers away from the body. The arms should support the body only lightly, like training wheels on a bicycle. The legs are together at an approximately 60-degree angle to the floor.

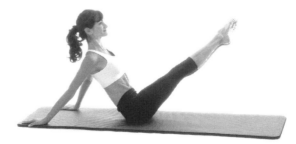

Inhale. Shift the pelvis and the legs as one unit to one side.

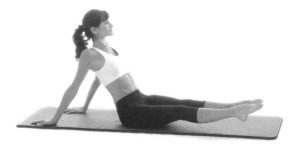

Exhale. Circle the legs down and around to the opposite side; the pelvis moves through the center to the opposite side, then the legs and pelvis return to the starting position as one unit.

Kneeling Side Kick

This exercise is an extension of the Mat Work: Side Kick (page 75), made more difficult by decreasing the base of support to one hand and the lower leg. The primary focus remains on trunk stabilization and hip flexion and extension. Remember to keep the swinging leg at the highest level possible even during the transition from front to back; this increases the abductor component exponentially. Keep the head aligned with the spine throughout to avoid any neck tension. A good way to test balance is by lifting the supporting hand slightly off the ground and balancing on only the lower leg. The body should be able to balance briefly, with a sense of lightness.

In advanced mat work, the role of the upper body becomes more prominent because it bears much of the weight. This can pose a problem for individuals with wrist problems or weak upper bodies.

The following are some recommendations for alleviating wrist pressure:

- Press the fingertips into the ground to engage the wrist flexors and slightly decrease wrist extension.
- Make a fist with the supporting hand, which again decreases or even eliminates wrist extension.
- Employ effective shoulder and trunk stabilization to help alleviate the weight bearing down on the wrist.

Imagery

Use the same imagery as the Mat Work: Side Kick (page 75), adding the feeling of being suspended like a bridge high off the ground.

- ☐ Maintain a neutral pelvis.
- ☐ Do not sink into the supporting shoulder or the underside of the rib cage.
- ☐ Try to keep the leg above hip height (as high as possible).

Muscle Focus

- Abdominal muscles
- Shoulder stabilizers
- Hip abductors, flexors, and extensors

Objectives

- To develop trunk stabilization
- To develop hip flexor and hip extensor control
- To improve hip flexor and hip extensor flexibility
- To strengthen the hip abductors

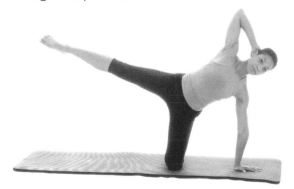

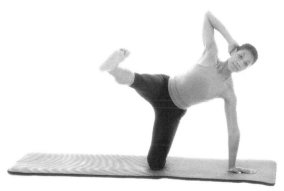

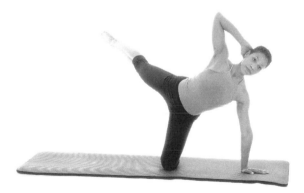

Inhale. Kneeling, shift the weight to one knee. Place the supporting hand (on the same side of the body as the weighted knee) on the floor directly under the shoulder, and lift the other leg to hip height or higher. Place the free hand behind the head and face the foot of the supporting leg directly back.

Exhale. Swing the top leg as far forward as possible, dorsiflexing the foot and avoiding a tuck (posterior tilt) of the pelvis. Perform two pulses together with the breath when the leg is at maximum forward reach.

Inhale. Swing the leg back as far as possible and plantarflex the foot; avoid hyperextending the lumbar spine and anteriorly tilting the pelvis. Elongate the leg backward, pausing at maximum reach before swinging it forward again. End the exercise with the leg reaching back.

Muscle Focus

- Abdominal muscles
- Hip, back, and shoulder extensors

Objectives

- To develop spinal articulation
- To improve trunk stabilization
- To strengthen the hip extensors

Jackknife

The jackknife is an extension of the Mat Work: Roll-Over (page 64) and should not be attempted until you have mastered that exercise. Initially the feet reach overhead and are parallel to the floor, then they are lowered down to the floor as with the roll-over. At this point rather than rolling down again, you recruit the hip and spinal extensors to reach the legs in a swooping action up toward the ceiling, creating a perpendicular line from the floor up through the shoulders, trunk, hips, legs, and feet. Using the shoulder extensors to assist in keeping the structure stable and upright and in alleviating pressure on the cervical spine in this position is legitimate. When rolling the spine down vertebra by vertebra, keep the feet above the face until the pelvis reaches the floor, then return the legs to the starting position.

Because of the weight that this exercise places on the cervical spine, people with neck problems may

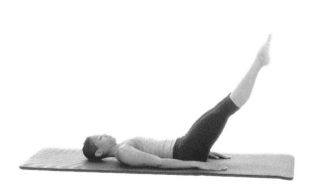

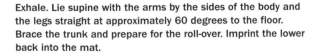

Exhale. Lie supine with the arms by the sides of the body and the legs straight at approximately 60 degrees to the floor. Brace the trunk and prepare for the roll-over. Imprint the lower back into the mat.

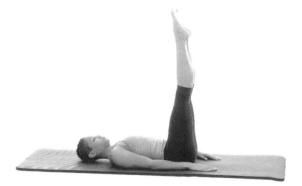

Inhale. Raise the legs to 90 degrees, anchoring the pelvis and continuing to sink the low back into the mat.

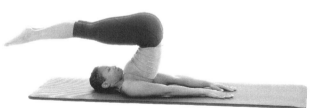

Exhale. Roll over, maximizing the flexion of the lumbar region and maintaining a 90-degree angle in the hip joint. Complete this phase with the legs parallel to the floor and the weight on the shoulders.

need to avoid it. Although the weight is distributed between the shoulders and the arms, and the pressure on the cervical spine is minimized, it still bears significant pressure.

Imagery

The jackknife should feel like a spring-loaded hinge or knife closing and opening in the hip joint with a swooping movement.

☐ Maximize flexion of the lumbar spine during the roll-over phase.

☐ Use the hip, shoulder, and back extensors to achieve maximum height of the legs and trunk.

☐ Roll down with the feet opposite the face (but held as high as possible rather than close to the face).

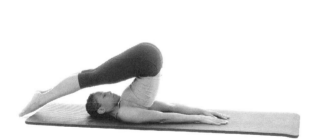

Inhale. Lower the legs toward the floor.

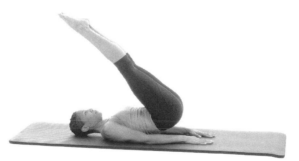

Still inhaling, lift the legs toward the ceiling. Move the pelvis forward and press the arms into the mat.

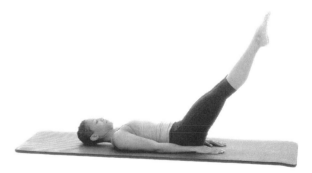

Exhale. Slowly roll down, articulating the spine and keeping the feet opposite the face. As the pelvis reaches the mat, anchor it with the legs at 90 degrees, then lower the legs to return to the starting position.

Side Bend

Muscle Focus

- Oblique abdominal muscles

Objectives

- To strengthen the oblique abdominal muscles and shoulders
- To improve oblique abdominal muscle flexibility
- To develop shoulder strength and stabilization

The side bend relies primarily on trunk and shoulder strength and stabilization. As you enter the realm of advanced-level work, the base of support becomes smaller, and in many cases, unstable. In this exercise, the pivot point around which much of the movement occurs is the shoulder joint, which is a very mobile, unstable joint. Therefore you must focus particular attention on correct shoulder mechanics. This exercise is quite challenging because the movement focuses on this unstable joint and the body is supported by only one shoulder. As the body arcs at the top position, the pelvis should lift as high as possible toward the ceiling while the free arm swoops over the body. The head must follow the line of the spine, focusing toward the hand on the floor. Resist the tendency to lift the head and look upward; doing so can produce neck tension.

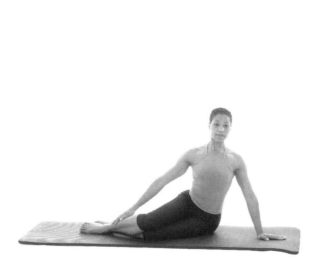
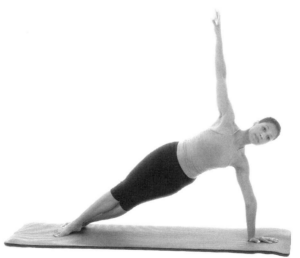
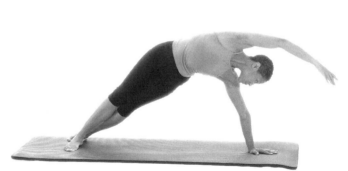

Exhale. Sit sideways with your weight on one side of the pelvis. Bend the legs and place the top foot in front of the bottom one. Rest the upper body weight on the supporting arm, maintaining shoulder stability and recruiting the abdominal obliques. The other arm rests on the side of the body.

Inhale. Lift the pelvis away from the floor while straightening the legs, and raise the upper arm to shoulder height, fingers pointing toward the ceiling. Reach a point where the body is in a straight diagonal line and the arms are in a straight line.

Exhale. Draw in the lateral muscles of the underside of the trunk and lift the pelvis higher toward the ceiling, creating an arc with the body as the upper arm reaches overhead.

The musculature should not relax between repetitions—you should keep a sense of continuous movement, even at the bottom "resting" position. There should be room enough for a piece of paper to pass between the pelvis and the mat. Tremendous support must come from the lateral aspect of the trunk, particularly the underside. The oblique abdominal muscles are the engine that drives this exercise.

Imagery

A wonderful image to aid in lifting and arcing the body is that of a dolphin leaping out of the water.

- ☐ Initiate the movement from the oblique abdominal muscles.
- ☐ Maintain abdominal engagement throughout the exercise.
- ☐ Keep the scapular stabilizers engaged throughout.

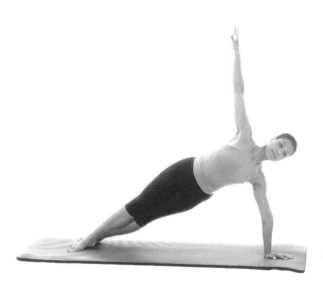

Inhale. Return to the previous position with the body in a straight diagonal line and the arms in a straight line.

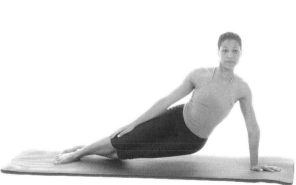

Exhale. Lower the body to the starting position (without touching the floor if possible).

Twist

Muscle Focus

- Oblique abdominal muscles

Objectives

- To strengthen the oblique abdominal muscles and shoulders
- To stretch the oblique abdominal muscles
- To develop shoulder stabilization

This exercise adds the element of rotation to the Mat Work: Side Bend (page 96), making the movement three-dimensional instead of two-dimensional. The rotation involves not only the trunk but also, significantly, the shoulder. A single shoulder supports the weight of the body in a suspended position and accommodates its rotation, with most of the movement occurring in the glenohumeral joint. This is a tall order for this small, relatively unstable, muscle-dependant joint.

As stated in chapter 3, the level of an exercise is determined by the complexity of its coordination, stabilization, and movement. The twist has it all. I like to teach the Mat Work: Side Bend before teaching the twist. Once both have been learned I often combine them, doing three repetitions of one and then three of the other.

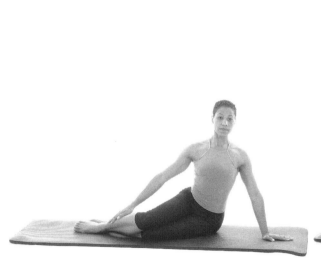

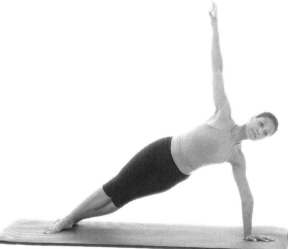

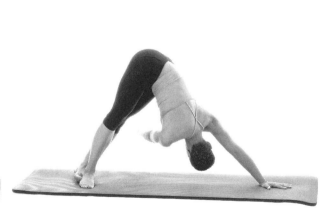

Exhale. Sit sideways with your weight on one side of the pelvis. Bend the legs and place the top foot in front of the bottom one. Rest the upper body weight on the supporting arm while maintaining shoulder stability and recruiting the abdominal obliques. The other arm rests on the side of the body.

Inhale. Lift the pelvis away from the floor while straightening the legs, and raise the upper arm to shoulder height, fingers pointing toward the ceiling. The body is in a straight diagonal line and the arms are straight and aligned with each other.

Exhale. Lift the pelvis as high as possible and rotate the trunk as the free arm reaches under the body.

Imagery

I use several images in this exercise. The visual I give for the top position of the twist is a flat pyramid—the trunk creates one side of the pyramid and the legs, as one unit, the other side. The movement of the free arm reaching under the body is like threading a needle. The return to the diagonal position should create a well-defined line. In this position, feel the strong energy line running through the body and a second line running through the arms from the floor up to the sky. Line is everything in this wonderful and challenging exercise.

- ☐ Minimize the use of the legs and maximize the activation of the trunk lateral flexors and rotators.
- ☐ Keep the scapula stable; rotate around the glenohumeral joint.
- ☐ Maintain correct alignment of the head with the spine.

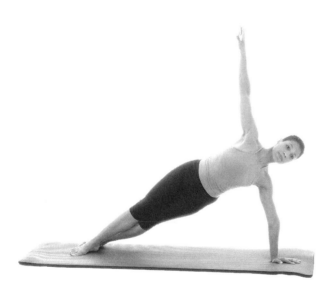

Inhale. Return to the previous position with the body in a straight diagonal line.

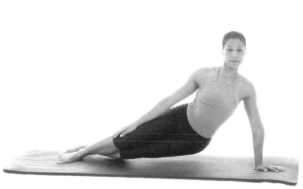

Exhale. Lower the body to the starting position, keeping the pelvis slightly off the mat (if possible) or placing it lightly on the mat.

Teaser Prep

Muscle Focus

- Abdominal muscles
- Back extensors

Objectives

- To strengthen the abdominal muscles and back extensors
- To prepare for the Mat Work: Teaser (page 101)

This exercise prepares you for advanced abdominal work. Here you use the principles of several more basic mat work exercises, such as the roll-up (page 52), rolling like a ball (page 54), and the open-leg rocker (page 69). However, this exercise is more difficult because it requires a high level of control and eliminates the support of the hands and the use of momentum as with rolling like a ball and the open-leg rocker. Find the point of equilibrium, using the back extensors, supported by the abdominals, to create a stable structure. Note that the legs should be still and the shins parallel to the floor. As with the earlier exercises, focus on articulation of the spine when transitioning from extension to flexion and vice versa.

Imagery

The image of a fishing line unwinding as the body rolls down, and then being reeled in as the body rolls back up, helps to give the feeling of continuous, seamless movement.

- ☐ Use the back extensors to complete the movement.
- ☐ Articulate the spine when lowering and lifting the trunk.
- ☐ Initiate the roll-down and roll-up with deep lumbar flexion.

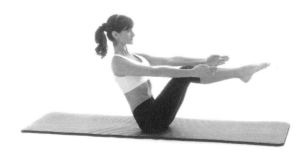

Inhale. Sit upright, balancing on the base of the pelvis (sit bones), arms reaching forward in front of the shoulders. Bend the knees with the shins parallel to the floor.

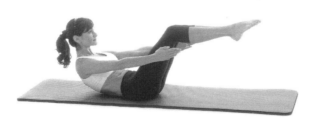

Exhale. Round the lower back and lower the spine to the floor. Go down only to the point where you can maintain complete control, no further than the base of the scapulae.

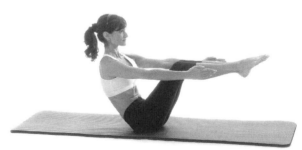

Inhale. Roll back up, maximizing the articulation of the spine. Complete the movement by extending the back and returning to the starting position.

Teaser

This is a combination of the abdominal exercises, particularly the teaser prep (page 100) and roll-up (page 52), and the balancing exercises, especially the open-leg rocker (page 69). The starting position is identical to that of the open-leg rocker except that it is performed with the arms overhead and the legs together. Roll down the spine without moving the legs and feet. After a complete roll-down with the arms reaching overhead, roll up as you would in the roll-up exercise, except that in this exercise the legs are in the air. Maintaining this leg position demands hip flexor recruitment and control, which in turn demands strong abdominal engagement to prevent hyperlordosis and an anterior tilt of the pelvis. Although this full-body exercise places great emphasis on the abdominal muscles, the strength of the back extensors and hip flexors contributes immensely to the control of the movement.

Imagery

See the roll-up (page 52), open-leg rocker (page 69), and teaser prep (page 100) for imagery ideas.

☐ Articulate the spine when rolling down and up.

☐ Initiate the roll-down and roll-up with deep lumbar flexion.

☐ Keep the legs at the same angle throughout the exercise; avoid swinging them up and down.

Muscle Focus

- Abdominal muscles
- Back extensors
- Hip flexors

Objectives

- To strengthen the abdominals and back extensors
- To develop control of the hip flexors
- To develop trunk stabilization
- To develop balance

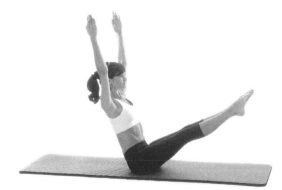

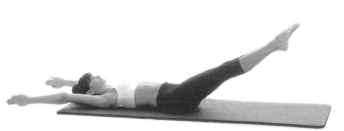

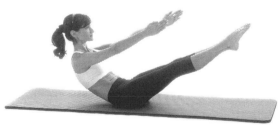

Inhale. Sit upright, balancing on the base of the pelvis (sit bones), with the legs straight at approximately 60 degrees to the floor, creating a V position with the body. Lift the arms overhead.

Exhale. Roll the body down onto the floor, lowering the arms to shoulder height and then reaching them overhead after rolling out the spine. Keep the legs still throughout the movement.

Inhale. Roll up, articulating through the spine. Emphasize lumbar flexion. Complete the movement with back extension, returning to the starting position.

Muscle Focus

- Abdominal muscles
- Back extensors

Objectives

- To strengthen the abdominal muscles and back extensors
- To develop hip flexor control
- To stretch the chest
- To develop balance

Boomerang

This is a high-level exercise because of its complexity. It also demonstrates the progression of exercises in Pilates, the logical methodology of one exercise building on another. The boomerang requires strength, flexibility, and, most important, coordination. It resembles the Reformer: Rowing Back I (page 182) in its movement pattern, and adds the Mat Work: Roll-Over and Teaser (pages 64 and 101). These aforementioned exercises should be mastered before embarking on the boomerang.

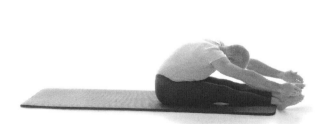

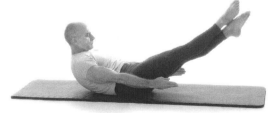

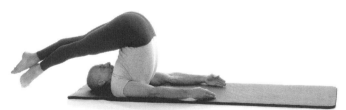

Exhale. Sit with the legs straight, forward, and crossed and with the feet plantar flexed. Round the trunk over the legs and reach the arms forward.

Inhale. Roll the body down, pausing when you reach the lumbar region. Hold the trunk and legs stable in this boomerang position.

Exhale. Lower the chest and head, then round the lower back further, rolling the legs and body up and over. Once you are over, lower the legs toward the mat (see roll-over, page 65).

Imagery

It takes awhile to understand why this exercise is called the boomerang, but once you achieve a flow it becomes apparent. At the point when the body rolls down, before the legs are taken overhead, the shape resembles a boomerang. After the legs change position overhead, the body springs back to the prior position before lifting into the teaser—and thus we have the boomerang.

☐ Keep the movement fluid.
☐ Open and stretch the chest as the arms reach back.
☐ Use trunk stabilization during the balance phase, keeping the legs as high as possible.

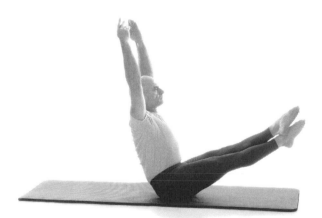

Inhale. Switch the crossed legs and then exhaling, take the legs back over to approximately a 60-degree angle and, while holding them stable, roll up into a teaser position (page 101).

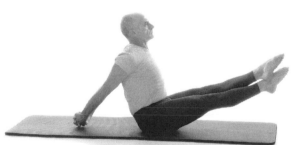

Inhale. Interlace the fingers behind the back as you lift the chest and extend the trunk further.

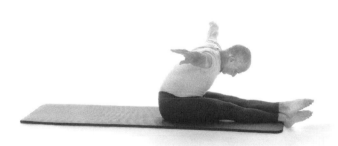

Exhale. Lower the legs and release the hands. Circle the arms around to the sides, bringing the body forward and returning to the starting position.

Swan Dive

Muscle Focus

- Back extensors
- Hip extensors

Objectives

- To strengthen the back and hip extensors
- To develop trunk stabilization
- To harness energy

The swan dive is a beautiful exercise to watch and a very difficult one to execute well. It embodies many of the movement principles of Pilates, particularly flow. This exercise is all about harnessing energy and keeping it moving. Although it appears to rely on back flexibility, this is a misconception. Flexibility is certainly important, but the essence of doing it well is stabilizing and activating the correct muscles in the correct sequence with immaculate timing.

You must hold the trunk in a firm position created by the back extensors and hip extensors and supported by the abdominals. I have seen many a young dancer who is blessed with a spine like rubber struggle and fail to do this exercise well, flopping around like an out-of-control puppy. Success comes from years of practice in harnessing the enormous energy that becomes available when the body is unleashed into the forward dive. Hold the body stable, keep all the necessary muscles activated, and maximize the range of every vertebra in the spine and the hip joint.

Imagery

Visualize a big, fully inflated tire rolling back and forth. If it is not inflated it will make jarring movements, getting stuck at certain points. So it is with the body: It will stop and start, even if the back extensors and hip extensors are engaged, if the abdominals are not engaged. The abdominals assist in providing a firm surface, as well as distributing the work through the entire back rather than solely in the lumbar spine.

- ☐ Engage the abdominal muscles throughout the exercise.
- ☐ Maximize momentum and fluidity of movement.
- ☐ Maintain the arc shape of the body.

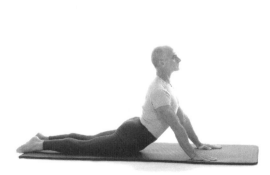

Inhale. Lie prone with the hands under the shoulders and the elbows on the mat. Contract the abdominals and extend the back. Keeping the elbows by the sides, straighten the arms and lift high into the arc position.

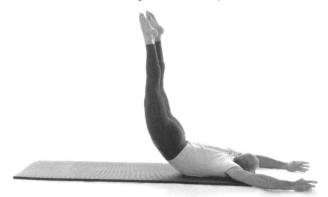

Exhale. Release the arms, dropping the body toward the mat. Reach the arms beyond the head in line with the ears and extend the legs back and up toward the ceiling.

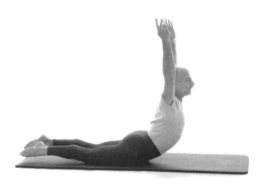

Inhale. Rock backward in an arc shape with the trunk upright, reaching the arms toward the ceiling and lowering the legs to the mat. Continue rocking, increasing the height of the legs and arms on each repetition. On the final repetition, place the arms down and return to the supported arc position before lowering the body to the prone position.

The seal puppy is often done at or near the end of a mat work routine as a form of stretching and relaxation. I encourage using this exercise to focus on the many movements that have been performed in the session and to allow the effort to culminate in this moment of flow and balance.

This exercise stretches the back (the trunk is held in deep flexion) and the shoulders (the shoulders are drawn down by the legs in this unique, folded-under position). As with Mat Work: Rolling Like a Ball (page 54) and Mat Work: Open-Leg Rocker (page 69), you should focus on the internal flow of energy and on the balance of the rolling action. The claps of the legs allow you to pause without stopping the flow of the movement.

Imagery

The image for this exercise is the same as for several of the rolling exercises, such as rolling like a ball—keeping the feeling of an inflated tire rolling back and forth without obstructions and jarring movements. In the balance position, I like to imagine that I am balancing on a precipice or floating on a cloud without any tension. This is the position in which I often do some relaxation, inner focusing, and meditation.

☐ Maintain a constant C curve of the spine.
☐ Keep the head aligned with the spine, and relax the shoulders.
☐ Place the inside of the legs as high up on the arms as possible.

Muscle Focus

- Abdominal muscles

Objectives

- To stabilize and develop control of the trunk
- To improve hip joint flexibility

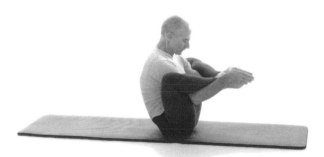

Exhale. Sit with the knees open and feet together. Lift one leg and place it over the arm on the same side. Reach the arm under the leg and wrap it around the lower leg, placing the palm on top of the foot. While balancing, do the same on the other side. Balance in this rounded-back position.

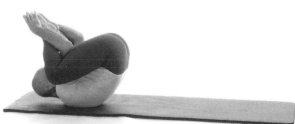

Inhale. Roll back and clap the feet together three times by moving the legs slightly in and out (not only moving the feet).

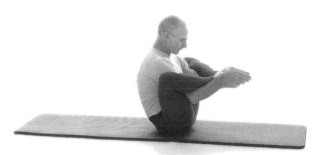

Exhale. Roll up to the balance position and again clap the feet together three times while balancing.

Crab

Muscle Focus

- Abdominal muscles

Objectives

- To stretch the neck and lower back
- To develop trunk stabilization

Although this exercise appears uncomfortable and even dangerous because it involves leaning forward onto the head and transferring weight onto the neck, it is enjoyable and beneficial as long as it is done correctly. The body's full weight should never be placed on the neck; instead, transfer the weight cautiously and with control. The remainder of the exercise is very similar to Mat Work: Rolling Like a Ball (page 54), with an element of coordination added. In addition, since the legs are held close to the body by the arms in the cross-legged position, the possibility of opening the legs and using them for momentum is diminished.

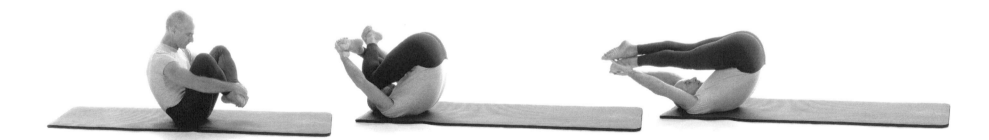

Inhale. Sit in a balanced position on the base of the pelvis with the body in a ball shape (see rolling like a ball, page 54). Cross the legs, reach the arms around the legs from the outside, and hold the feet.

Exhale. Roll back onto the shoulders.

Inhale. Straighten the legs and switch them. Bend the knees and take hold of the feet again, tucking back into a ball shape.

Imagery

I have never been able to relate this exercise to a crab, despite spending hours observing them on beaches. I find using the image of a rolling wheel, keeping a smooth flow back and forth, more beneficial.

- ☐ Transfer weight cautiously onto the neck.
- ☐ Maximize lumbar flexion when rolling.
- ☐ Keep the legs close to the body.

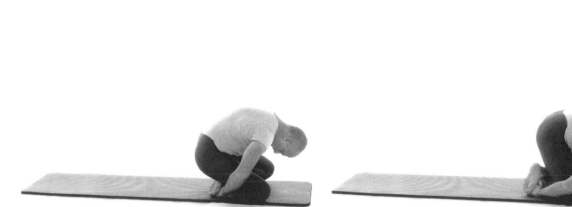

Exhale. Roll forward, transferring the weight over the legs.

Inhale. Place the head on the floor and, slowly rolling over the head, cautiously transfer the weight toward the neck and stretch the neck extensors. Return to the starting position.

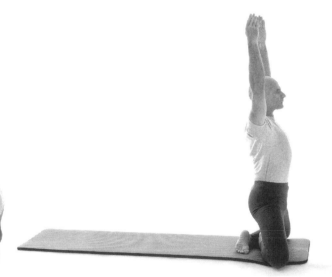

I have choreographed an alternative ending for those who cannot or do not want to place any pressure on the head and neck. This position demands good balance and core strength.

CHAPTER 5

Universal Reformer

The universal reformer, commonly known as just the reformer, is undoubtedly the most recognizable and popular piece of equipment in the Pilates menagerie. It is versatile beyond all imagination. The scope of this piece of equipment is infinite and is only limited by our own imagination and knowledge. It is the creation of a genius—a man way ahead of his time. The movements performed on the reformer range from fundamental to extremely advanced, movements that are performed in every conceivable position and for every possible purpose.

Each piece of Pilates apparatus has specific advantages and features that are unique. Just as a good carpenter would not use a screwdriver when a hammer is called for, so it is with the choice of Pilates apparatus—it should be well suited to the task at hand. For instance, the reformer is perhaps the most user-friendly apparatus on which to perform the foot work; it places the body in a comfortable, nonweight-bearing supine position and recruits the muscles in a balanced fashion. Performing the foot work on the reformer is easier initially than the same exercises are on the cadillac or wunda chair, and the stabilization of the pelvis and trunk, although of course emphasized throughout, is less of a challenge. The reformer also provides the teacher with a good vantage point to observe and correct alignment and muscle action.

The stretches performed on the reformer for the hip flexor, hamstring, and adductor muscles cannot be duplicated as effectively on the other apparatus. The reformer offers the most variety of movements, particularly relating to the upper body. The jumping series is unique to this piece of apparatus, and the reformer readily accommodates movement in a full range of motion, rather than the limited range offered by some of the other pieces.

Foot Work

Foot work is a fundamental section in the Pilates workout that can be done on the reformer, cadillac, and wunda chair. In order to be consistent I teach the same comprehensive foot work routine on each of the pieces of equipment. Within my block system, the foot work typically follows the warm-up because I see the foot work as part of the warm-up, aiding the transition into the main body of the session. Although I label it foot work, it clearly involves the entire leg. In fact it involves the entire body. Focus is first given to the positioning of the pelvis and the spine.

The position of the pelvis and trunk is essentially the same throughout the foot work. The aspect that changes is the positioning of the legs. The musculature of the lower body is challenged in subtly different ways while the core remains constant. I recommend a pelvis-neutral spine position throughout. However, this *ideal* cannot always be achieved. Therefore in specific cases it is best to deviate from neutral in order to achieve correct muscle activation or muscle relaxation.

The thrust of the muscle activation in this block is the hip extensors and knee extensors, with particular bias toward the hamstrings. This is due to the overpowering quality of the quadriceps (being a larger muscle group) and the need to ensure that the hamstrings engage. I prefer that the gluteals, which are also hip extensors, be relaxed during this series of exercises. This allows smooth, unrestricted hip movement and a higher probability of maintaining a neutral pelvic position.

It is important to focus on both the concentric and eccentric contraction as the legs straighten and bend. The eccentric contraction, as the legs bend, is often overlooked. Striving to balance the concentric and eccentric contractions is among the factors that make Pilates such an excellent vehicle for functional training.

It is also important to straighten the legs completely. There is a tendency to stop short of fully straightening the legs out of fear of locking the knees. This can lead to problems, both muscular and neuromuscular. A person loses the sensation of completely straightening the leg and *almost* straight begins to feel like *completely* straight. The knee joint was built to reach *full* extension and it should be used to its maximum potential.

In the foot work, I often speak of straightening the legs from the abdominals. Anatomically this is clearly not the case—there is no physical muscular connection between the abdominals and the legs. Yet, conceptually, visualizing pushing the legs from deep in the pelvic bowl by contracting the muscles of the ISS helps ensure a stable foundation and smooth, flowing movement. I like to visualize the ISS as a steam engine and the legs as cranks being driven by the engine. This visualization helps create not only the desired movement pattern but also a sensation of warming up.

There is a tendency among some students to drop the heel as the leg straightens, releasing the resistance, and then lift it, placing the foot in full plantarflexion as the leg bends. This typically occurs when there is a lack of strength, and it should be avoided by keeping the heel

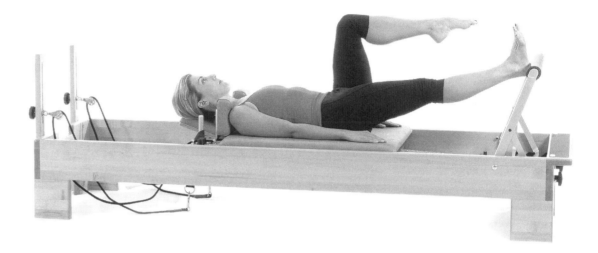

still. Working with less resistance in order to maintain the correct foot position is preferable to loading on the weight and compromising the foundation of this movement.

The foot work offers the teacher and the student a great deal of information regarding strength, flexibility, stabilization, alignment, and movement patterning. In many ways the foot work resembles the gait cycle and as such gives insight into the way a person walks and runs. It is a fascinating area of study and should be observed from various different angles.

Parallel Heels

Muscle Focus

- Hamstrings
- Quadriceps

Objectives

- To strengthen the hip extensors and knee extensors
- To warm up by using the larger muscle groups
- To develop pelvic–lumbar stabilization

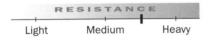

RESISTANCE

Light   Medium   Heavy

This heel position has two major benefits. The first is that it allows you to align and use the legs while initially taking the complex alignment of the foot partially out of the picture. Although the foot is the foundation, it remains still; the movement occurs primarily in the ankle, knee, and hip joints. The second benefit of bearing weight on the heel is that you can more readily connect with the hamstrings when extending the hip and knee (i.e., straightening the leg).

When using the various heel positions, the foot should remain still. The pivot point is the ankle joint; in contrast, if the foot were in full dorsiflexion, the ankle would be stable and the movement would resemble a rocking back and forth on the heel.

Imagery

Visualize a rubber band connecting the heel to the sit bones. As the leg straightens, the band stretches, creating a strong pull between the heel and sit bones; as the leg bends, resist the movement as if you were

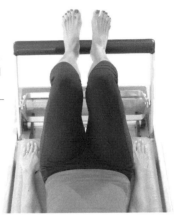

The parallel heels position allows full use of the ankle, knee, and hip joints.

trying to keep the leg straight. This internal resistance increases the work in the muscles, maximizing the eccentric contraction.

- ☐ Maintain a neutral pelvis throughout the series.
- ☐ Initiate the movement with the hamstrings.
- ☐ Keep the feet partially dorsiflexed and still, as if standing on the floor.
- ☐ Use the ankle as the pivot point of the movement.

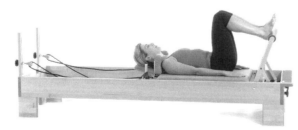

Inhale. Lie supine with a neutral spine position, placing the heels on the foot bar 2 to 4 inches (5 to 10 centimeters) apart with the legs parallel. Relax the arms by the sides of the body. The shoulders gently touch the shoulder rests. Place the head on the headrest (adjusted to provide optimal spinal alignment, free of tension).

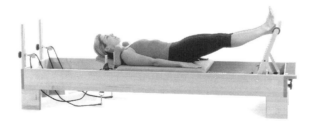

Exhale. Straighten the legs completely, extending the hips and knees while maintaining stability in the remainder of the body. Reach the farthest point possible.

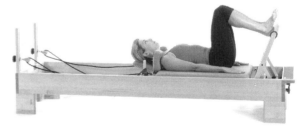

Inhale. Bend the knees and flex the hips, returning toward the stopper without hitting it or halting the movement.

During foot work exercises in the toe positions on the reformer, cadillac, or wunda chair, the foot should remain active, pivoting at the ankle joint (not the metatarsal–phalange joint) and maintaining a constant degree of plantarflexion (the maximum amount that can be achieved when the knees are fully extended). As the knees bend, maintain this same angle of the foot to the foot bar, keeping the heel still. There is a tendency, to maintain maximum plantarflexion throughout the movement. This results in a rocking back and forth on the ball of the foot, eliminating the ankle as the pivot point.

Pressure should be evenly distributed throughout the front of the foot when pushing off the ball of the foot and the toes. The toes wrap gently over the bar.

The toe positions are more challenging than the heel positions. Not only are they more complex, with more joints involved, but the amount of resistance also increases due to the added height of the foot.

To correct a tendency to roll the foot out (supinate), adjust the subtalar joint, placing slightly more weight on the inner aspect of the foot, and engage the peroneal muscles more fully. Do the opposite if the foot rolls in.

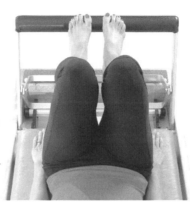

Imagery

The imagery described for the parallel heels exercise (page 112) works for all the foot work positions. When pushing off the toes you should feel a lifted sensation, as if you were pushing off a springboard.

☐ Initiate the movement from the hamstrings.

☐ Keep the heels still and the angle of the feet consistent throughout the movement.

Muscle Focus

- Hamstrings
- Quadriceps

Objectives

- To strengthen the hip extensors, knee extensors, and feet
- To warm up, using the larger muscle groups
- To align the foot, the leg, and the related joints
- To develop pelvic–lumbar stabilization

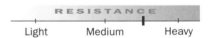

RESISTANCE

Light　　Medium　　Heavy

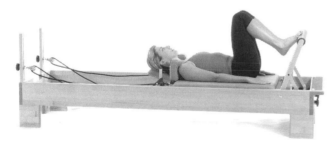

Inhale. Lie supine in a neutral spine position, placing the toes on the foot bar 2 to 4 inches apart, keeping the legs parallel and gently wrapping the bar with the toes. Relax the arms by the sides of the body. The shoulders gently touch the shoulder rests. Place the head on the headrest.

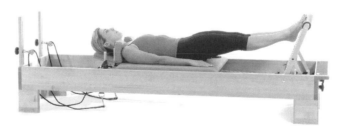

Exhale. Straighten the legs completely, extending the hips and knees while keeping the rest of the body stable. Reach the farthest point possible. Inhale. Bend the knees and flex the hips, returning toward the stopper without hitting it or halting the movement.

V-Position Toes

Muscle Focus

- Hamstrings
- Quadriceps

Objectives

- To strengthen the hip extensors and knee extensors
- To warm up, using the larger muscle groups
- To develop ankle control

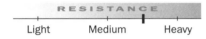

RESISTANCE

Light   Medium   Heavy

The degree of external rotation of the hips in this exercise is not great, no more than 30 degrees, although this will be somewhat individual. Dancers who are accustomed to working with much greater hip external rotation (turnout) should not compare this position to first position in ballet—it is not. It is a classic Pilates position that can be more accurately compared to a military stance. (Dancers can add exercises that are specifically adapted to incorporate turnout.)

The exact position can be achieved when transitioning from the parallel toes position by simply bringing the heels together without adjusting the width between the feet. Note that this position is typically done on the toes only, making the transition from the previous position seamless.

Imagery

Imagine straightening the legs and squeezing them together at the same time, as if you were holding a big ball or balloon between the legs.

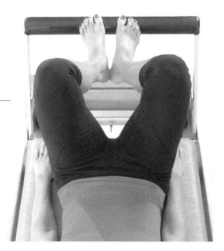

The V position offers comfortable, rather than maximal, external rotation.

- ☐ Initiate the movement from the hamstrings.
- ☐ Keep the heels still while squeezing them together.
- ☐ Straighten the legs completely, focusing on the co-contraction of the quadriceps and the hamstrings.

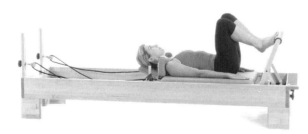

Inhale. Lie supine in a neutral spine position, placing the toes on the foot bar 2 to 4 inches apart. Bring the heels together to make a V position. Relax the arms by the sides and gently touch the shoulder rests with the shoulders. Place the head on the headrest.

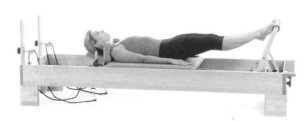

Exhale. Straighten the legs completely, extending the hips and knees while maintaining stability in the remainder of the body. Reach the farthest point possible.

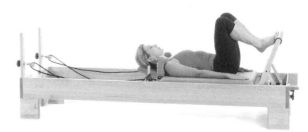

Inhale. Bend the knees and flex the hips, returning toward the stopper without hitting it or halting the movement.

Open V-Position Heels

The wide V positions, both on the heels and toes, are not from the classic Pilates repertoire but offer valuable benefits. They take the hip joint into a wider, more challenging range of motion than most people are used to, in terms of both hip abduction and external rotation. I encourage you to explore this "unused" range to maintain optimal function of the hip joint. These positions also allow dancers (and other athletes who use similar movements) to simulate positions that are used extensively in dance in order to correct their technique and develop strength.

Imagery

As with the V-position toes (page 114), imagine straightening the legs and simultaneously squeezing them together, emphasizing the involvement of the hip adductors as the legs straighten and bend. When the knees bend, visualize them reaching out to the sides of the body along a constant diagonal energy line.

To find the most comfortable position, duplicate the shape of the V-position toes and then open the legs wider, placing the feet toward the outside of the foot bar.

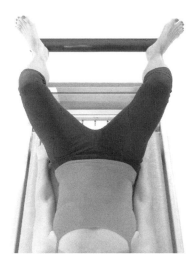

☐ Focus on engaging the adductors.

☐ Keep the feet partially dorsiflexed and still, as if standing on a floor.

☐ Maintain correct tracking of the leg, aligning the hip, knee, and foot.

Muscle Focus

- Hamstrings
- Quadriceps
- Hip adductors

Objectives

- To strengthen the hip extensors and knee extensors
- To control the hip adductors
- To increase the range of motion of the hip joints
- To warm up, using the larger muscle groups

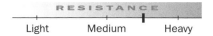

RESISTANCE

Light   Medium   Heavy

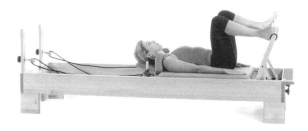

Inhale. Lie supine with a neutral spine, placing the heels on the ends of the foot bar. Relax the arms by the sides and gently touch the shoulder rests with the shoulders. Place the head on the headrest.

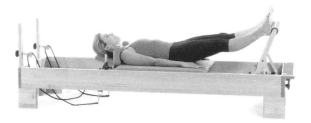

Exhale. Straighten the legs completely, extending the hips and knees while maintaining stability in the remainder of the body. Reach the farthest point possible.

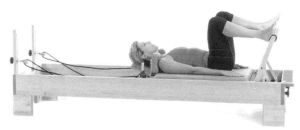

Inhale. Return toward the stopper without hitting it or halting the movement. Maintain the same degree of hip external rotation throughout.

115

Open V-Position Toes

Muscle Focus

- Hamstrings
- Quadriceps
- Hip adductors

Objectives

- To strengthen the hip extensors and knee extensors
- To develop adductor and foot control
- To warm up, using the larger muscle groups

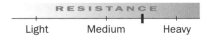

RESISTANCE

Light · Medium · Heavy

This wide V position on the toes is possibly the most complex position in the foot work block because it requires tremendous control of the hip and knee joints and also the foot. In addition, it offers the most stretch in the hip joint and a unique angle of challenge for the hamstrings and quadriceps.

Imagery

Employ the same images used for the previous foot positions (pages 112 to 115). In addition, the image of an open-leg squat may help you release tension in the hip joint and create a sensation of the pelvis opening and relaxing.

- ☐ Straighten the legs completely.
- ☐ Keep the heels still throughout the movement.
- ☐ Maintain correct tracking of the leg, aligning the hip, knee, and foot.

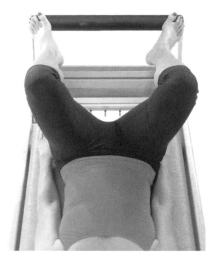

The vastus medialis oblique muscle (VMO) can be distinctly felt and strengthened (often a goal in corrective work of the knee) during this exercise.

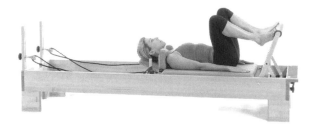

Inhale. Lie supine with a neutral spine, placing the toes toward the outside of the foot bar so that they form a wide V. Relax the arms by the sides and gently touch the shoulder rests with the shoulders. Place the head on the headrest.

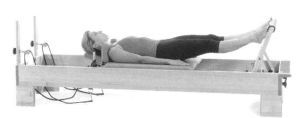

Exhale. Straighten the legs completely, extending the hips and knees while maintaining stability in the remainder of the body. Reach the farthest point possible.

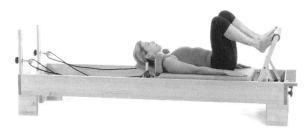

Inhale. Return toward the stopper without hitting it or halting the movement, keeping the heels still.

Calf Raises

This is an exceptional exercise for increasing functional range of motion and strength of the foot, including the many joints involved in its movement. It also allows you to focus on correcting foot alignment, which is so important in walking and other everyday movements and many athletic pursuits. You can imagine the importance of exact and efficient foot movement for a marathon runner who repeats the same movement pattern thousands of times in one event, not to mention in the hundreds of hours of training.

Pay particular attention to the eccentric contraction as you lower the heel. You should not succumb to the pull of the springs by dropping the heel; instead, resist them as you lower the heel and actively dorsiflex the foot at the end range. Some people tend to roll onto the outside of the foot as they reach the maximum plantarflexion. Limiting the range of the ankle joint and maintaining correct alignment, with weight evenly distributed through the toes, is preferable to going higher and deviating from the centerline.

Imagery

The image of pushing the foot bar away from the body helps to achieve the desired amount of plantarflexion. The more stable the body is, particularly the pelvis, the more powerful each thrust will be. Picture 50 percent of the weight concentrated around the big toe and the remaining 50 percent distributed through the other toes proportionately, according to the size of the toe. This is an approximation but provides a good image.

☐ Use the full range of motion of the ankle.

☐ Maintain correct tracking of the hip, knee, and foot.

☐ Align the foot correctly, focusing on the subtalar joint.

Muscle Focus

▪ Foot plantarflexors

Objectives

▪ To strengthen the foot plantarflexors

▪ To develop foot control and correct alignment

▪ To warm up the muscles of the lower leg

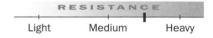

RESISTANCE

Light   Medium   Heavy

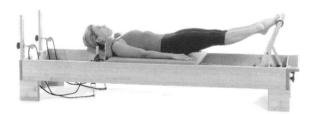

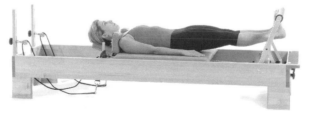

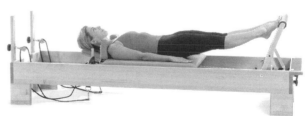

Inhale. Lie supine with a neutral spine, placing the toes on the foot bar approximately 2 to 4 inches apart with the legs parallel. Gently wrap the toes over the foot bar and plantarflex the feet. Relax the arms by the sides and gently touch the shoulder rests with the shoulders. Place the head on the headrest.

Exhale. Dorsiflex the feet, pressing the heels under the foot bar.

Inhale. Plantarflex the feet.

Prances

Muscle Focus

- Foot plantarflexors

Objectives

- To strengthen and stretch the foot plantarflexors
- To develop pelvic–lumbar stabilization
- To warm up the muscles of the lower leg

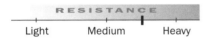

RESISTANCE

Light   Medium   Heavy

This exercise starts in the same position as the Reformer: Calf Raises (page 117), with the legs straight and the feet in maximum plantarflexion. One foot then dorsiflexes while the other plantarflexes. As the feet switch, it is important to pass through the beginning position with both feet in maximal plantarflexion and to achieve a sense of height and elongation through each cycle. The stability of the pelvis and the profound work of the feet give this exercise the desired sense of flow and lightness.

Imagery

This is a movement used often in dance training, and the image of a horse prancing is commonly used. Aim to achieve the same grace, flow, and proud, upright feeling of a beautiful dancer or horse, barely touching the ground. Imagine also the foot bar as a trampoline, emphasizing the upward movement, adding lift and buoyancy.

- ☐ Maintain a stable pelvis throughout the movement.
- ☐ Work both feet equally in their respective full ranges of motion; as one lifts into plantarflexion, the other presses down into dorsiflexion.

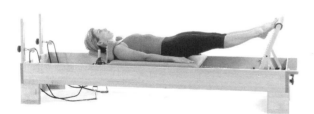

Inhale. Lie supine with a neutral spine, placing the toes on the foot bar approximately 2 to 4 inches apart with the legs parallel. Gently wrap the toes around the foot bar and plantarflex the feet. Relax the arms by the sides and gently touch the shoulder rests with the shoulders. Place the head on the headrest.

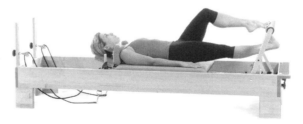

Exhale. Dorsiflex one foot and plantarflex the other. Switch the feet while moving through the starting position.

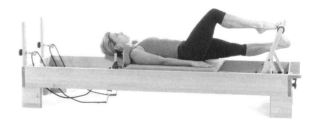

Inhale. Repeat the cycle twice as above. Continue for 10 complete cycles.

Single-Leg Heel

Working a single leg is invaluable for several reasons. First, it allows each leg to work independently without relying on the other. Often one leg is dominant and will take over the work. This is particularly common following an injury or surgery. Working unilaterally (typically starting with the weaker side) will strengthen the weaker leg in an endeavor to create balance. It will also magnify compensations and misalignments, making them easier to detect. Finally, exercising a single leg increases the challenge of keeping the pelvis stable. Clearly this series should be included in your workout if at all possible.

Imagery

Imagine that both legs are on the bar and that everything is the same as in the double-leg positions. Visualizing the invisible leg helps keep the structure stable and balanced.

☐ Keep the working foot dorsiflexed as if standing on the floor.

☐ Keep the supporting leg stable.

☐ Maintain correct alignment and stability of the pelvis.

Muscle Focus

- Hamstrings
- Quadriceps

Objectives

- To strengthen the hip extensors and knee extensors
- To develop pelvic–lumbar stabilization
- To warm up, using the larger muscle groups

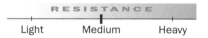

RESISTANCE

Light   Medium   Heavy

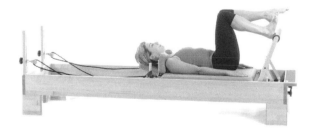

Inhale. Lie supine with a neutral spine, placing the heels on the foot bar approximately 2 to 4 inches apart with the legs parallel. Lift one leg and hold it in a tabletop position. Relax the arms by the sides and gently touch the shoulder rests with the shoulders. Place the head on the headrest.

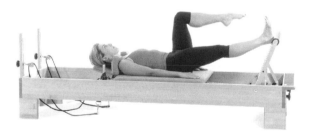

Exhale. Straighten the leg that is on the foot bar completely, extending the hips and knees while maintaining stability in the remainder of the body. Reach the farthest point possible.

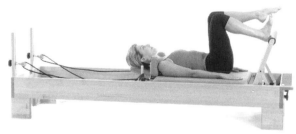

Inhale. Bend the leg, returning toward the stopper without hitting it or halting the movement.

Single-Leg Toes

Muscle Focus

- Hamstrings
- Quadriceps

Objectives

- To strengthen the hip extensors and knee extensors
- To strengthen the plantarflexors
- To warm up, using the larger muscle groups

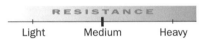

RESISTANCE

Light   Medium   Heavy

The instructions pertaining to the Reformer: Single-Leg Heel (page 119) apply to this exercise. The position of the foot is described in Reformer: Parallel Toes (page 113). This is the most challenging position in the foot work series in terms of load. Remember, working with a lighter load and correct alignment is always preferable to compromising good form for the sake of load. However, once you have achieved good form and control, increasing the load to challenge the musculature and improve strength is valuable.

Imagery

The desired sense of elongation of the movement is easier to feel in the toes position than in the heel position (see also single-leg heel, page 119).

- ☐ Keep the heel of the working foot still.
- ☐ Straighten the working leg completely with each repetition.
- ☐ Keep the supporting leg stable.
- ☐ Maintain correct alignment of the foot and stability of the pelvis.

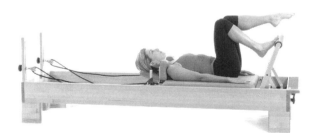

Inhale. Lie supine with a neutral spine, placing the toes on the foot bar approximately 2 to 4 inches apart with the legs parallel. Lift one leg and hold it in a tabletop position. Relax the arms by the sides and gently touch the shoulder rests with the shoulders. Place the head on the headrest (adjusted to provide optimal spinal alignment, free of tension).

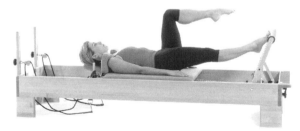

Exhale. Straighten the leg that is on the foot bar completely, extending the hips and knees while maintaining stability in the remainder of the body. Reach the farthest point possible.

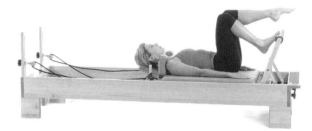

Inhale. Bend the leg, returning toward the stopper without hitting it or halting the movement.

The prehensile position is one of the classic Pilates positions. At the same time, I regard it as a unique and specialized position, and I don't necessarily offer it to students early in their training. Because of the unusual position of the foot and a relatively complex movement pattern, it is difficult to execute well. When used appropriately, it is certainly a very valuable position. Its benefits include providing a specific stretch for the foot and its intrinsic muscles.

Imagery

The most effective image is a bird wrapping its feet around a branch and holding it firmly.

☐ Keep reaching the heels under the foot bar throughout the movement to maximize the calf stretch.

☐ Wrap the toes around the foot bar, stretching the top of the foot

☐ Keep the toes spread out as opposed to clenching up

The prehensile position places pressure on points that correlate with reflexology pressure points.

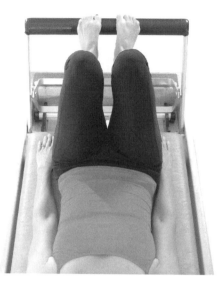

Muscle Focus

- Hamstrings
- Quadriceps

Objectives

- To strengthen the hip extensors and knee extensors
- To stretch the calf muscles
- To stretch the intrinsic muscles of the foot

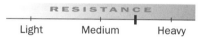

RESISTANCE

Light   Medium   Heavy

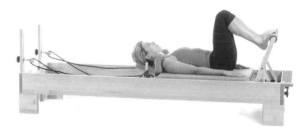

Inhale. Lie supine with a neutral spine and place the balls of the feet on the foot bar 2 to 4 inches apart with the legs parallel. Wrap the front part of the foot, including the toes, around the bar. Relax the arms by the sides and gently touch the shoulder rests with the shoulders. Place the head on the headrest.

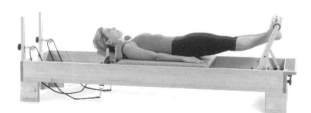

Exhale. Straighten the legs while pushing the heels under the foot bar.

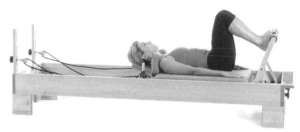

Inhale. Bend the knees, returning toward the stopper without hitting it or halting the movement. Continue pushing the heels under the foot bar.

Abdominal Work

In Pilates, it is difficult to overemphasize the abdominal work. At the same time, you must remember that the abdominals are only part of the whole and not the entire picture. Because of the focus on abdominal work, at times Pilates teachers view abdominal exercises as the "be all and end all" of this system. They are not! A healthy balance is the goal, and therefore it is important to create some guidelines from the outset.

There are four layers of abdominal muscle, the most superficial being the external obliques, followed by the rectus abdominis, the internal obliques, and finally the deepest layer, the transverse abdominis (TA). The TA is a fundamental ingredient in the "powerhouse" concept, which is part of every movement in Pilates. Therefore, the TA should be engaged throughout the Pilates session because it plays a fundamental role in stabilization and thus the protection of the spine. The TA is particularly pertinent when performing abdominal work in order to achieve the desired effect and the correct quality of movement.

It is interesting to compare, for instance, the typical abdominal crunch to the Mat Work: Chest Lift (page 48). They are seemingly so similar, yet the quality and the outcome of each exercise are entirely different, in large part because of the emphasis on TA engagement in the chest lift. The emphasis on the TA should not in any way devalue the importance of the other abdominal muscles, which when working together as an integrated complex serve as both an immaculate brace for the trunk and a powerful motivator for any trunk movement. I have witnessed many tough and seasoned athletes who were accustomed to performing hundreds of repetitions of abdominal crunches crumble after attempting 10 good chest lifts.

When compiling the abdominal section of the Pilates session, take care to use both isometric and isotonic exercises as well as a balance between sequences that develop strength versus those that develop muscle endurance. Finally, remember that it is not only during forward flexion that the abdominals are recruited and trained but in fact during all ranges of motion, including trunk extension.

An image commonly used in Pilates work to achieve the correct recruitment of the abdominal muscles is that of hollowing the midsection (abdominal cavity) of the body. It is this drawing in the navel to the spine that encourages the recruitment of the TA. I like to visualize a hollow, deep, carved-out wooden bowl. This image appears as firm and stable, able to hold large amounts of energy and life force within it.

Hundred Prep

The hundred prep is simple and very effective. You can immediately feel the abdominal muscles working and sense the synergy between the trunk flexors and the shoulder extensors. This exercise is a challenge for people of every fitness level, and it has many variations to meet different goals. It serves as an excellent preparation for the more advanced Reformer: Hundred (page 124) and Reformer: Coordination (page 125) as it includes elements of both. Hundred prep is an isotonic exercise, which complements many isometric abdominal exercises. I recommend that a balanced abdominal program include isotonic and isometric exercises; each type of exercise develops the muscles differently and is important for optimal function.

Imagery

This exercise begs the image of a seesaw lifting up and lowering as one unit. Achieving this integrated feeling early in the abdominal work is important because it is a recurring theme throughout the abdominal series and Pilates in general.

☐ Maintain a stable position of the pelvis throughout the exercise.

☐ Avoid hyperlordosis and bulging of the abdominal region.

☐ Keep the head aligned with the spine.

☐ Engage the abdominal muscles throughout the exercise.

Muscle Focus

- Abdominal muscles

Objectives

- To strengthen the abdominal muscles and shoulder extensors
- To develop the pelvic–lumbar stabilization

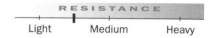

RESISTANCE

Light   Medium   Heavy

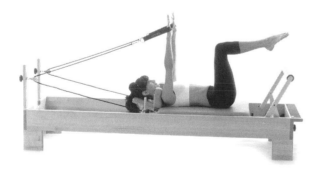

Inhale. Lie supine on the reformer with the legs in a tabletop position (hips and knees at a 90-degree angle). Place the hands in the straps with the arms perpendicular to the body, maintaining slight tension in the straps. At this point the spine should be in a neutral position.

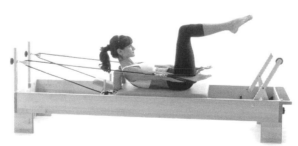

Exhale. Lift the head and chest, simultaneously pressing the arms down to the sides of the body and keeping the legs in the tabletop position. Coordinate the movement by first contracting the abdominals, then lifting the upper body while extending the arms.

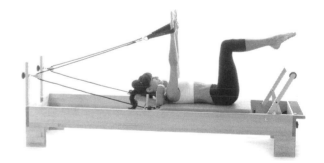

Inhale. Lower the body to the starting position.

Hundred

Muscle Focus

■ Abdominal muscles

Objectives

■ To strengthen the abdominal muscles
■ To develop pelvic–lumbar stabilization

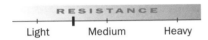

```
         RESISTANCE
    |_____|_____|
   Light    Medium     Heavy
```

Like the hundred prep, this exercise emphasizes integration of the abdominals and shoulder extensors. The slight up-and-down beating motion of the arms adds movement to the isometric activity of the abdominals and stimulates circulation and deep breathing.

To make the exercise easier on the abdominals and alleviate potential strain on the low back, raise the legs toward a 90-degree angle in the hip joint. If the exercise still proves too challenging, bend the knees and flex the hips into a tabletop position.

The hundred is a signature exercise of the classic Pilates repertoire (see page 50). This challenging exercise demands a high level of awareness, control, abdominal strength, and understanding of the concept of the internal support system (ISS; pages 17-19). The hundred and several other exercises involve isometric contraction of the abdominal muscles in the same position, so supplementing them with isotonic exercises is important in creating a complete abdominal strengthening program.

Imagery

Visualize the pumping action of the arms as a generator creating energy that gushes through the body, with the epicenter in the abdominal region. The hollow bowl image mentioned in the Mat Work: Chest Lift (page 48) also helps to fortify the position of the trunk.

☐ Imprint the lower back into the mat throughout the exercise.

☐ Keep the head aligned with the spine and the eyes focused forward.

☐ Keep the carriage as still as possible as the arms pump up and down with small, calm movements.

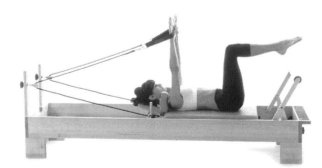

Inhale. Lie supine on the reformer with the legs in a tabletop position. Place the hands in the straps with the arms perpendicular to the body, maintaining slight tension in the straps. At this point the spine should be in a neutral position.

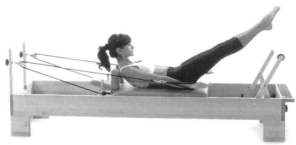

Exhale. Lift the head and chest, straightening the legs and keeping the feet at eye level. Simultaneously extend the arms down to the sides of the body. Inhale. Pause, deepening the abdominal contraction.

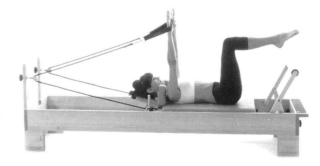

Exhale. Pump the arms up and down in a small rhythmic motion for five counts. Inhale and continue pumping the arms up and down for five counts. Focus on the stabilization of the trunk and pelvis, maintaining forward flexion. Repeat for 10 breath cycles and return to the starting position.

The name of this exercise suggests the complexity of its movements. Coordinating the breath with the movement in itself presents a challenge. Although coordinating four distinct breaths with four movements might seem to make more intuitive sense and be easier to coordinate, I prefer to use two breaths for the four movements. Doing so creates better flow and continuity and encourages deeper breathing with more active use of the respiratory muscles. It also challenges the coordination even further.

During the movement, the body can either stay up in trunk flexion or the trunk and head can be lowered after each repetition. Each version has its benefits; the former being an isometric exercise for the abdominals, the latter an isotonic exercise. However, the head should never go halfway up or down (an area I call *the danger zone*) because this position will inevitably create tension in the neck.

Imagery

This exercise is a rub-your-stomach-while-patting-your-head type of motion. Picture a closed-loop mechanical toy that repeatedly goes through an identical sequence of movements. However, making your actions too mechanical will sacrifice the dynamic of the exercise and flow of the movement. The motion should be smooth, with the opening and closing of the legs a little sharper in dynamic than the lifting and lowering of the body.

☐ Keep the feet opposite the eyes when the legs straighten, imprinting the lower back into the mat.

☐ Draw the knees in toward the chest before lifting the arms and lowering the trunk.

Muscle Focus

- Abdominal muscles

Objectives

- To strengthen the abdominal muscles
- To increase pelvic–lumbar stabilization
- To improve coordination

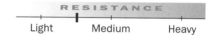

RESISTANCE

Light   Medium   Heavy

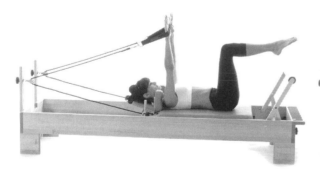

Inhale. Lie supine on the reformer with the legs in the tabletop position. Place the hands in the straps with the arms perpendicular to the body, maintaining slight tension in the straps. At this point the spine should be in a neutral position.

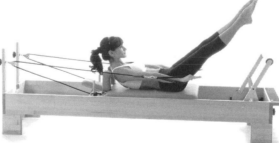

Exhale. Lift the head and chest, straightening the legs and keeping the feet above eye level. Simultaneously extend the arms down to the sides of the body. Continue to exhale, opening and closing the legs (no wider than the foot bar) in a brisk motion.

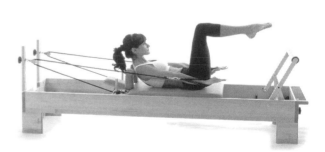

Inhale. Bend the legs to the tabletop position, then lift the arms and lower the head and trunk to the starting position.

Muscle Focus

- Abdominals

Objectives

- To strengthen the abdominals
- To develop hip flexor control

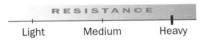

RESISTANCE

Light   Medium   Heavy

Round Back

The round back exercise introduces the short box series on the reformer, which also includes the flat back (page 127), climb-a-tree (page 128), tilt (page 195), twist (page 196), and round-about (which does not appear in this book). The term short box refers to the Pilates box being placed on the reformer sideways to the carriage. Each exercise in the series uses the abdominals in a slightly different way, and certain exercises fit comfortably into more than one block. "Borrowing" exercises from the series to fulfill a different block is quite legitimate; for instance, the tilt and twist exercises have been allocated as part of the lateral flexion and rotation block as they include lateral flexion and rotation, respectively.

The round back comprises two distinct positions: the initial upright position and the round back C curve. Drawing in the abdominals while focusing the flexion in the lumbar spine creates the desired C curve. Then take the trunk back, pivoting at the hip joint, ideally to the point where the lower back rests on the box. Then lift it again, returning to the position in which the shoulders are above the hips. At this point, extend the trunk into the upright position. These two positions of the trunk, upright and round back, form the basis of many of the abdominal exercises.

Imagery

In the sitting position, the placement of the shoulders is above the hips. As the trunk is rounded, imagine that the spine is being stretched from the back like a rubber band, creating the C curve. Visualizing that the round position opens the vertebrae, making the spine feel "longer," will help avoid collapsing the spine. You should feel even more lifted and taller in the round back position than in the upright position. Once established, the round back position then tips back in an action that resembles pouring tea from a teapot.

☐ Establish the round back position prior to tipping back.

☐ Maintain the stable round position of the trunk as it tips back and then lifts up again.

☐ Straighten into an upright position to conclude the exercise only after the shoulders are over the hips.

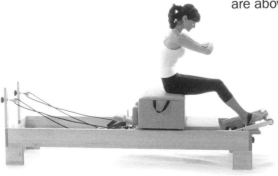

Inhale. Sit upright on the box close to the front. Place the feet under the foot strap, bend the knees, and cross the arms. Exhale. Round the trunk, simultaneously lifting the arms away from the chest.

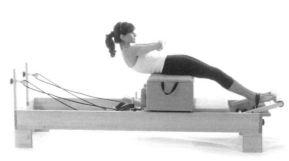

Still exhaling, lower the body backward with the trunk in the rounded position. Inhale and pause in this position.

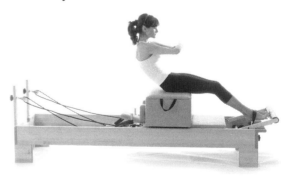

Exhale. Raise the body so the shoulders are level with the hips, maintaining the C curve of the trunk. Then inhale as you return to the starting position.

Flat Back

The flat back exercise has similarities to the Reformer: Round Back (page 126) in terms of the action of the abdominals and the hip joint being the pivot point of the movement. Both exercises work the abdominal muscles, maintain a stable trunk as the body is lowered and lifted, and feature movement in the same plane of motion. However the action of the abdominals is different in that in the flat back they contract isometrically together with the back extensors, holding the body in a neutral spine position as it is lowered and lifted. In the round back exercise, it is primarily the abdominals that maintain the C-curve position as the body is lowered and lifted. In both cases the hip flexors play an important role, contracting eccentrically as the body is lowered and concentrically as it returns to the upright position. Yet, the load on the hip flexors is even greater in the flat back.

The movement of the trunk is relatively contained and should not exceed 45 degrees when lunging back. Beyond this angle there is a high risk of hyperextending the back; to avoid this the pelvis and the trunk must move as one unit, hinging at the hip joint. If the pelvis stops and the upper body continues to tilt back, the result is hyperextension and pressure on the lower back.

Imagery

The image of a closed door lying flat, opening slightly on its hinge and then closing again, helps achieve the correct movement.

☐ Co-contract the abdominals and back extensors.
☐ Move the pelvis and trunk as one unit, hinging at the hip joint.
☐ Keep the head aligned with the spine.

Muscle Focus

- Abdominals
- Back extensors

Objectives

- To strengthen the abdominal muscles
- To develop control of the back extensors
- To develop control of the hip flexors
- To develop trunk stabilization

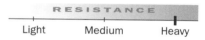
RESISTANCE
Light   Medium   Heavy

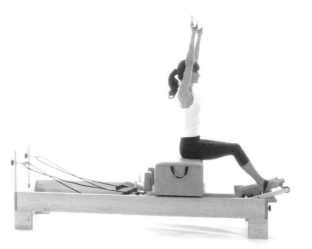

Exhale. Sit upright on the box close to the front. Place the feet under the foot strap, bend the knees, and interlace the fingers behind the head or hold a pole overhead with the arms straight and shoulder-width apart.

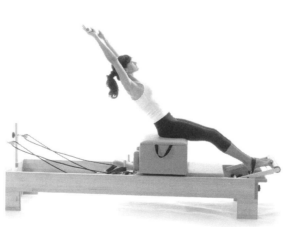

Inhale. Lunge back, moving the trunk and pelvis as one unit.

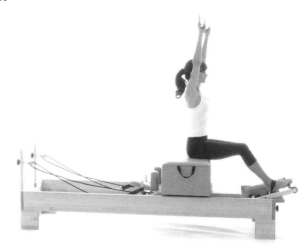

Exhale. Lift the trunk, returning to the starting position.

Climb-a-Tree

Muscle Focus

- Abdominal muscles

Objectives

- To strengthen the abdominal muscles
- To develop control of the back extensors
- To stretch the hamstrings

Although this exercise in its classic form is performed on the short box (the box is placed on the reformer sideways to the carriage), I recommend learning it (and prefer practicing it) with the box in the long box position. The long box offers far more support for the lower back and provides a better stretch for the thoracic region.

I encourage maximizing the stretch of the hamstrings when the leg is straight in the sitting position (initial and final phases of the exercise) by keeping the back extensors engaged and the trunk as upright as possible. It is important to maintain abdominal contraction throughout the exercise, particularly during the arm circle phase because of the tendency to hyperextend the lower back at this point. Achieve deep flexion of the trunk as you climb down and then up the "tree" (leg), again highlighting abdominal activation. As with the other exercises in the short box series, for safety reasons all the springs should be in place to prevent the carriage from moving.

RESISTANCE
Light   Medium   Heavy

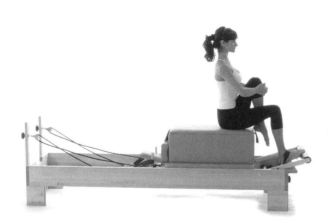

Inhale. Sit upright at the front edge of the box with one foot placed securely under the strap and the knee bent. Bend the other leg, drawing the thigh to the chest. Hold the knee and extend the back. Exhale. Pump the thigh to the chest three times, elongating the back and sitting more upright with each pump.

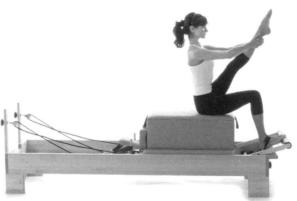

Inhale. Holding the ankle, straighten the leg while keeping the back as upright as possible.

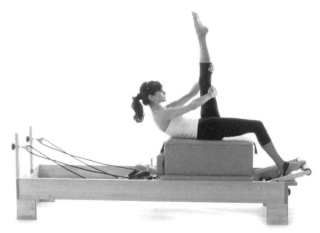

Exhale. Walk the hands down the leg, lowering the trunk to the box in deep flexion. The upright leg moves to a position perpendicular to the box and holds still (like a tree trunk).

Imagery

Imagine climbing down and then up a tree, keeping the body close to the trunk of the tree by maximizing spinal flexion.

☐ Begin the movement by sitting upright with the back extensors engaged.

☐ Emphasize trunk flexion when "climbing" down and up the leg.

☐ Avoid arching the back and thrusting the ribs forward during the arm circle phase.

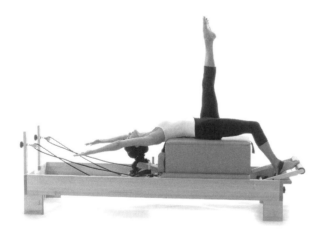

Inhale. Arch the mid- and upper back over the box, circling the arms overhead and around.

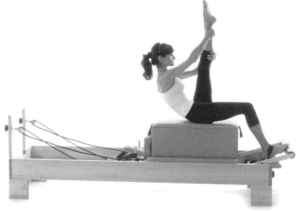

Exhale. Return to trunk flexion and place the hands back on the leg. Climb up the leg, maintaining deep abdominal work.

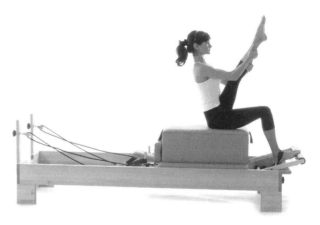

Inhale. Restack and extend the spine while keeping the leg straight. Still inhaling, bend the leg and return to the starting position.

Backstroke

Muscle Focus

- Abdominal muscles

Objectives

- To strengthen the abdominal muscles
- To develop pelvic–lumbar stabilization
- To develop shoulder control

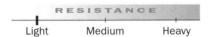

RESISTANCE

Light   Medium   Heavy

The backstroke is a complex, high-level exercise that demands coordination and strength. The potential for undue neck strain is great in this exercise because of the perched position on the box, along with the added resistance from the straps. This results in an enormous demand on the abdominals. Keeping a stable trunk and head as the arms and legs move independently is the key to the success of this exercise. In many instances, introducing this exercise on the mat or box without the straps is advantageous, adding resistance only when good coordination, muscle recruitment, and strength have been achieved.

Imagery

Use the image of the hollow bowl for the abdominals, and think of the legs and arms moving in a circular, backstroke (or more precisely, breaststroke on the back) motion. The pause following the circling of the arms and legs places the body in a streamlined position, and you should feel as if you were gliding through the water after a powerful stroke of the legs and arms.

- ☐ Align the edge of the box with the base of the scapulae.
- ☐ Keep the eyes focused directly forward throughout the exercise.
- ☐ Maintain maximum trunk flexion with the head aligned with the spine.
- ☐ Synchronize the movement of the arms and legs.

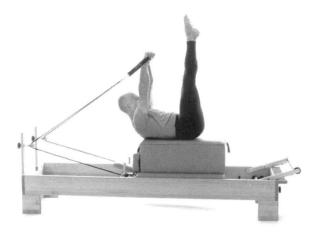

Exhale. Lie supine on the long box, facing the foot bar with the shoulders slightly beyond the back edge of the box. Lift the trunk into maximal spinal flexion with the legs in the tabletop position. Hold the straps with the hands in a fist position, and the elbows pointing outward. Inhale. Straighten the arms and legs directly up toward the ceiling.

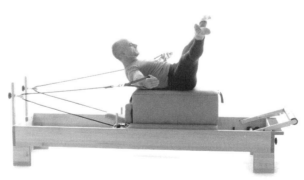

Externally rotate (turn out) the legs. Exhale. Circle the arms and legs out and around.

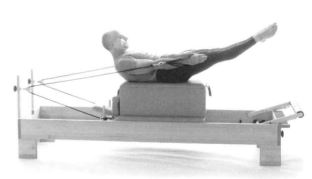

Still exhaling, pause when the legs are straight ahead and the arms are pressing against the outer thighs, then return to the starting position.

Abdominals With Legs in Straps

The Reformer: Scooter (page 155) and Reformer: Knee Stretch, Round Back (page 156) exercises, plus an understanding of the concepts of trunk stabilization and hip disassociation, are prerequisites to proper execution of this exercise, which is essentially the knee stretch in a supine position. Viewing it in this way enables you to relate to a previously learned movement pattern.

Because of the significant load on the hip flexors, this exercise can create potentially hazardous stresses on the spine, particularly if the spinal stabilization provided largely by the abdominals is insufficient. This makes the exercise very challenging. Developing hip flexor strength along with abdominal strength is important in creating a good strength ratio between these two muscle groups. Problems arise when one group (usually the hip flexors) overpowers the other.

Focus on using the iliopsoas, a single-joint hip flexor, over the rectus femoris, a two-joint hop flexor. To encourage use of the iliopsoas, the movement should come from deep in the abdominal bowl rather than pulling with the legs. It sometimes helps to imagine the legs feeling almost weightless and being pulled in by the abdominals.

Imagery

Combine two images: the abdominal muscles creating a hollow bowl, anchored into the carriage, and the legs moving like pistons pumping in and out (with the emphasis on the "in" toward the body phase). The feet remain at eye level, moving along a horizontal plane.

☐ Draw the knees in toward the forehead.

☐ Move the feet along a horizontal line.

☐ Maintain pelvic–lumbar stabilization while imprinting the lower back into the carriage.

Muscle Focus

- Abdominal muscles

Objectives

- To strengthen the abdominal muscles and hip flexors
- To develop pelvic–lumbar stabilization

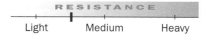

RESISTANCE

Light   Medium   Heavy

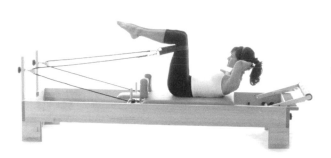

Inhale. Lie supine with the head close to the foot bar and the pelvis in front of the shoulder rests, touching the shoulder rests with the tips of the fingers. Thread the legs through the straps, placing them just above the knees, and bring the legs into a tabletop position. Hold the trunk in forward flexion and place the hands behind the head.

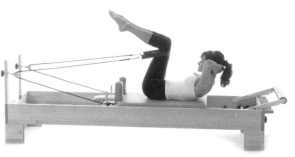

Exhale. Draw the thighs toward the chest.

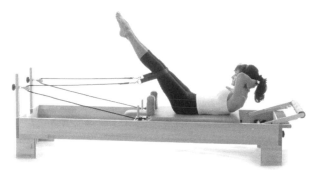

Inhale. Straighten the legs, maintaining pelvic–lumbar stability. Exhale. Return to the starting position after 5 to 10 repetitions.

Oblique Abdominals With Legs in Straps

Muscle Focus

- Oblique abdominal muscles

Objectives

- To strengthen the oblique abdominals and hip flexors
- To develop pelvic–lumbar stabilization

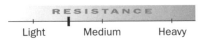

RESISTANCE

Light   Medium   Heavy

This exercise is identical to the Reformer: Abdominals With Legs in Straps but has the added component of trunk rotation, keeping the pelvis stable. The element of rotation increases the challenge of maintaining pelvic stability—achieved with strong, efficient abdominal recruitment. The upper body should move as one unit, with the elbows pointing outward in a stable and constant position. Although the rotation of the vertebrae occurs largely in the thoracic spine, the sense should be that the upper body moves as a unit while the lower body is stable; the movement occurs in the area of the waist. Similar to rotating disks, the lower disk (the pelvis in this case) is stable while the upper disk rotates, the center being the waist. Mastery of the Mat Work: Criss-Cross (page 58) is a recommended prerequisite for this variation.

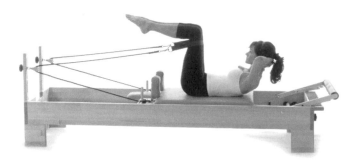

Inhale. Lie supine with the head close to the foot bar (facing the back of the reformer), the pelvis in front of the shoulder rests, and the legs in a tabletop position. Thread the legs through the straps and place the straps just above the knees. Hold the trunk in forward flexion and place the hands behind the head.

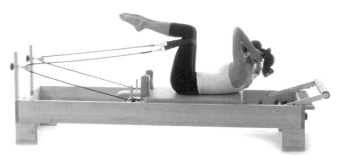

Exhale. Draw the thighs toward the chest as the trunk rotates, bringing one shoulder toward the opposite knee.

Imagery

See Reformer: Abdominals With Legs in Straps, page 131.

☐ Rotate the trunk as opposed to swiveling it (lateral flexion).

☐ Try to keep the lower scapulae off the carriage during the rotation.

☐ Keep the elbows wide and still and the shoulders relaxed.

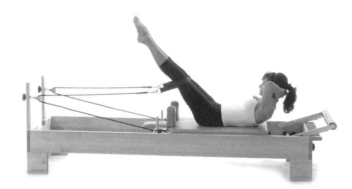

Inhale. Straighten the legs and keep the feet level as you bring the trunk back to center, preparing to rotate to the opposite side.

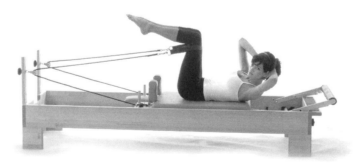

Exhale. Draw the thighs toward the chest as the trunk rotates to the other side. Continue alternating sides, straightening the legs and bringing the upper body to center prior to each rotation. Return to the starting position after 5 to 10 repetitions.

Hip Work

The hip joint deserves special consideration and has earned a block unto itself because of its close proximity to and profound influence on the pelvis, which in turn affects the whole body, up and down the kinetic chain. The hips are fundamentally involved in the gait cycle and many other daily activities, from climbing stairs to sitting down and rising up from a chair. The many muscle groups that act on the hip joint are prone to imbalance. For instance the gluteus medius, so vital in hip support and pelvic alignment, tends to be weak in relation to the other gluteals. The hip flexors often become tight while the hip extensors become relatively weak, due in part to a modern lifestyle in which we spend many hours a day sitting. Imbalances of the musculature are further compounded by certain activities such as dance, particularly classical ballet, in which the hip joint is trained for much of the time in external rotation (turn out).

A concept that is emphasized in the hip work block is *hip disassociation*—in which a smooth, uninterrupted movement of the hip joint is executed while stability of the pelvis is maintained. Mastering the concept of disassociation is important not only in relation to the hip joint, but also to many other parts of the body, such as the shoulder joint.

The hip joint can be viewed as a big spoon in a pot. The action used when stirring a pot is similar to the smooth action desired when mobilizing the hip joint. The balance of the musculature is critical, and a good choice of imagery can assist in achieving the often intricate process of activating and stabilizing different muscle groups.

Frog

The frog resembles the V-Position Toes in the foot work (page 114): Stability and alignment of the trunk and pelvis are maintained, and the basic action of the legs is the same. However, in this exercise the focus changes from the knee extensors and hip extensors to the hip adductors. This challenging series demands a higher degree of stabilization since the feet are in the straps instead of on the stable foot bar. Note that the resistance is light, orienting the work toward stabilization as opposed to strength and requiring that the weaker muscle groups of the hip joint do more of the work. When the resistance is higher the larger, stronger, and more superficial muscles such as the quadriceps tend to take over.

Imagery

The image of a frog jumping works well, although the dynamic of the exercise is relatively slow. Focus on squeezing the legs together as you straighten the knees, as if you were holding a big balloon between the legs. This is important in order to encourage activation of the hip adductors (rather than emphasizing the knee extensors).

☐ Stabilize the pelvic–lumbar region throughout the exercise.

☐ Avoid bringing the knees too close to the chest, which causes the tailbone to lift.

☐ Squeeze the heels together continuously.

Muscle Focus

- Hip adductors

Objectives

- To strengthen the hip adductors
- To develop pelvic–lumbar stabilization

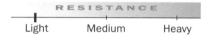

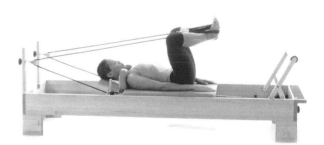

Inhale. Lie supine with the spine in a neutral position. Place the feet in the straps and bend the knees out to the sides, with the hips externally rotated. Softly dorsiflex the feet and press the heels together.

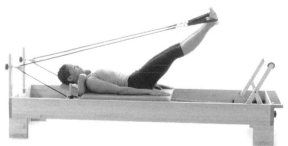

Exhale. Straighten the legs on a diagonal line at an approximately 45-degree angle to the carriage.

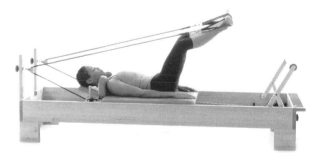

Inhale. Bend the knees and return to the starting position.

Down Circles

Muscle Focus

- Hip adductors
- Hip extensors

Objectives

- To strengthen the hip adductors and hip extensors
- To develop pelvic–lumbar stabilization

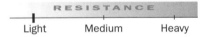

RESISTANCE

Light   Medium   Heavy

The hip circles highlight the skill of hip disassociation. They also activate the hip adductors profoundly, emphasizing control and precision. Softening or even bending the knees slightly can be beneficial, in order to deemphasize the quadriceps and emphasize the hip adductors. Keeping the pelvis stable and in a neutral position encourages correct muscle activation with a good balance between the hip adductors and the hamstrings. The hamstrings tend to overpower the adductors at certain points in the exercise, possibly because most people are more familiar with using them and because they are generally better conditioned.

Imagery

Imagine drawing the desired circular shape (two back-to-back semicircles as opposed to two true circles) in space with the feet. The legs squeeze together as they draw a line down the center and then part as they trace the semicircles, meeting again at the top. The size of the circle may be increased as more control is gained. The movement should be fluid and the lines of the drawing smooth and continuous.

☐ Maximize the hip adductor work.

☐ Engage the hamstrings together with the adductors as the legs are lowered down the center.

☐ Maintain a stable neutral pelvis.

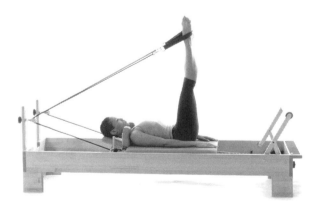

Inhale. Lie supine with the spine in a neutral position. Place the feet in the straps and straighten the legs toward the ceiling, creating as close to a 90-degree angle of the hip as possible without tilting the pelvis. Externally rotate (turn out) the hips and softly point the feet.

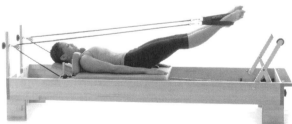

Exhale. Press the legs straight down the center.

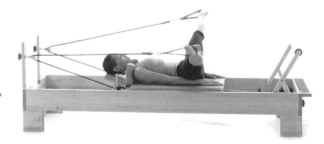

Inhale. Open the legs and circle them around and up to the starting position.

It is often easier to feel the adductors working as the legs circle in this direction. The load on the adductors is clearly felt as the legs come together, pressing against the resistance of the springs during the concentric contraction. In the Reformer: Down Circles (page 136) the adductors work eccentrically during this phase, resisting the pull of the springs as they open. In both versions, the adductors should work isometrically as the legs press against each other when moving up and down the centerline.

Imagery

See Reformer: Down Circles (page 136). An image that I often use here is that of a big spoon stirring thick syrup or porridge, the spoon being the femur and head of the femur. This encourages a smooth, fluid motion devoid of tension, which often binds and restricts the hip. Note that if the movement of the hip joint is restricted, the pelvis will tend to move around in order to compensate for the limitation of motion in the hip.

☐ Maximize the hip adductor work.

☐ Engage the hamstrings with the adductors as the legs are lifted up the center.

☐ Maintain a stable neutral pelvis.

Muscle Focus

▪ Hip adductors
▪ Hip extensors

Objectives

▪ To strengthen the hip adductors and hip extensors
▪ To develop pelvic–lumbar stabilization

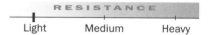

RESISTANCE

Light   Medium   Heavy

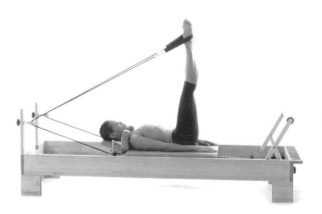

Exhale. Lie supine with the spine in a neutral position. Place the feet in the straps and straighten the legs toward the ceiling, creating as close to a 90-degree angle of the hips as possible without tilting the pelvis. Externally rotate the hips and softly point the feet.

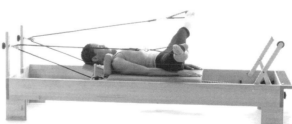

Inhale. Open the legs to the sides.

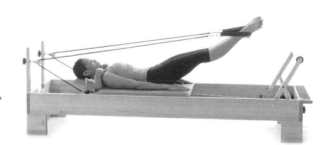

Exhale and circle the legs down and around to connect with each other. Inhale and lift the legs up to the starting position.

Openings

Muscle Focus

- Hip adductors

Objectives

- To strengthen the hip adductors
- To develop hip adductor flexibility
- To develop pelvic–lumbar stabilization

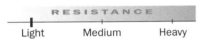

RESISTANCE

Light   Medium   Heavy

This exercise is a particularly valuable part of the feet-in-straps series because it places the body in an optimal position to explore the hip joint's functional range of motion (ROM)—the maximum ROM in which the joint is well supported by the musculature and the pelvis and spine are held in good alignment. This exercise has the potential to develop control and strength in the extreme ranges, which is particularly important for dancers, figure skaters, and gymnasts.

Imagery

Imagine squeezing the legs against a large balloon.

- ☐ Keep the legs well supported so that they do not drop toward the floor.
- ☐ Keep the pelvis in a neutral position.
- ☐ Maximize hip adductor activation.

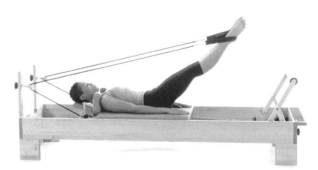

Exhale. Lie supine with the spine in a neutral position. Place the feet in the straps and straighten the legs to an approximately 60-degree angle (halfway between the low and high points of the leg circles exercises). Externally rotate the hips and gently plantarflex the feet, keeping the knees soft.

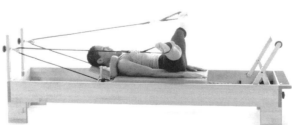

Inhale. Open the legs wide toward the line of the pelvis.

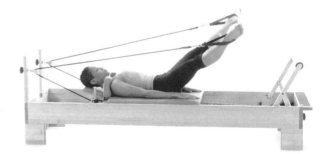

Exhale. Adduct the legs to the starting position.

Extended Frog

The extended frog combines the Reformer: Frog (page 135) with Reformer: Openings (page 138) but requires more control and coordination than either exercise. Keeping tension in the straps as the legs bend into the frog position from the open-leg position is important. (Do this by keeping the hamstrings engaged and the carriage still.) I like to think of the movement as circular rather than linear, originating in the hip joints. The positioning and stability of the pelvis is critical; it provides a foundation for the exercise and accommodates the stretch by serving as a solid anchor.

Imagery

You should feel as if you were stirring an enormous pot with the feet while the legs perform a circular motion.

☐ Keep the carriage still as the legs bend in from the open position.

☐ Keep the pelvis in a stable neutral position throughout the movement.

☐ Maintain hip extensor engagement as the legs bend to prevent their coming too close to the chest.

Muscle Focus

▪ Hip adductors

Objectives

▪ To strengthen the hip adductors
▪ To develop hip adductor flexibility
▪ To develop pelvic–lumbar stabilization

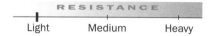

RESISTANCE

Light   Medium   Heavy

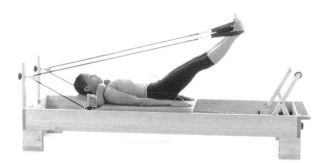

Exhale. Lie supine with the spine in a neutral position. Place the feet in the straps and straighten the legs at an approximately 60-degree angle. Externally rotate the hips and dorsiflex the feet.

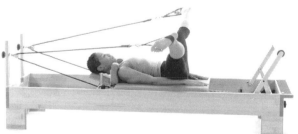

Inhale. Open the legs as in openings (page 138).

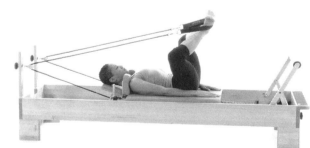

Exhale. Bend the knees, bringing the heels together to the frog position (page 135), maintaining tension in the straps. As the heels connect, straighten the legs to the starting position.

139

Extended Frog Reverse

Muscle Focus

- Hip adductors

Objectives

- To strengthen the hip adductors
- To develop hip adductor flexibility
- To develop pelvic–lumbar stabilization

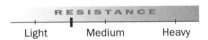

The extended frog reverse, although very similar to its sibling, the extended frog, feels quite different. The stretch in the adductors is more intense as the legs are straightened out to the sides, and the work of the adductors is more challenging as the legs are brought together. Keeping tension in the straps and the carriage is still important as the legs straighten from the frog position to the open position. Maintaining hamstring engagement helps keep tension in the straps. Emphasize the circular action that occurs in the hip joints. The position and stability of the pelvis should not be compromised—if it tilts, the full potential of the adductor stretch will be lost.

Imagery

See Reformer: Extended Frog (page 139).

- ☐ Keep the carriage still as the legs straighten out to the sides.
- ☐ Keep the knees soft as the legs close.
- ☐ Maintain pelvic stability, in a neutral position, throughout the movement.

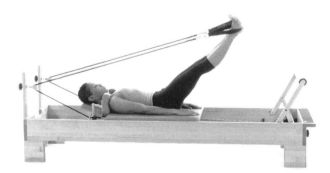

Exhale. Lie supine with the spine in a neutral position. Place the feet in the straps and straighten the legs at approximately a 60-degree angle. Externally rotate the hips and dorsiflex the feet.

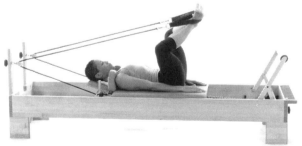

Inhale. Bend the knees, bringing the heels together to a frog position.

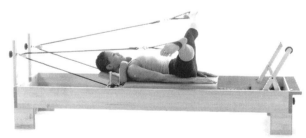

Exhale. Without moving the carriage, straighten the legs out to the sides in an open position, then draw the legs together to the starting position.

Spinal Articulation

The spinal articulation block incorporates the principles and targets the muscle groups that are fundamental to Pilates. The spine is the central pillar of the body, not only in terms of bone structure but also in terms of muscular support and neurological well being. As Joseph Pilates wrote in *Return to Life Through Contrology,* "If your spine is inflexibly stiff at 30, you are old; if it is completely flexible at 60, you are young." Cultivating awareness and control of the intricate intersegmental movements of the spine is a lifelong journey and an ever-exciting process. Joseph Pilates specifically addresses the vertebra-by-vertebra movement of the spine in *Return to Life* and claims that this "rolling" and "unrolling" movement "gradually but surely restores the spine to its normal at-birth position with its corresponding increased flexibility."

In order to achieve the desired flowing movement, you must be acutely aware of the small intervertebral muscles and be able to control them. Breath is also an important component in spinal articulation; not only does it provide a rhythm to the movement, but it also encourages the recruitment of the correct muscles. In addition, spinal articulation enhances the breathing process by "wringing" the lungs out as you would a sponge, which in turn allows them to fill to their full capacity.

It is true that the majority of the spinal articulation exercises move through spinal flexion, and it is typically this range of motion that we think of when we hear the term *spinal articulation.* However, at times you may reap great benefits by visualizing spinal articulation as the spine extends. This is not prudent in all back extension exercises, but when used at the right time it can serve as an invaluable cue. It is also true that whenever you perform spinal articulation, the abdominals play a prominent role, whether it is articulation through flexion, in which the abdominals function as movers, or spinal extension, in which the abdominals function as stabilizers. Whatever the case, good abdominal control is a required ingredient for successful spinal articulation. Furthermore, the TA has a particularly profound role in facilitating efficient spinal articulation. Spinal articulation should be practiced and mastered at all levels of Pilates work.

Being a man who loves the ocean—I swim, surf, and windsurf—any image relating to water inspires me. The image of a rolling wave describes spinal articulation exceptionally well. It conjures up not only the image but also the feeling of the continuous flow of the waves.

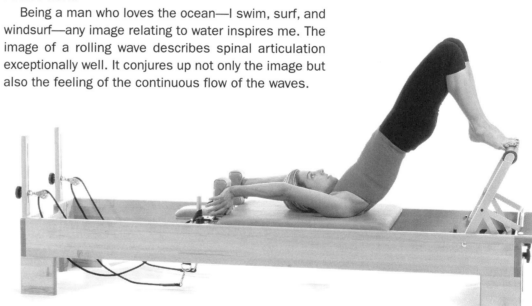

Bottom Lift

Muscle Focus

- Abdominal muscles
- Hamstrings

Objectives

- To develop spinal articulation
- To strengthen the hip extensors

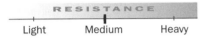

RESISTANCE

Light   Medium   Heavy

The introductory exercise in the spinal articulation block, the bottom lift, is essentially a pelvic curl (typically the first exercise in the mat work). However, the element of instability (because of the mobile carriage) makes it more challenging than the mat work version. In addition, the range of motion is greater because the feet are placed much higher. Pelvic stabilization and spinal articulation should be mastered on the mat before proceeding to the bottom lift. The hamstrings, which are crucial to the lifting and lowering of the body, play an even greater role in this version. The movement of the carriage should be minimal; strive to keep it still and close to the stopper (a task made more difficult as the spring tension is decreased).

Note that the weight is on the balls of the feet, which demands foot stability and exceptional control to maintain good alignment.

Imagery

Use the image of a banana peel being peeled off the fruit, just as the spine is peeled off the reformer.

- ☐ Minimize movement of the carriage.
- ☐ Align the feet, keeping the heels still throughout the exercise.
- ☐ Keep the legs parallel and the adductors engaged.

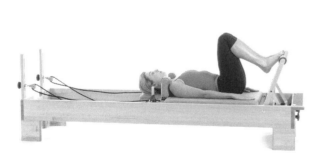

Inhale. Lie supine in a neutral spine position with the headrest down. Place the balls of the feet on the foot bar with the legs parallel and the knees bent.

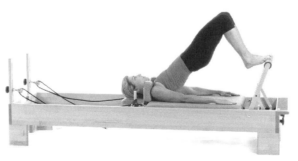

Exhale. Draw in the abdominal muscles and tilt the pelvis in a posterior direction. Continue curling the pelvis and articulating the spine one vertebra at a time, extending the hips and lifting onto the shoulder girdle. Create a straight line from the shoulders through the trunk to the knees avoiding hyperlordosis. Inhale while holding this position.

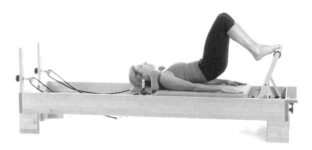

Exhale. Articulate the spine down to the starting position.

Adding extension to the bottom lift accentuates the hip extensor component of the exercise and requires more pelvic–lumbar stabilization. Hip extensor activation, assisted by the knee extensors, facilitates the extension of the legs, creating a suspended bridge position. Although the gluteal muscles may be recruited to help support the position, they are not the prime focus and an effort should be made to engage the hamstrings prior to the gluteals during hip extension as there is a tendency for the gluteals to overpower the other muscles.

Avoid straightening the legs completely as this can place undue strain on the lower back. When returning to the stopper, maintain the strong energy line from shoulders through the trunk to the knees; this helps protect against the natural tendency to drop the pelvis and flex at the hip joint.

Imagery

The extended position resembles a suspension bridge—well supported and stable, with no breaks in the line of the body from feet to shoulders.

☐ Keep the heels still throughout the movement.
☐ Keep the knees soft; do not extend them completely.
☐ Lift the pelvis and extend the hips as you return the carriage toward the stopper.

Muscle Focus

- Abdominal muscles
- Hamstrings

Objectives

- To develop spinal articulation
- To strengthen the hip extensors

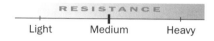

RESISTANCE

Light   Medium   Heavy

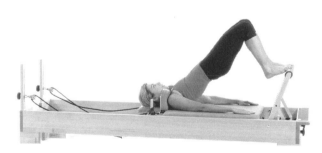

Inhale. Start in the same neutral spine position as the bottom lift (page 142). The exhale. Draw in the abdominal muscles and tilt the pelvis in a posterior direction. Articulate the spine upward, one vertebra at a time, extending the hips and lifting onto the shoulder girdle. Form a straight line from the shoulders to the knees. Inhale and pause.

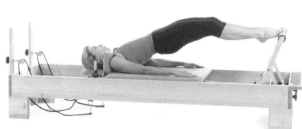

Exhale. Extend the knees (without straightening them completely) and the hips without dropping the pelvis.

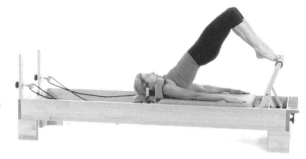

Inhale. Bend the knees, keeping the pelvis high and the legs parallel. Repeat this movement 5 to 10 times. Then exhale and articulate the spine down to the starting position.

Semicircle

Muscle Focus

- Abdominal muscles
- Hamstrings

Objectives

- To develop spinal articulation
- To strengthen the hip extensors
- To increase upper back and shoulder flexibility

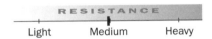

RESISTANCE

Light   Medium   Heavy

The semicircle is a progression of the Reformer: Bottom Lift With Extension (page 143), demanding not only greater control but also the recruitment of several additional muscle groups. The raised position of the pelvis and V position of the legs requires increased hip adductor and extensor control to keep the hip flexors stretched and the legs well aligned. (Often the legs tend to splay out because of tight hip flexors or overuse of the gluteal muscles.) Keeping the pelvis lifted as the carriage returns toward the stopper ensures an effective stretch of the hip flexors.

This exercise benefits the upper body as well as the lower body. It emphasizes shoulder stability and flexibility as well as extension of the thoracic spine. This stretch of the thoracic region is particularly beneficial for people who have tight shoulder and chest muscles and the rounded-shoulder posture that is so prevalent in modern society.

The direction of this sequence can be reversed. From the starting position, extend the knees (not completely). Roll the spine down, placing the pelvis close to the springs, without moving the carriage.

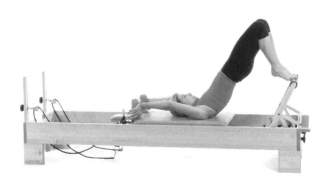

Inhale. Lie on the carriage with the feet in a small V position, toes on the foot bar and heels together. Lift the pelvis and fully extend the hips. Press the hands against the shoulder rests and straighten the arms, lifting onto the shoulder girdle and keeping the pelvis elevated.

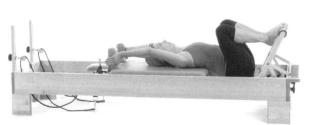

Exhale. Articulate the spine downward, beginning the movement from the top of the thoracic spine and continuing until the pelvis is touching the springs and the spine is hyperextended. Keep the carriage as still as possible during this phase.

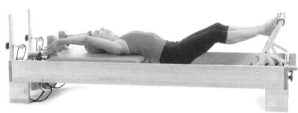

Inhale. Extend the knees (not completely), keeping the pelvis just above the springs and the spine hyperextended.

Then bend the knees, bringing the carriage in, and roll up to the starting position.

Imagery

The movement of the semicircle should feel like a rolling wave. The sensation of flow is wonderful, and it is a beautiful exercise to do and watch.

☐ Minimize the movement of the carriage when articulating the spine up and down.

☐ Squeeze the heels together throughout the exercise, maintaining a small V position of the feet.

☐ Keep the arms straight.

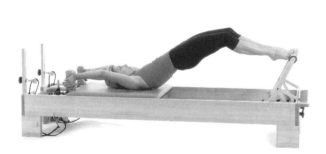

Exhale. Draw in the abdominal muscles, tilt the pelvis in a posterior direction, and articulate the spine upward one vertebra at a time as you lift onto the shoulder girdle to the point of full hip extension. Keep the carriage as still as possible during this phase.

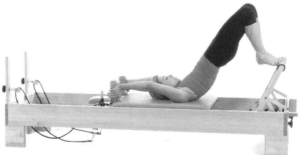

Inhale. Return to the starting position.

Muscle Focus

- Abdominal muscles

Objectives

- To develop spinal articulation
- To increase flexibility in the lower back and hamstrings

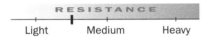

RESISTANCE

Light Medium Heavy

Short Spine

This variation of the short spine is slightly different from the exercise performed by Joseph Pilates. In the classic version, the roll-up was performed as the carriage moved toward the stopper; here, the roll-up onto the shoulders is performed with the carriage still and positioned against the stopper. Not relying on the springs or straps during the roll-up requires greater abdominal control and a flexible spine. In addition, you will achieve a more effective hamstring stretch as you bring the legs over the face, taking the carriage all the way to the stopper. During this phase, keep the pelvis as stable as possible and the sacrum anchored. Most people find it impossible to keep the pelvis in its neutral position; however, the fact that the sacrum is being anchored ensures a significant hamstring stretch.

Keep the feet positioned above the face and the legs in a diamond shape as the spine rolls down through deep flexion onto the carriage after the shoulder stand. This provides a wonderful stretch for the lower back. Focus on maintaining the diamond shape of the legs without further bending of the knee as you return the starting position and place the pelvis in neutral (use the hip extensors).

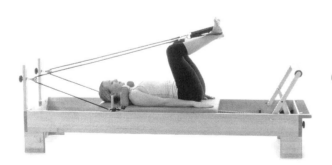

Inhale. Lie supine with the feet in the straps in the frog position (page 135), feet dorsiflexed. Note that the headrest must be down.

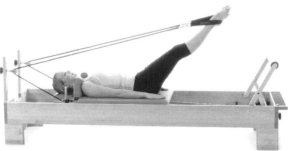

Exhale. Straighten the legs and plantarflex the feet.

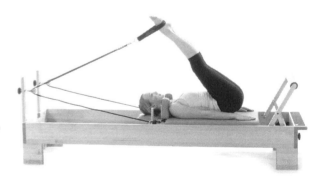

Inhale. Bring the legs overhead, moving the carriage to the stopper.

Note that the extreme flexion created in this position, plus the potential weight placed on the cervical spine, precludes those with back and neck problems (particularly when discs are involved) from performing this exercise.

Imagery

The flow or wavelike motion of this exercise is similar to the Reformer: Semicircle (page 144).

☐ Bring the carriage all the way to the stopper before rolling up.

☐ Keep tension in the straps when up on the shoulders and bending the legs into the diamond shape.

☐ Maintain the diamond shape of the legs during the final phase, emphasizing hip extension rather than bending the knees.

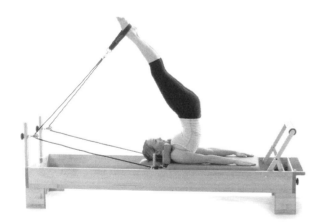

Exhale. Articulate the spine, rolling up onto the shoulders.

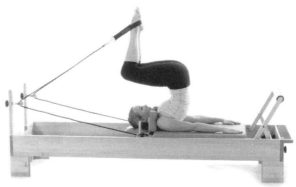

Inhale. Bend the knees, creating a diamond shape with the legs. Exhale. Articulate the spine downward, keeping the feet above the face.

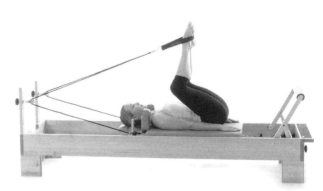

Inhale. Dorsiflex the feet, draw the sacrum toward the carriage, and return to the starting position.

Long Spine

Muscle Focus

- Abdominal muscles
- Hamstrings

Objectives

- To develop spinal articulation
- To develop hip extensor control

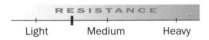

RESISTANCE

Light   Medium   Heavy

This variation of the long spine differs slightly from the classic Pilates exercise in which the carriage is stationary against the stopper during the roll-up onto the shoulders and the straps are lengthened to accommodate this position. In this version, the focus is on balance and stabilization during the roll-up and the roll-down. The carriage is kept still, with the springs in a tensioned state, which demands tremendous control of the ISS and the hip extensors.

Maintaining the straight upright position of the legs, perpendicular to the floor, requires great control on the way up and even more on the way down. In the down phase, the eccentric contraction of the hip extensors allows smooth articulation of the spine without any movement of the carriage. This is a formidable challenge, particularly when the resistance is light.

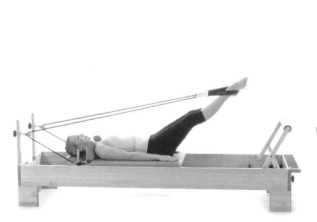

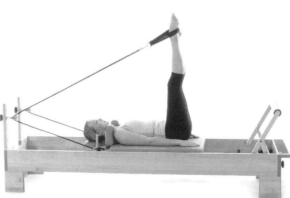

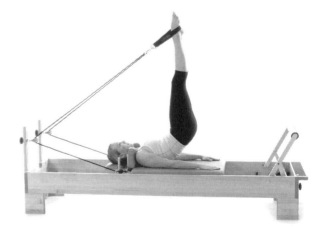

Exhale. Lie supine on the carriage with the feet in the straps and the legs straight and together at approximately a 60-degree angle. The headrest must be down.

Inhale. Lift the legs to a 90-degree angle, keeping the sacrum anchored on the carriage.

Exhale. Roll up onto the shoulder girdle, articulating the spine. Keep the carriage still during this phase.

Imagery

Imagine the legs being pulled up a boat's mast like a sail. Once at the top, the body remains as straight as the mast.

☐ Keep the carriage still while articulating the spine up and down.

☐ Use the hamstrings eccentrically during the roll-down phase.

☐ Place the pelvis down firmly, anchoring the sacrum on the carriage before returning to the starting position

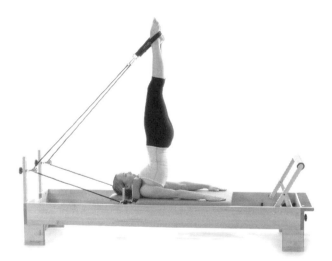

Inhale. Abduct the legs slightly, maintaining the upright position of the body.

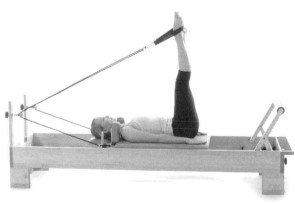

Exhale. Roll down to the carriage, articulating the spine. Keep the carriage still during this phase.

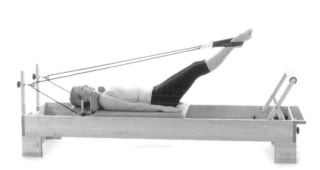

Still exhaling, anchor the sacrum and then circle the legs around to the starting position.

Stretches

Few would argue that flexibility is an important aspect of any fitness and conditioning regimen. This block of stretches should always be included in a well-balanced session. It is up to you to decide what part of the body should be emphasized in terms of flexibility. I suggest, if at all possible, always including a stretch for the hip flexors and hamstrings because these two muscle groups tend to be tight in most people and because they have a profound influence on the pelvis. Clearly, balance in the pelvic area is crucial.

Another area that deserves particular attention in terms of flexibility is the shoulder girdle. The shoulders tend to get tight, which severely affects the upper body and the neck, leading to deterioration in function and at times pain and discomfort. I often add a stretching regimen for this area to a session.

Of course, flexibility of the spine is addressed in the spinal articulation block. Flexibility in general, but particularly that of the spine, deteriorates with age, making this an element of fitness that must be addressed. For optimal function at any level of activity, flexibility and functional range of motion are key.

Because stretches need to be held for an extended period of time to achieve relaxation of both the muscle being stretched and the body in general, using visual imagery depicting the muscle elongating like an elastic band can be extremely advantageous. In addition, focusing on long and deep breaths is invaluable in achieving relaxation and a sensation of a deep stretch in the muscle.

The length of time a stretch should be held is somewhat controversial. I recommend holding a stretch for the duration of three to five breath cycles. Most important is that there should not be pain or tension—only elongation.

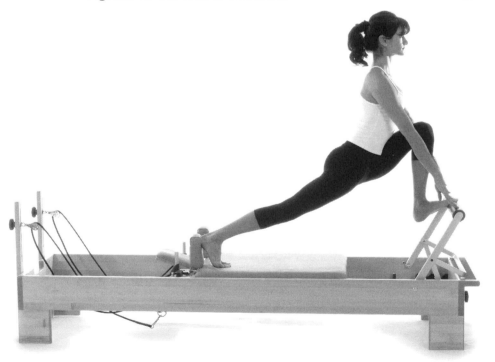

Hamstring Stretch Standing Lunge

This is the first in a series of three hamstring–hip flexor stretches. Flexibility is accomplished through two phases: a hip flexor stretch and a hamstring stretch. Coordinated action of these two muscle groups helps create a balance in pelvic function. During the hip flexor stretch, angle the pelvis slightly posteriorly by contracting the abdominal muscles (in this case, particularly the rectus abdominis) and the hamstrings. This position increases the stretch of the hip flexors and alleviates pressure on the lower back.

Throughout the hamstring stretch, contract the back extensors, drawing the pelvis in an anterior direction and creating a deeper stretch of the hamstrings. This strengthens the muscles of the back, particularly the mid-back, which are so important for healthy posture. Note that the front knee never advances beyond the ankle and that the pelvis should travel along a consistent horizontal line (without dropping or lifting) as the front leg straightens and the hamstrings stretch.

Imagery

The basis of all stretches is a stable anchor point. For the hip flexors and the hamstrings, the anchor point is the pelvis. However, for each muscle group the pelvis is anchored in the opposite direction in order to maximize the stretch: posterior for the hip flexors, creating the feeling of a strong force pulling the pelvis up the front of the body and resulting in an arch shape; anterior for the hamstrings, imagining a straight energy line emanating from the back of the pelvis and running up through the spine and out the top of the head.

☐ Tilt the pelvis posteriorly and extend the upper back during the hip flexor stretch.

☐ Travel along a horizontal line with the pelvis when straightening the front leg.

☐ Tilt the pelvis anteriorly, keeping the back flat and the head aligned with the spine during the hamstring stretch.

Muscle Focus

- Hamstrings
- Hip flexors

Objectives

- To increase hamstring and hip flexor flexibility
- To improve control of the back extensors

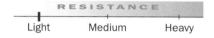

RESISTANCE		
Light	Medium	Heavy

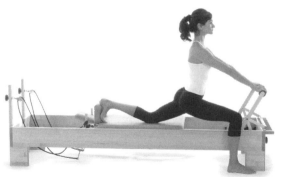

Stand beside the reformer with the hands on the foot bar, shoulder-width apart, and the arms straight. Place the outside foot on the floor in line with the foot bar and the other leg on the carriage with the foot against the shoulder rest. Bend the knee of the standing leg so that it is directly over the ankle, and maintain an upright position of the trunk. Focus on the hip flexor stretch of the kneeling leg and hold the position for three to five breath cycles.

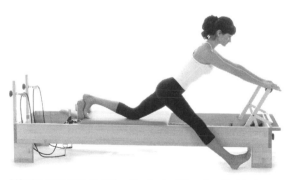

Lift the toes and dorsiflex the foot of the standing leg; straighten the knee, keeping the pelvis on the same horizontal line as it travels back, and hinge the trunk forward. Keep the back extensors engaged, focusing on the hamstring stretch, and hold the position for three to five breath cycles.

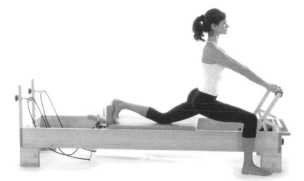

Return to the starting position. Repeat the sequence twice on the same side before changing to the other side and again repeating the sequence twice.

Hamstring Stretch Kneeling Lunge

Muscle Focus

- Hamstrings
- Hip flexors

Objectives:

- To increase hamstring and hip flexor flexibility

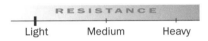

RESISTANCE

Light   Medium   Heavy

The primary principles of the hamstring–hip flexor stretches are consistent throughout the series. During the hip flexor stretch, the focus is on maximizing the stretch to the hip flexors by activating the abdominals and tilting the pelvis posteriorly and on activating the upper back extensors, extending the thoracic spine and creating an arc shape from the lower knee through the thigh, pelvis, trunk, and head. During the hamstring stretch, the focus is on maximizing the stretch to the hamstrings by activating the lower back extensors, tilting the pelvis anteriorly, and on keeping the pelvis and trunk square. Keeping the spine aligned along the centerline (rather than trying to place it over the straightening leg) is important.

Note also that in the initial position the knee is aligned directly above the ankle. As the body transitions into the hamstring stretch, the pelvis travels along a consistent horizontal line and does not drop toward the carriage; at the same time the angle of the kneeling leg to the carriage also remains constant. The kneeling lunge position necessitates even greater pelvic stability and more flexibility than the standing lunge. A misaligned, unstable pelvis compromises the pelvis' effectiveness as an anchor and subsequently compromises the stretch as well.

Imagery

See imagery for the Reformer: Hamstring Stretch Standing Lunge (page 151).

☐ Slightly tilt the pelvis posteriorly and extend the upper back during the hip flexor stretch.

☐ Keep the plane of the pelvis consistent when straightening the front leg.

☐ Keep the back extensors engaged and the head aligned with the spine during the hamstring stretch.

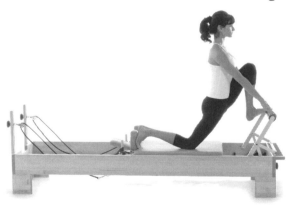

Kneel on the carriage and place one foot on the foot bar with the knee directly over the ankle. Keep the other knee on the carriage with the foot against the shoulder rest. Place the hands on the foot bar, shoulder-width apart, and maintain an upright position of the trunk. Focus on the hip flexor stretch of the kneeling leg and hold the position for three to five breath cycles.

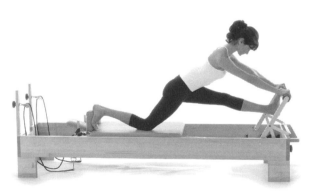

Straighten the leg on the foot bar, moving the pelvis along a consistent horizontal line and hinging forward with the trunk to create a "crease" between the back leg and the pelvis at the hip joint. The angle of the back leg to the carriage should remain consistent. Keeping the back extensors engaged, focus on the hamstring stretch and hold the position for three to five breath cycles.

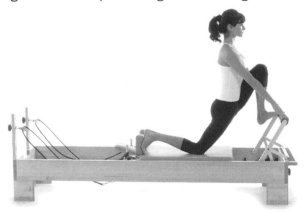

Return to the starting position.

Hamstring Stretch Full Lunge

This third stretch of the series is very challenging. It adds an element of balance; take advantage of it by practicing letting go of the foot bar and balancing in an upright trunk position. This develops control, strong awareness of the core, and functional strength and flexibility of the hamstrings and hip flexors.

Note again that in the hip flexor stretch the knee is aligned above the ankle and the back leg is completely straight. As the body transitions into the hamstring stretch, the pelvis travels along a consistent horizontal line and does not drop or rise (which often occurs when the hamstrings are tight). This variation is particularly difficult to control for hypermobile people, such as dancers and gymnasts, who are very flexible but may lack the strength to support large ranges of motion. Such an imbalance can cause injuries. The full lunge develops strength and flexibility concurrently, resulting in a healthy balance between the two.

During the hamstring stretch, emphasize engaging the back extensors, slightly tilting the pelvis anteriorly, and keeping the pelvis and the trunk square. The spine and head must be aligned on the centerline of the body as opposed to reaching over the straightening leg.

Imagery

See imagery for the Reformer: Hamstring Stretch Standing Lunge (page 151).

☐ Press the heel of the back leg against the shoulder rest.

☐ Keep the knee of the back leg straight throughout the exercise.

☐ Align the front foot with the hip joint on the same side.

Muscle Focus

- Hamstrings
- Hip flexors

Objective

- To increase hamstring and hip flexor flexibility
- To develop hamstring and hip flexor control

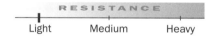

RESISTANCE

Light   Medium   Heavy

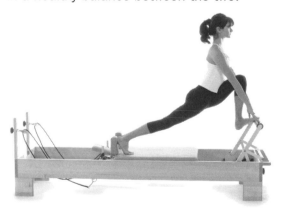

Stand on the carriage with the hands on the foot bar, shoulder-width apart. Place one foot against the shoulder rest and the other on the foot bar with the front knee directly over the ankle. Maintain an upright position of the trunk and keep the back leg straight. Focus on the hip flexor stretch of the back leg and hold the position for three to five breath cycles.

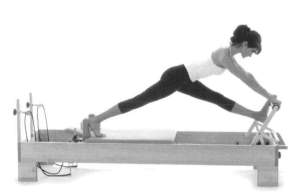

Straighten the front leg, hinging the trunk forward. Keeping the back extensors engaged, focus on the hamstring stretch and hold the position for three to five breath cycles.

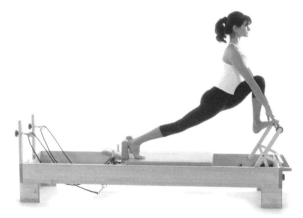

Return to the starting position.

Full Body Integration

This block exemplifies the Pilates philosophy possibly better than any other. It is about the whole, about the body working as an integrated machine—well lubricated and well calibrated. It is true that all Pilates exercises are about full body integration, yet the exercises in this block are those that defy categorization according to a single region of the body. The exercises in this block rely on the integration of the whole body for performance.

Because there are many exercises in this block, they have been further broken down according to level of difficulty and complexity. Full body integration I (FBI I) includes the fundamental to intermediate level exercises. The dynamic of many of the FBI I exercises emphasize the

in (forward) phase of the movement. As you pull the leg forward and draw in the abdominals against resistance (imagined or real), the breath pattern dictates that you exhale. Full body integration II (FBI II) includes the higher intermediate to advanced and master level exercises. All exercises in FBI I should be mastered before proceeding to the higher level exercises of FBI II. Please remember that Pilates is not about learning the higher level work and then never again doing the more fundamental exercises. Sessions should vary continuously and should be a combination of different levels of the work.

The FBI exercises demand a high level of body awareness. The better the understanding of the work, the deeper and more profound the results.

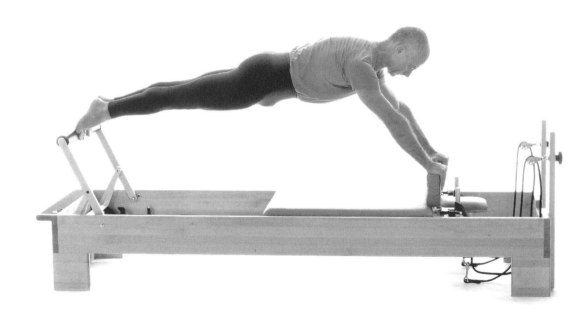

The scooter highlights the concept of disassociation, in which one region of the body remains stable while supporting another part of the body that is moving. In this exercise, the trunk, supporting leg, and pelvis remain stable while the opposite leg moves back and forth. The intention is to extend the moving leg to the point of full hip extension without compromising pelvic stability. Given the positioning of the pelvis, this may mean that the knee does not straighten completely, depending on the flexibility of the hip flexors.

In establishing the position of the trunk, the first step is to draw in the abdominals and round the back. The focus of the flexion is in the lumbar spine, although the entire trunk is in fact in forward flexion. Initiating the flexion from the lumbar region and allowing the pelvis, upper back, and head to respond to this action creates the desired shape.

There is a tendency to recruit the gluteal muscles excessively as a result of the positioning of the pelvis. Excessive gluteal recruitment often inhibits the movement of the hip joint, which must move freely in this exer-

cise. Also, there is a tendency to round the upper back excessively as a result of the natural inclination of the thoracic spine. This should be avoided as it diminishes the focus on the lumbar region and abdominal recruitment, encourages shoulder elevation, and reinforces the undesired round-shoulder position.

Increasing the tension of the springs emphasizes the leg work and strengthens the knee and hip extensors, whereas decreasing the tension highlights trunk stabilization.

Imagery

The position for the scooter resembles a runner preparing for a sprint race, pushing back into the starting block. It exemplifies power about to be unleashed.

☐ Maintain lumbar flexion and the resulting curve of the spine.

☐ Avoid elevating the shoulders.

☐ Focus on hip disassociation and pelvic stability.

Muscle Focus

- Abdominal muscles
- Hip and knee extensors

Objectives

- To develop trunk stabilization
- To strengthen the hip and knee extensors

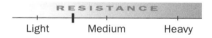

RESISTANCE

Light   Medium   Heavy

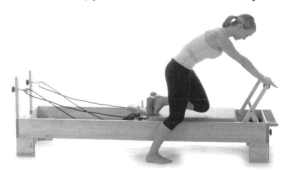

Exhale. Place the hands on the foot bar, shoulder-width apart, with the arms straight. Press one foot against the shoulder rest with the knee slightly above the carriage. Place the other foot on the ground, aligning the heels, and slightly bend the knee. Draw in the abdominal muscles and round the trunk.

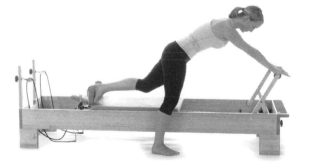

Inhale. Extend the leg that is on the carriage, moving the carriage away from the stopper. Pause before the point at which the pelvis would start to move in an anterior direction.

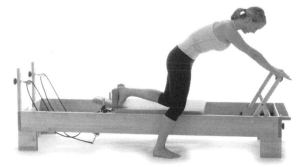

Exhale. Draw the leg back to the starting position, emphasizing the inward motion and maintaining stability of the shoulders, trunk, and pelvis.

Knee Stretch, Round Back

Muscle Focus

- Abdominal muscles

Objectives

- To develop trunk stabilization
- To strengthen the hip extensors and knee extensors

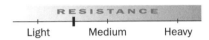

RESISTANCE

Light   Medium   Heavy

This exercise also utilizes the concept of disassociation, with the trunk in exactly the same position as the Reformer: Scooter (page 155), except that now both legs are moving. The body is no longer anchored by having one foot on the floor. This makes for a much less stable position, significantly increasing the difficulty of the exercise. Control of the trunk position, as the legs move backward and forward, is crucial.

Achieving the desired alignment of the spine, as with the scooter, involves rounding (flexing) the lumbar spine and allowing the upper back and pelvis to respond, resulting in a gentle curve of the entire spine (including the head). I advise not tucking the pelvis or contracting the gluteals; doing so restricts the movement in the hip joint, which in turn transfers the pivot point of the movement from the hip to the lumbar spine.

Imagery

Imagine the legs swinging back and forth like a pendulum that is placed on a slight diagonal. As the pendulum swings against gravity the movement is slightly slower, and as it returns with gravity assisting, the movement becomes more dynamic.

- ☐ Maintain lumbar flexion and the resulting curve of the spine.
- ☐ Emphasize the inward phase of the movement.
- ☐ Draw the carriage forward as close to the stopper as possible.

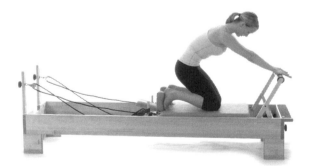

Exhale. Kneel on the carriage and sit on the heels with the feet against the shoulder rests. Place the hands on the foot bar, shoulder-width apart, with the arms straight. Draw in the abdominal muscles, round the trunk, and lift the pelvis slightly off the heels.

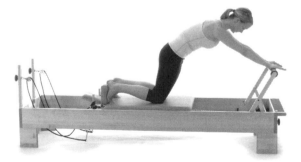

Inhale. Extend the legs, moving the carriage away from the stopper and keeping the arms and trunk stable.

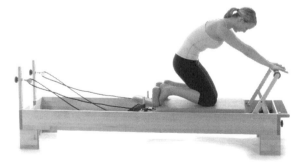

Exhale. Draw the legs forward, bringing the carriage toward the stopper.

In this exercise, *flat back* translates to a neutral spine position as opposed to an actual flat back in which the natural curves of the spine would be eliminated. Co-contraction of the abdominal muscles and the back extensors keeps the spine in a neutral position (as opposed to flexion of the spine seen in the Reformer: Knee Stretch, Round Back (page 156). However, all other aspects illustrated in that exercise remain the same, particularly the emphasis on trunk stability and hip joint disassociation. There is a strong sense of an energy line extending from head to tailbone, which helps maintain stability and alignment of the spine.

Imagery

Imagine a donkey kicking its hind legs back while balancing on its front legs with the upper body stationary, and then drawing the legs back in vigorously.

☐ Maintain a neutral spine position.

☐ Emphasize the hinging action of the legs from the hip joints.

☐ Keep the wrists neutral and firm with thumbs and fingers together and straight.

Muscle Focus

▪ Abdominal muscles
▪ Back extensors

Objectives

▪ To develop trunk stabilization
▪ To strengthen the hip extensors and knee extensors

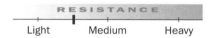

RESISTANCE

Light   Medium   Heavy

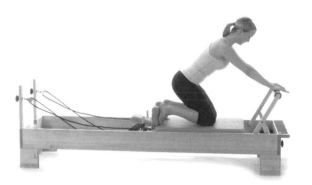

Exhale. Kneel on the carriage, sitting on the heels with the feet against the shoulder rests. Place the hands on the foot bar, shoulder-width apart, with the arms straight. Stabilize the shoulders, maintain a neutral spine, and lift the pelvis slightly off the heels.

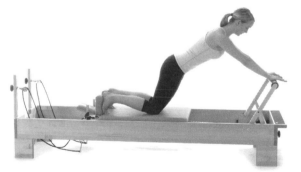

Inhale. Extend the legs, moving the carriage away from the stopper and keeping the arms and trunk stable.

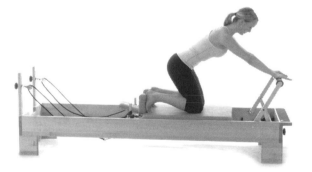

Exhale. Draw the legs forward, bringing the carriage toward the stopper.

Stomach Massage, Round Back

Muscle Focus

- Abdominal muscles
- Back extensors

Objectives

- To develop trunk stabilization
- To strengthen the knee extensors and foot plantarflexors

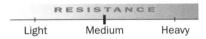

RESISTANCE

Light   Medium   Heavy

This exercise features vigorous, intense work of the legs (including the feet) while the trunk remains stable. The sitting position (as opposed to the supine position in the foot work) intensifies the demand on the abdominal muscles and back extensors, making it very challenging. With the trunk in an upright position, the exercise is more functional than when supine—the muscles are used in a way that more closely simulates common upright movements and enhances postural muscle development. Daily activities such as sitting in a chair, walking, and running are performed frequently without adequate attention to proper muscle activation and support, resulting in misalignment of the trunk and muscle strain. Proper execution of this exercise develops the stabilizers of the trunk and creates awareness of correct spinal alignment.

Imagery

Push the foot bar away from you as if you were pushing away a heavy box or catapulting a heavy load into the air with your legs.

- ☐ Press the hands gently against the front of the carriage.
- ☐ Maintain a moderate C curve of the trunk with the head following the line of the spine.
- ☐ Keep the shoulders above the hips throughout the exercise.

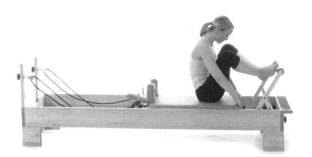

Inhale. Sit on the reformer facing the foot bar; position yourself on the sit bones. Place the feet on the foot bar in a V position on the toes. Press the hands against the front of the carriage and round the trunk, positioning the shoulders directly above the hips.

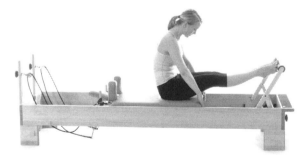

Exhale. Straighten the legs completely. Dorsiflex and then plantarflex the feet.

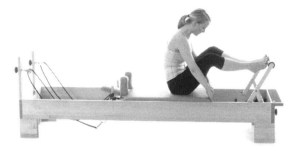

Inhale. Bend the knees, returning to the starting position.

Stomach Massage, Flat Back

This version of the stomach massage shares the movement sequence of the Reformer: Stomach Massage, Round Back (page 158), pressing the feet against the foot bar, straightening the legs, dorsiflexing and plantarflexing the feet, and maintaining a stable trunk throughout the motion. However, the flat back changes the position of the trunk. In this context *flat back* translates to a neutral spine position. The trunk should be fully supported by the musculature rather than the arms. The arm position simply creates a frame for the body, offering support like flying buttresses of a bridge and adding a stretch across the front of the chest (also felt in the anterior aspect of the shoulder). Keep the elbows pointing directly back, parallel to each other and slightly bent.

Imagery

The imagery from the Reformer: Stomach Massage, Round Back (page 158) is useful here. In fact the image is enhanced by the flat back position, which could be likened to leaning against a wall and pushing a large load away or lying supine on the floor and catapulting a big bag up into the air with the legs.

☐ Maximize the co-contraction of the back extensors and abdominal muscles.

☐ Keep the elbows parallel, slightly bent, and reaching backward.

☐ Keep the trunk stable and upright throughout the movement.

Muscle Focus

- Back extensors
- Abdominal muscles

Objectives

- To develop trunk stabilization
- To strengthen the back extensors, knee extensors, and foot plantarflexors

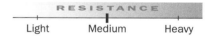

RESISTANCE

Light   Medium   Heavy

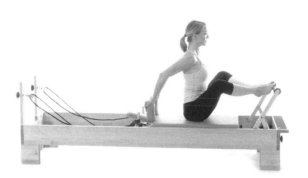

Inhale. Sit on the reformer facing the foot bar; position yourself on the sit bones. Place the feet on the foot bar in a V position on the toes. Place the hands on the shoulder rests with the fingers and elbows facing back and the elbows slightly bent. Keep the trunk upright in as close to a neutral spine position as possible.

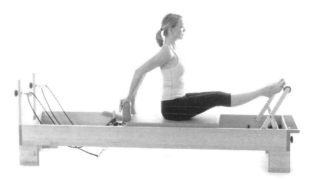

Exhale. Straighten the legs completely. Dorsiflex and then plantarflex the feet.

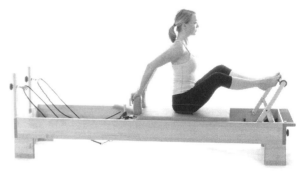

Inhale. Bend the knees, returning to the starting position. To add challenge to the exercise, reach the arms up and forward on a diagonal. By eliminating arm support, this position intensifies the work of the trunk stabilizers.

Reverse Knee Stretch

Muscle Focus

- Abdominal muscles
- Hip flexors

Objectives

- To develop trunk stabilization
- To strengthen the abdominal muscles and hip flexors

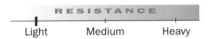

This exercise focuses on three core principles: pelvic–lumbar stabilization, shoulder girdle stabilization, and hip flexor activation. The abdominal support is crucial to prevent excessively loading the lower back and to keep the pelvis and trunk stable. The juxtaposed actions—the legs move forward and back while the upper body and the pelvis remain still—facilitate effective hip disassociation. As with all Pilates exercises, this one can be broken down to the stabilization of one area, utilizing isometric contraction, and the movement of another, using both concentric and eccentric contractions.

In this exercise executing the concentric phase (with the legs coming forward toward the chest) is easier than doing the eccentric phase (in which the legs move backward and the hip flexors elongate). The latter phase demands strong abdominal support to achieve the desired pelvic–lumbar stabilization and to counteract the pull of the legs moving backward. Use caution when executing this exercise because the hip flexors are being loaded with resistance, which can potentially stress the lower back. For this reason I prefer to do this exercise in spinal flexion, which gives a mechanical advantage to the abdominals in protecting the spine.

Imagery

The legs move back and forth like pistons of an engine, with the driving action on the forward motion and the control on the return. The fuel of the engine is the powerhouse, the core strength of the body.

- ☐ Maintain spinal flexion throughout the exercise.
- ☐ Avoid elevating the scapulae.
- ☐ Support the arms on a slight diagonal with the shoulders forward of the hands.

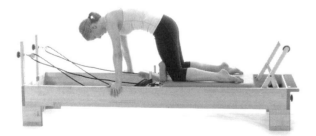

Inhale. Kneel in a quadruped position, placing the knees against the shoulder rests and the hands on the frame of the reformer with the fingers on the outside of the rail. Position the shoulders slightly forward of the hands. Stabilize the shoulder girdle and round the trunk.

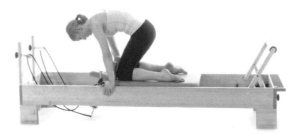

Exhale. Draw the knees toward the chest; keeping the pelvis still and maintaining the C curve of the trunk.

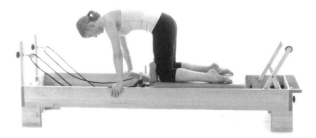

Inhale. Return the legs to the starting position without changing the position of the spine or pelvis.

Down Stretch

Although this exercise appears relatively simple, it demands considerable control and strength. It highlights the concept of trunk stabilization coupled with scapular and pelvic control. The hip is in an extended position, the abdominal muscles (which draw the pubic symphysis up) working together with the hamstrings (which draw the sit bones down) to keep the pelvis stable in a slight posterior tilt. The posterior tilt of the pelvis, together with strong abdominal work, protects the lumbar spine from excessive pressure, prevents hyperlordosis, and magnifies the stretch of the hip flexors.

The shoulder joint acts as a pivot point for the movement. The shoulder extensors lift the body from the downward phase (with the assistance of the springs) to the stopper. Emphasize extension of the thoracic spine, particularly in the upward phase. Note that the lighter the resistance, the more challenging the exercise becomes.

Imagery

An image I have used in this exercise for many years is the figurehead of an old wooden ship. Imagine it rolling up and down as the ship sails over huge swells in the ocean. Also, I like to visualize a fishing line connected to the sternum that helps lift the body, particularly the chest, on the return movement toward the stopper.

☐ Maintain a slight arc shape with the body.

☐ Keep the back, hip, and shoulder extensors working throughout the exercise.

☐ Press the feet against the shoulder rests, keeping the legs parallel.

Muscle Focus

▪ Abdominal muscles
▪ Upper back extensors

Objectives

▪ To develop trunk stabilization
▪ To develop shoulder extensor and upper back extensor control

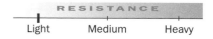

RESISTANCE

Light   Medium   Heavy

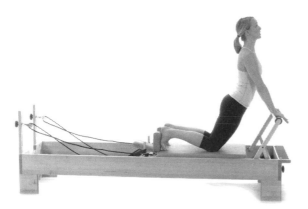

Inhale. Kneel on the carriage facing the foot bar; place the hands on the foot bar, shoulder-width apart, with arms straight. Place the feet against the shoulder rests with the legs parallel. Establish a line that runs from the knees through the thighs, hips, trunk, and shoulders and out the top of the head.

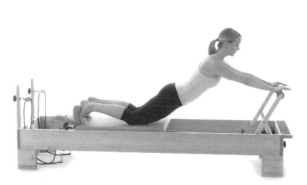

Exhale. Push the carriage back, pivoting from the shoulders and maintaining the arc shape of the body.

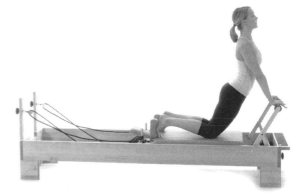

Inhale. Extend the shoulders, pressing down onto the foot bar. Bring the body up to return to the starting position, and hold the carriage against the stopper momentarily before repeating.

Elephant

Muscle Focus

- Abdominal muscles
- Back extensors

Objectives

- To develop trunk stabilization
- To improve hamstring and shoulder flexibility
- To develop core strength

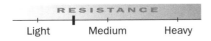

RESISTANCE

Light   Medium   Heavy

The elephant and the Reformer: Up Stretch (page 163) are almost identical except that the elephant is performed with the feet flat. This adjustment increases the stretch down the back of the legs, which can be further enhanced by lifting the toes. Although this exercise is sometimes performed with a round back, my preference is to keep the spine extended, establishing one long line from the hip joints through the trunk, shoulders, arms, and hands. This ensures strong work of the back extensors (in co-contraction with the abdominal muscles), particularly those of the mid- and upper back. It also accommodates a deep stretch of the shoulders and, by activating the back extensors, pulls the pelvis in an anterior direction, accentuating the hamstring stretch.

The legs should move back and forth fluidly, emphasizing the inward phase. The range of motion of the hip joint and the distance the carriage travels should be relatively small. Two energy lines are present throughout: one runs from the hips through the trunk, shoulders, and arms and the other runs from the hips down the legs and through the heels. They form a pyramid, with the tailbone, reaching up toward the ceiling, as the top point.

Imagery

The legs move like a pendulum swinging from the hip joints. The movement should be disassociated from the pelvis and the trunk. The image of using the abdominal muscles to pull in the legs deepens the abdominal work. Be aware, however, that physiologically the abdominals do not pull the legs in; they help stabilize the trunk.

- ☐ Maintain stability of the arms, shoulders, and trunk.
- ☐ Align the head with the spine and maintain the pyramid shape throughout the exercise.
- ☐ Keep the weight on the heels to maximize the stretch down the back of the legs.

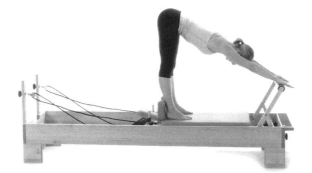

Exhale. Stand on the carriage with the body in a pyramid shape, pelvis high in the air and hands on the foot bar, shoulder-width apart. Place the heels against the shoulder rests with the feet flat on the carriage, and lift the toes slightly.

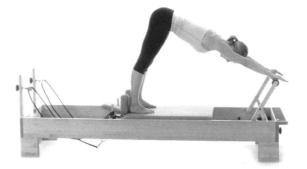

Inhale. Move the carriage back, hinging at the hip joint.

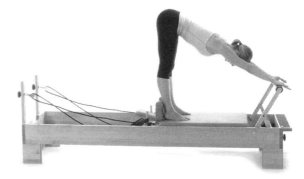

Exhale. Draw the abdominal muscles in and hinge at the hip joint, bringing the carriage forward toward the stopper, returning to the starting position.

Up Stretch

This exercise and its many variations, all based on the pyramid position, are about creating straight lines and pivoting from specific joints. The line of the body extends from the hips through the trunk, shoulders, arms, and hands. With this line serving as a solid foundation, the legs merely move in and out like a pendulum, creating a second straight line. Trunk stabilization and core strength are the essence of this exercise, with a coordinated contraction of the abdominal muscles (which prevent hyperlordosis as the carriage moves out) and the back extensors (which prevent spinal flexion as the carriage returns toward the stopper). The shoulders should remain firm and stable, establishing a strong connection to the trunk.

As with most of the FBI exercises, using less resistance increases the level of difficulty, particularly challenging the body's core strength and stabilization.

Imagery

As with the Reformer: Elephant (page 162), there is a sense of pulling the legs in with the abdominal muscles. I like to visualize a pyramid (which is what I often call this exercise), with the tailbone as its tip and the feet and hands as its base. As the legs go back and forth the size of the base changes, but the pyramid shape remains constant with the tailbone reaching skyward.

☐ Maintain the stability of the arms, shoulders, and trunk.

☐ Align the head with the spine.

☐ Press the heels into the shoulder rests.

Muscle Focus

▪ Abdominal muscles
▪ Back extensors

Objectives

▪ To develop trunk and shoulder stabilization
▪ To improve hamstring and shoulder flexibility
▪ To develop core strength

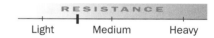

RESISTANCE

Light   Medium   Heavy

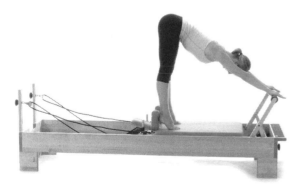

Exhale. Stand on the carriage and place the hands on the foot bar, shoulder-width apart. The pelvis is high in the air and the feet are in front of the shoulder rests, with the heels pressing into them halfway up.

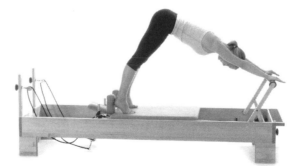

Inhale. Move the carriage back, stabilizing the trunk and shoulders and hinging at the hip joint.

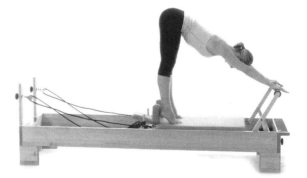

Exhale. Draw the abdominal muscles in, hinging at the hip joint, bringing the carriage forward towards the stopper, and returning to the starting position.

Long Stretch

Muscle Focus

- Abdominal muscles
- Scapular stabilizers

Objectives

- To develop trunk and scapular stabilization
- To develop core strength
- To strengthen the shoulder flexors

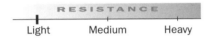

RESISTANCE

Light   Medium   Heavy

The long stretch begins in the Reformer: Up Stretch (page 163) position. Lower the pelvis from this high point to a Mat Work: Front Support position (page 83), commonly regarded as a push-up position, keeping the arms stable and pivoting from the shoulder and hip joints. Without altering the position of the body and with only the arms generating the movement, glide the body forward over the foot bar, moving the carriage all the way to the stopper and then back to the starting position.

Fitness enthusiasts who have grown up doing hundreds of push-ups will soon recognize that this exercise takes the common push-up to a whole new level of difficulty. The precision, control, and core strength achieved in the long stretch can then be incorporated into all forms of the push-up, heightening both its integrity and intensity.

Imagery

Imagine the feeling of being catapulted out of a cannon. This powerful image initially feels unstable and perhaps frightening. But once you establish a strong, stable platform with the body, your confidence—and your enjoyment of performing this challenging movement—will grow.

- ☐ Maintain scapular depression and abduction.
- ☐ Align the head with the spine.
- ☐ Assume a slight posterior tilt of the pelvis to ensure abdominal engagement and to protect the lower back.

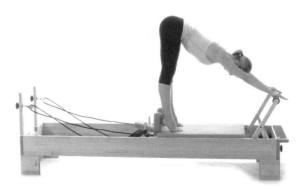

Exhale. Start in the pyramid position (see up stretch, page 163): pelvis high in the air, hands on the foot bar and shoulder-width apart, and feet in front of the shoulder rests with the heels pressing against them midway up.

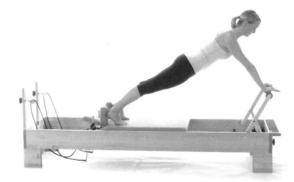

Still exhaling, lower the body to a push-up position without altering the angle of the arms or shifting the shoulders. Inhale. Glide the body forward over the foot bar until the carriage reaches the stopper.

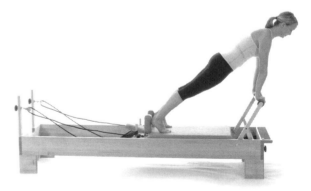

Exhale. Push the carriage back to the starting position.

This exercise resembles the Reformer: Long Stretch (page 164). However, it places the body in a more unstable and somewhat precarious position, which raises the level of difficulty considerably. Co-contraction of the abdominal muscles and the back extensors creates the necessary stabilization and support for the movement and exemplifies the meaning of core strength. In addition, proper form in this exercise demands shoulder stabilization and immaculate mechanics of the shoulder girdle.

I recommend orienting the pelvis toward a posterior tilt, which provides a mechanical advantage to the abdominal muscles and prevents the pelvis from sinking. Dropping the pelvis places pressure on the lower back, compromises the stability of the entire structure, and may result in injury. Likewise, depression and abduction of the scapulae reinforces the stability of the upper body, and allowing this area to collapse may result in strain or other injuries. To increase the challenge and create a beautiful line, I have added plantarflexion of the feet to the positioning of this exercise, which is classically performed with the feet either in a neutral position or dorsiflexed.

Imagery

Visualize the body suspended like a drawbridge. The movement of the arms, like the mobile section of the bridge, occurs independently of the rest of the body. There should be a sensation of floating—the more relaxed you can feel, the better. In addition, visualize one strong energy line running through the body from the tips of the toes to the top of the head, and a second line running from the shoulders through the arms, hands, and fingers.

☐ Stabilize the trunk.
☐ Minimize movement of the scapulae.
☐ Keep the feet plantarflexed.

Muscle Focus

▪ Abdominal muscles
▪ Scapular abductors

Objectives

▪ To develop trunk and scapular stabilization
▪ To develop core strength
▪ To strengthen the shoulder flexors

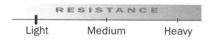

RESISTANCE

Light   Medium   Heavy

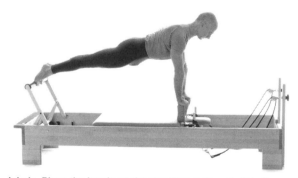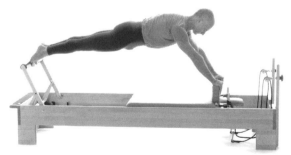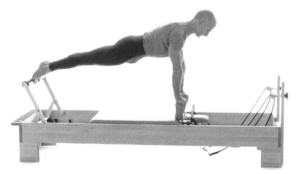

Inhale. Place the hands on the shoulder rests and align the shoulders directly above them. Stabilize the upper body and place one foot on the foot bar in a plantarflexed position. Straighten the leg and lower the body into a plank position, then position the other foot on the foot bar with minimal shifting of weight. Ensure that the body is in one straight line.

Exhale. Flex the shoulders, pushing the carriage toward the back of the reformer and hinging at the shoulder joints while maintaining the stable, planklike position of the body.

Inhale. Control the carriage as it moves back to the starting position.

Balance Control Back Prep

Muscle Focus

- Back extensors
- Shoulder extensors
- Elbow extensors

Objectives

- To develop trunk and scapular stabilization
- To strengthen the shoulder and elbow extensors
- To develop hip extensor control

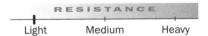

RESISTANCE

Light — Medium — Heavy

This exercise divides the body into two separate units in terms of function: the upper section, the trunk; and the lower section, the legs. The hinging action occurs at the hip and shoulder joints. The movement is relatively small and the focus is primarily on maintaining an L shape of the trunk and legs. The L shape opens slightly as the shoulders extend and the carriage is moved back, but it soon returns to position as the carriage moves forward toward the stopper.

The back extensors and scapular depressors, fortified by the abdominals, stabilize the trunk. The movement is initiated by the shoulder extensors. The hip extensors also play an important role in stabilizing the lower body; they should remain engaged throughout the exercise. A common tendency, particularly when the pectorals are tight, is to round the trunk, which eliminates the L shape and the upright trunk. Avoid rounding even if it means minimizing the degree of movement. To take this exercise one step further to a Reformer: Balance Control Back, lift the pelvis up so that the body forms a straight line as in Mat Work: Back Support (page 88).

Imagery

The letter L provides a good image to help achieve the initial position. Visualize two spring-loaded hinges: one in the shoulder joint and one in the hip joint. These joints open slightly and then spring back to position.

- ☐ Maintain a neutral spine position.
- ☐ Keep the back extensors activated.
- ☐ Emphasize scapular depression.

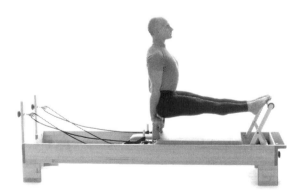

Inhale. Face the foot bar and place the hands on the shoulder rests. Set the feet on the foot bar with the legs parallel. Establish an L position with the legs and the trunk.

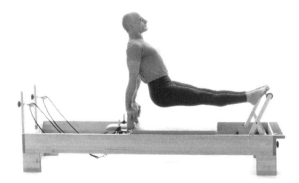

Exhale. Extend the shoulders as you push the carriage back, keeping the back straight.

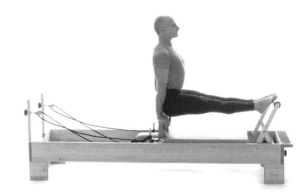

Inhale. Control the carriage as it returns to the starting position.

Arm Work

There are myriad choices of upper body exercises in Pilates. Probably this is because Joe Pilates was a man, and men often focus their physical training on the upper body. I have arranged the many arm work exercises into series or groupings to simplify the choices and enhance the organization of the session. Rather than choosing from individual exercises, you can choose whole series, which are formulated in such a way that each one offers a well-balanced upper body workout that challenges the body in different ways and offers variety in both execution and effect.

A crucial element in arm work is clearly the shoulder. The shoulder is a wonderfully mobile joint, but at the same time it is very unstable. It relies mostly on the musculature for support and thus is often called a *muscle-dependent joint*. Immaculate shoulder mechanics are required to reap the benefits of the arm work. As the movements become more difficult and you enter into the advanced or master level repertoire, this fact becomes even more pertinent, as the vast majority of the higher level work relies heavily on shoulder support.

Correct shoulder mechanics involve a coordinated, linked movement of the humerus and scapula termed the *scapulohumeral rhythm*. Many of the movements of the arm require intricate coordination of the muscles of the scapulae to prevent undesired movements and provide a stable base on which the arms can work. Furthermore, coordinated use of the rotator cuff when elevating the arms is essential to prevent undesired upward motion of the head of the humerus into the overlying structures (impingement). Without correct mechanics, it is likely that at some point problems will occur in the shoulder, the neck, or even the back.

I like to advance the notion of one area stabilizing the body while another area moves freely (disassociation). In the case of the shoulder, the scapulae provide support as the arms (glenohumeral joint) move uninterrupted. The scapulae should move in relation to the movement of the arm, but the amount and direction of the movement must be proportional. The degree and direction of movement, or the lack thereof, is determined by the synergists. The image (used in the hip work) of a spoon stirring a pot of syrup can also be used with the shoulder. The movement of the arm should be smooth and uninterrupted, as the scapulae make small intricate adjustments to accommodate the movement of the arm.

Supine Arm Extension

Muscle Focus

- Latissimus dorsi

Objectives

- To strengthen the shoulder extensors
- To develop trunk and scapular stabilization

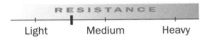

RESISTANCE

Light   Medium   Heavy

The supine arms series is performed in a supine position with the spine in neutral, requiring extensive use of the core stabilizers. Emphasize developing a rhythmic coordination of the shoulder stabilizers, specifically the lower trapezius (which helps maintain scapular depression) and the serratus anterior (which helps maintain scapular abduction) with the muscles that move the shoulder. The scapulohumeral rhythm helps prevent excessive elevation and adduction of the scapulae during the arm movements.

This series is particularly valuable because it places the body in a safe, comfortable, nonweight-bearing position, developing arm and shoulder strength together with trunk stabilization. All of the work occurs in a range of motion below shoulder height, which is valuable for people who have painful conditions such as impingement syndrome, in which lifting the arm higher than the shoulder is often contraindicated.

Imagery

Imagine that you are swimming on your back and your arms are like large fins, pushing the water and propelling the body with each movement of the arms. Keep the movement smooth and integrated with the stabilizers of the body. I always say, *the better the stabilization, the better the mobilization*. In this case the focus of the movement is in the glenohumeral joint and the stabilization is in the trunk and scapulae.

- ☐ Maintain pelvic–lumbar and scapular stabilization.
- ☐ Use a smooth and even dynamic during both the concentric and eccentric phases.
- ☐ Keep the arms straight without placing excessive force on the elbow.

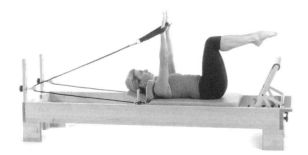

Inhale. Lie supine on the reformer with a neutral spine, knees and hips in a tabletop position. Hold the arms perpendicular to the carriage, with the shoulders stable and the hands in the straps. Maintain slight tension in the straps, with the palms facing the knees.

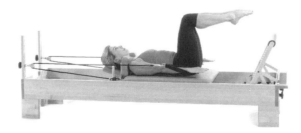

Exhale. Extend the arms straight down toward the carriage, pausing when they reach the sides of the body, in line with the shoulders and parallel to the carriage.

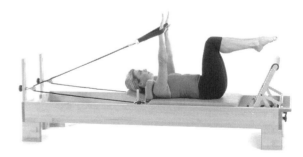

Inhale. Return to the starting position.

Supine Arm Adduction

This exercise is similar to the Reformer: Supine Arm Extension (page 168), except that the arms adduct to the sides of the trunk. Emphasize the same points as in the shoulder extension exercise, including the neutral spine, trunk stabilization, and scapular depression and abduction. In this exercise the scapulae naturally tend to adduct, or squeeze together. Lying supine enables you to feel the scapulae against the carriage and keep them spread out.

Imagery

Use an image similar to that for the supine arm extension. The feeling with each arm movement toward the body should be one of propelling the body through water or soft gel.

☐ Maintain pelvic–lumbar stabilization.

☐ Avoid elevating and adducting the scapulae.

☐ Face the palms toward the hips.

☐ Keep the arms straight without excessive force on the elbows.

Muscle Focus

▪ Latissimus dorsi

Objectives

▪ To strengthen the shoulder adductors
▪ To develop trunk and scapular stabilization

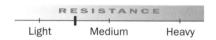

RESISTANCE

Light   Medium   Heavy

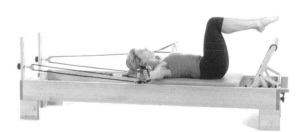 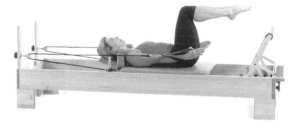 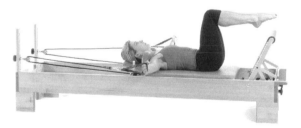

Inhale. Lie supine on the reformer with a neutral spine and the knees and hips in a tabletop position. Hold the arms out to the sides in a T position, with the shoulders stable and the hands in the straps. Maintain slight tension in the straps, with the palms facing the sides of the body.

Exhale. Adduct the arms and gently press them against the sides of the body.

Inhale. Return to the starting position.

Supine Arm Circles

Muscle Focus

- Latissimus dorsi

Objectives

- To strengthen the shoulder extensors and adductors
- To develop trunk and scapular stabilization
- To improve shoulder mobility

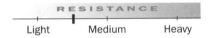

RESISTANCE

Light   Medium   Heavy

The circles are a combination of the Reformer: Supine Arm Extension and Reformer: Supine Arm Adduction exercises (pages 168 and 169). The name can be misleading. Rather than tracing a true circle, the arms move in an elliptical pattern created by joining the lines of movement of the prior two exercises. By drawing the pattern as large as possible you will achieve maximum range of motion of the glenohumeral joint.

This movement can also be performed in reverse (called *circles reverse*). Observe the same principles of maximizing the range of motion.

Imagery

The arm movement in the circles should be fluid and as large as possible, reaching each point of the pattern and rotating accordingly. The feeling should be like moving through gel, providing a sense of resistance throughout. There should be no difference in sensation or presentation between the concentric phases and eccentric phases.

☐ Do not raise the arms above shoulder height.

☐ Maintain flowing movement.

☐ Define exact points that describe the shape of the pattern.

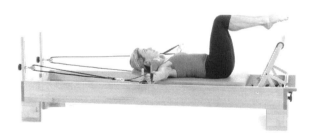

Inhale. Lie supine on the reformer with a neutral spine and the knees and hips in a tabletop position. Hold the arms out to the sides in a T position, keeping the shoulders stable and placing the hands in the straps. Maintain slight tension in the straps, with the palms facing the sides of the body.

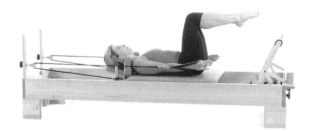

Exhale. Adduct the arms and gently press them against the sides of the body. Internally rotate the arms so that the palms face the carriage.

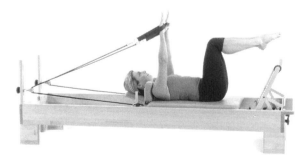

Inhale. Lift the arms up to a position perpendicular to the carriage. Return the arms to the starting T position.

Supine Triceps

The motion in this exercise focuses solely on the forearm, isolating the movement of the elbow. The wrist must remain straight and firm, creating a line from the elbow through the fingers. The arms should press into the sides of the body throughout to assist in keeping the shoulders stable and maintaining good alignment. The movement commences with the elbow at a 90-degree angle and the fingers pointing straight up toward the ceiling. It ends with the elbow at 180 degrees, with the arms and fingers forming a straight line with the shoulders. The arms stay parallel to the floor and in line with the shoulders rather than pushing down onto the carriage. (Pushing down onto the carriage with the elbows, a common mistake, often results in adduction of the scapulae and thrusting the ribs forward.)

Imagery

Imagine pushing through water and propelling yourself forward with only your forearms, like an upside down dog paddle.

☐ Hold the arms parallel to the carriage, in line with the shoulder, in the final position.

☐ Press the elbows against the sides of the body and keep the upper arms still throughout the exercise.

☐ Keep the wrists stable in a neutral position.

Muscle Focus

▪ Triceps

Objectives

▪ To strengthen the elbow extensors
▪ To develop trunk and scapular stabilization

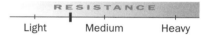

RESISTANCE

Light   Medium   Heavy

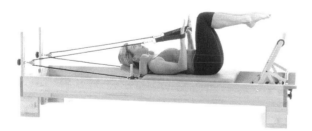

Inhale. Lie supine on the reformer with a neutral spine and the knees and hips in a tabletop position. Place the arms by the sides of the body with the elbows at a 90-degree angle. Maintain slight tension in the straps, with the palms facing the foot bar.

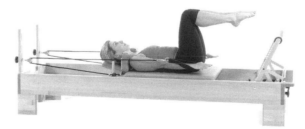

Exhale. Extend the elbows, pressing the hands down toward the carriage. Pause when the arms are in a straight line parallel to the carriage.

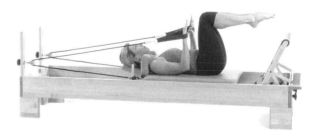

Inhale. Return to the starting position.

Muscle Focus

- Latissimus dorsi

Objectives

- To strengthen the shoulder extensors
- To develop trunk stabilization

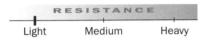

RESISTANCE

Light   Medium   Heavy

Seated Chest Expansion

The foundation of this series is keeping the trunk upright and as close to neutral alignment as possible. Avoid the common tendency to round the upper body or to thrust the ribs forward and hyperextend the lumbar spine. As the arms move toward the foot bar, the shoulders extend beyond the centerline of the body by a small amount. (How far is dictated by strength, flexibility, and the ability to maintain correct trunk alignment. Once alignment is compromised, the exercise has exceeded its functional range of motion.) Extending the shoulders beyond this range of motion causes compensations, including shoulder elevation and incorrect muscle recruitment.

Imagery

Many people visualize a horizontal back-and-forth motion of the arms in this exercise. I prefer to imagine the fingertips reaching down to the floor while the head simultaneously reaches up toward the ceiling.

☐ Keep the trunk upright and stable.
☐ Focus on the fingertips reaching toward the floor.
☐ Avoid thrusting the ribs forward.

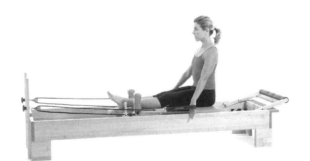

Inhale. Sit upright at the edge of the carriage (closest to the foot bar) facing the back of the reformer, with the legs straight and between the shoulder rests. Hold the straps with the palms facing back and fingertips reaching toward the floor. Keep the arms close to the sides of the body, approximately 20 to 30 degrees forward of the plumb line.

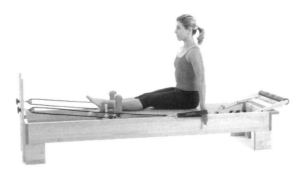

Exhale. Extend the shoulders as far back as possible without compromising the upright alignment of the trunk (10 to 20 degrees past the plumb line).

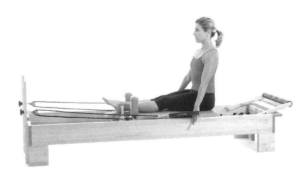

Inhale. Return to the starting position.

Seated Biceps

As with the Reformer: Seated Chest Expansion (page 172), maintain a strong, balanced neutral spine position with correct upright alignment. Avoid leaning back, which is a common mistake in this exercise. You should feel all the trunk stabilizers working.

The upper arms play a crucial role in the proper execution of this exercise. Reach directly forward and keep them absolutely stable and parallel to the floor, not dropping down or lifting up. Any deviation involves improper muscle recruitment and possible undesired elevation of the shoulders. This in turn compromises the isolated motion of the elbows and contraction of the biceps.

Imagery

The trunk and upper arm should create a stable platform for the lower arm to move on. The sensation should be like resting the upper arms on a table; the movement of the lower arms is completely disassociated from the upper arms. This image counters the tendency to lift the arms, resulting in shoulder flexion as opposed to isolated flexion of the elbows.

☐ Keep the upper arms parallel to the carriage and to each other throughout the exercise.

☐ Straighten the elbows completely after each repetition.

☐ Maintain the upright alignment of the trunk.

Muscle Focus

▪ Biceps

Objectives

▪ To strengthen the elbow flexors
▪ To develop trunk stabilization

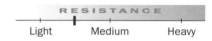

RESISTANCE

Light   Medium   Heavy

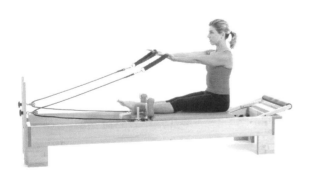

Inhale. Sit upright at the edge of the carriage (closest to the foot bar) facing the back of the reformer, with the legs straight and between the shoulder rests. Straighten the arms forward at shoulder height parallel to the carriage, and hold the straps with the palms facing up.

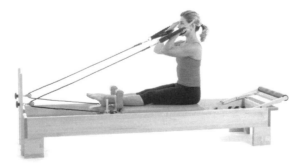

Exhale. Bend the elbows to 90 degrees or beyond (as long as correct alignment can be maintained), keeping the upper arms at a consistent level.

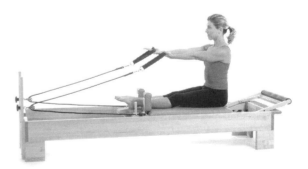

Inhale. Return to the starting position.

Muscle Focus

- Posterior deltoid
- Rhomboids

Objectives

- To strengthen the shoulder horizontal abductors
- To develop trunk stabilization

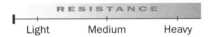

Seated Rhomboids

Although the name of this exercise singles out the rhomboids, the emphasis is initially on scapular stabilization and horizontal abduction of the shoulders. As in the Reformer: Seated Biceps (page 173), focus on keeping the upper arm at a right angle to the body and parallel to the carriage. Horizontally abduct the arms only to the point where the scapulae are about to retract. Be aware, however, of the rhomboids (located between the scapulae) and focus the energy there.

At a later stage, when good form and control have been achieved, you can add scapular adduction. The adduction occurs once you have reached the end point of glenohumeral horizontal abduction. This should be viewed as an isolated motion of the scapulae and not part of the movement of the humerus. After the scapular adduction, the scapulae then abduct before the arms return to the starting position.

Imagery

The palms are like two spotlights shining beams of light toward the face. The more stable the arm position is, and the more isolated the movement in the glenohumeral joint is, the better.

- ☐ Externally rotate the shoulders slightly to avoid internal rotation.
- ☐ Keep the humerus parallel to the floor at all times.
- ☐ Avoid elevating the shoulders.

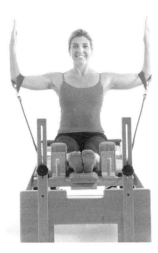

Remember to keep the palms facing in toward the head at all times.

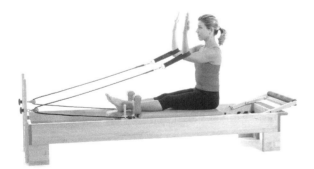

Inhale. Sit upright at the edge of the carriage, facing the back of the reformer with the legs straight and between the shoulder rests. Thread the arms through the straps and place them on the forearms, bending the elbows to a 90-degree angle. Make sure the upper arms are at shoulder height, parallel to the carriage and to each other, with the palms facing the body.

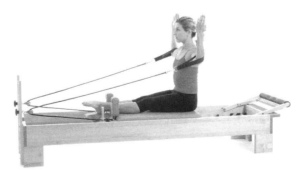

Exhale. Keeping the elbows on the same horizontal line and holding the 90-degree angle, horizontally abduct the arms.

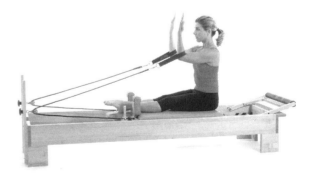

Inhale. Return to the starting position.

Seated Hug-a-Tree

The image of hugging a tree often results in rounding the arms and shoulders, which is contrary to the goals of this exercise. As the arms are horizontally adducted, I advise focusing on the mid- and upper back extensors, which prevents flexion and collapse of the upper thoracic spine. Elongating the arms out to the sides rather than rounding them encourages correct muscle recruitment, keeps the resistance engaged throughout the range of motion, and creates a long lever arm, which makes the exercise more challenging. I cannot emphasize enough the importance of a strong upright position and a stable trunk.

Imagery

Imagine sitting inside a barrel with the arms reaching out to touch its sides. The tree image works well for the trunk of the body, which should feel like the strong, sturdy trunk of a tree.

☐ Keep the back and shoulders broad and the scapulae open (abducted).

☐ Keep the hands within your peripheral vision.

☐ Externally rotate the shoulders slightly, leading the movement with the small finger.

Muscle Focus

- Pectorals

Objectives

- To strengthen the shoulder horizontal adductors
- To develop trunk stabilization

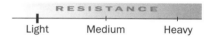

RESISTANCE

Light   Medium   Heavy

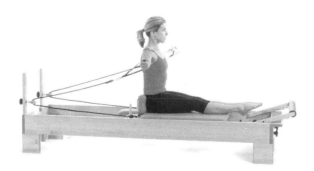

Inhale. Sit upright on the carriage with the back of the pelvis against the shoulder rests, facing the front of the reformer with the legs directly forward. Hold the arms out to the sides in a T position, keeping the elbows straight but not locked.

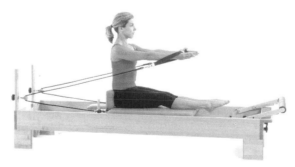

Exhale. Draw the arms toward each other until they are parallel to each other and in line with the shoulders.

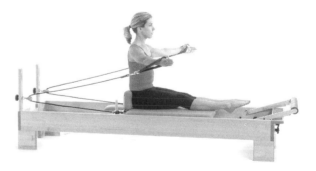

Inhale. Maximize the eccentric contraction of the horizontal adductors of the shoulders as the arms return to a T position without moving the scapulae.

Muscle Focus

■ Triceps

Objectives

■ To strengthen the elbow extensors
■ To develop trunk and scapular stabilization

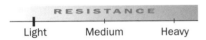

RESISTANCE

Light   Medium   Heavy

Seated Salute

Although the focus of this exercise is the triceps, this series emphasizes trunk stabilization and correct positioning of the scapulae. Avoid the tendency to round the upper body and elevate the shoulders. A good indication of the correct height of the arms is for the ropes to be slightly above the shoulders but not touching them. The arms will travel on a slight diagonal.

Imagery

Imagine the arms gliding along a ramp slightly above the horizon. Envisioning the horizon encourages a long, seemingly infinite line.

☐ Maintain scapular depression throughout the exercise.
☐ Keep the elbows lifted and reaching out to the sides when bent.
☐ Direct the fingers along the line of the movement.

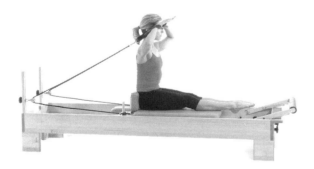

Inhale. Sit upright on the carriage with the back of the pelvis against the shoulder rests. Face the front of the reformer with the legs directly forward. Place the hands in the straps with the elbows out to the sides. Align the hands with the temples, fingertips facing forward in the direction of the movement.

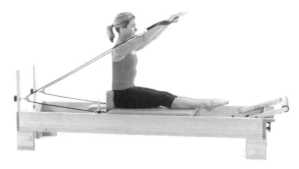

Exhale. Straighten the arms forward on the diagonal, 20 to 30 degrees above horizontal.

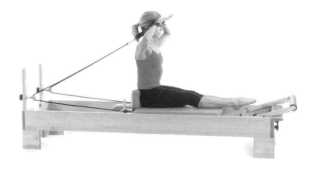

Inhale. Bend the elbows out and return to the starting position, with the fingers still facing forward.

Kneeling Chest Expansion

This exercise is far more challenging than the seated version (page 172), the standing version on the cadillac (page 228), or the version on the arm chair (page 295), primarily due to the element of instability. It requires a very high degree of trunk stabilization, balance, control, and focus. The control manifests particularly in the eccentric phase of the exercise, as the arms return to the starting position. If this phase is done too quickly, the carriage slides back to the stopper and the body lunges forward, which can cause injury.

Although a neutral spine is the ideal position, I often tilt the pelvis slightly posteriorly, which encourages abdominal activation. This in turn counters the tendency to flex at the hips, tilt the pelvis anteriorly, thrust the ribs forward, and hyperextend the back. Move the arms back toward the foot bar, extending the shoulders slightly beyond the plumb line. Once you have mastered the movement of the arms and stabilization of the trunk, you can add a rotation of the head to one side and then the other, bringing it back to center before returning the arms forward to the starting position. Alternate the side the head first turns to with each repetition.

Imagery

The trunk should feel like the trunk of a tree—tall, upright, and able to adapt to the subtle shifts as the arms move back and forth. As with the seated version, imagine the fingertips reaching down to the floor while the head simultaneously reaches up toward the ceiling. The head should then turn from side to side like a well-lubricated ball on ball bearings.

☐ Keep the trunk upright and stable.

☐ Keep the hip flexors stretched, sensing an elongation through the thighs.

☐ Avoid thrusting the ribs forward.

Muscle Focus

▪ Latissimus dorsi

Objectives

▪ To strengthen the shoulder extensors
▪ To strengthen the triceps
▪ To develop trunk stabilization

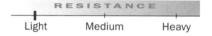

RESISTANCE

Light   Medium   Heavy

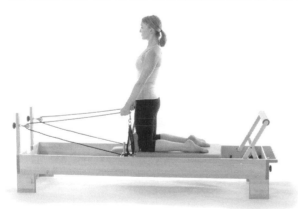

Inhale. Kneel facing the back of the reformer with the knees against the shoulder rests and the body upright. Hold the ropes in the hands, just above the straps, with the palms facing each other. Place the arms close to the sides of the body, approximately 20 to 30 degrees forward of the plumb line.

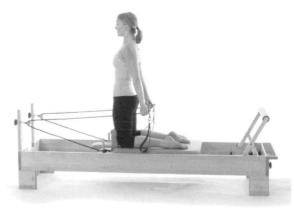

Exhale. Extend the shoulders as far back as possible without compromising the upright alignment of the trunk (10 to 20 degrees past the plumb line). In this position you may also rotate the head from side to side and back to center.

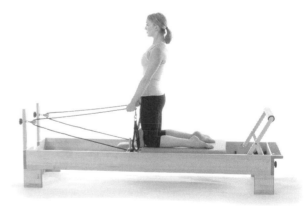

Inhale. Return to the starting position.

Kneeling Arm Circles

Muscle Focus

- Shoulder flexors (forward circles)
- Shoulder abductors (reverse circles)

Objectives

- To strengthen the shoulder flexors (forward) and the shoulder abductors (reverse)
- To develop control of the scapulae
- To develop trunk stabilization

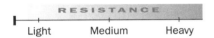

RESISTANCE

Light   Medium   Heavy

Few series of exercises challenge the upper body together with the trunk as profoundly as the arms kneeling series. I have given these exercises to athletes of many disciplines and they have all found them challenging and extremely beneficial. Swimmers in particular enjoy doing them as they address muscles and patterns fundamental to swimming.

There is a tendency to overuse the quadriceps and often the comment is that the legs are tiring more than the arms. As you learn to utilize the muscles of the core and the trunk becomes more stable, there will be less need to rely on the legs for support. As with the Reformer: Kneeling Chest Expansion (page 177), tilt the pelvis slightly posteriorly and focus on elongating the hip flexors and thighs. Avoid elevating the arms higher than the flexibility of the shoulders allows as this will result in scapular elevation and tension in the neck.

Due to the kneeling position, the center of gravity of the body is high and the lever arm (the trunk) is long; also the resistance is relatively light, making the carriage unstable. All this results in a precarious position of the body. The fact that the body is situated in the balance offers great biofeedback. Believe me, you only need to feel that you are being catapulted forward once and the body learns very quickly how to control the movement and stabilize. I avoid doing this particular series with pregnant women due to their changing center of gravity, added weight, diminished balance, and the obvious associated danger of falling.

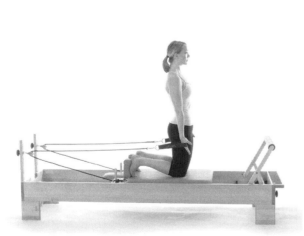

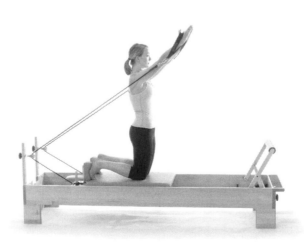

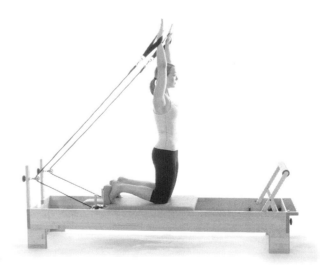

Inhale. Kneel facing the foot bar with the feet up against the shoulder rests and the trunk upright. Hold the straps with the palms facing forward and the arms by the sides of the body.

Exhale. Reach the arms forward and upward, flexing the shoulders, the palms continuing to face upward.

Inhale. Rotate the arms as they reach overhead so the palms face the front.

You can also perform this exercise in the reverse direction. This adds to the challenge of stabilizing and works the shoulder abductors profoundly. It is surprising how much more difficult this variation is than standard circles, and it may require that you reduce the resistance.

Imagery

In the initial phase I like to imagine that there is a large light beach ball in each hand that I am lifting up as if to toss them high into the air. The arms rotate at the top, and the palms face front, small finger leading the way down to the sides of the body. This encourages a light and effortless feel in the arms.

☐ Face the palms upward during shoulder flexion (as the arms move from directly in front of the shoulders to overhead).

☐ Face the palms forward during shoulder abduction (as the arms reach out to the sides and up overhead).

☐ Keep arms within peripheral vision as they circle around to the sides.

☐ Avoid elevating the scapulae as the arms rise above shoulder height.

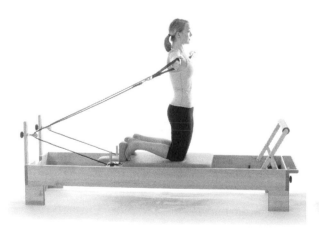

Still inhaling, circle the arms around.

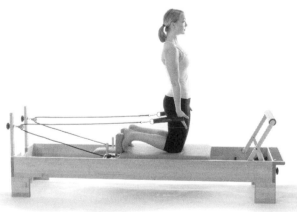

Exhale. Return the arms to the sides of the body.

Kneeling Salute

Muscle Focus

- Triceps

Objectives

- To strengthen the elbow extensors and shoulder abductors
- To develop trunk stabilization

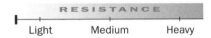

The focus of this exercise, as with the seated version (page 176) and the version performed on the arm chair (page 298), is the triceps. But given the unstable position, the shoulder girdle being higher up, and the hands traveling upward rather than forward, creating more pull on the springs and thus more resistance, it is a great deal more challenging. There is a strong tendency to round the upper body, elevate the shoulders, and move the arms forward. This should be avoided at all costs.

Imagery

Imagine the hands shaving the back of the head as the arms straighten and bend. The triangular shape created by the fingers should appear as a spearhead leading the movement.

- ☐ Maintain scapular depression throughout the exercise.
- ☐ Keep the elbows lifted and facing out.
- ☐ Direct the fingers along the line of movement.

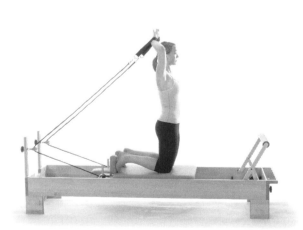

Inhale. Kneel facing the foot bar with the feet up against the shoulder rests and the trunk upright. Hold the straps with the hands behind the head, thumbs and index fingers touching, creating a triangle with the fingers. The elbows remain wide, reaching out to the sides.

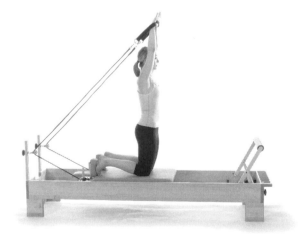

Exhale. Straighten the elbows, abducting the shoulders and keeping the fingers touching while reaching up to the ceiling.

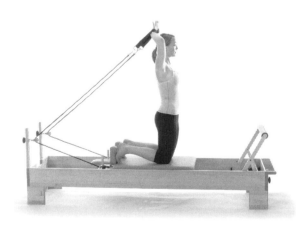

Inhale. Bend the elbows returning to the starting position.

This exercise is similar in many ways to the Cadillac: Standing Biceps (page 231) in that both impart a feeling of a profound stretch across the chest. In addition the long head of the biceps is held in a fully stretched position adding to the challenge and to the flexibility of the arms and shoulders.

Imagery

Although the trunk is upright rather than leaning forward as in the standing biceps, the same imagery can be employed—that of the body being likened to the masthead of an old wooden ship, the figurine at the front of these majestic boats. With each bend of the arms the chest should open more, with a feeling of reaching the chest forward (without thrusting the ribs out).

☐ Keep the upper arms still throughout the movement.

☐ Keep the arms parallel to each other.

☐ Maintain scapular stability.

Muscle Focus

▪ Biceps

Objectives

▪ To strengthen the elbow flexors
▪ To stretch the chest and anterior aspect of the shoulder
▪ To develop trunk stabilization

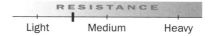

RESISTANCE

Light   Medium   Heavy

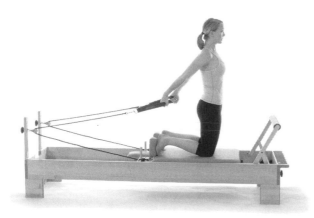

Inhale. Kneel facing the foot bar with the feet up against the shoulder rests and the trunk upright. Hold the straps with the arms reaching back.

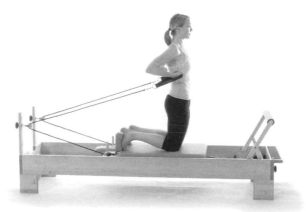

Exhale. Bend the elbows, keeping the upper arms absolutely still.

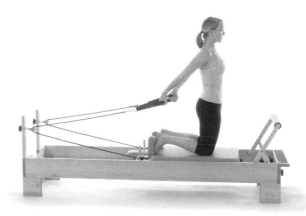

Inhale. Straighten the elbows, returning to the starting position.

Rowing Back I

The rowing series, beginning with this exercise, effectively integrates and displays all the wonderful elements of Pilates. When viewing someone doing this series, you can readily assess their competence and understanding of the method's intricacies. The coordinated muscle activation in this exercise is key. The combination of upper body support and shoulder mobility with maximal stability of the trunk illuminates the principle of functional range of motion. Avoid neck tension and shoulder elevation, which often occur because of the enormous amount of control required of the upper body. Above all, this exercise is about flow.

Muscle Focus

- Posterior deltoid and rhomboids

Objectives

- To strengthen the shoulder horizontal abductors
- To develop shoulder mobility and scapular stability
- To increase abdominal control

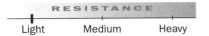

RESISTANCE		
Light	Medium	Heavy

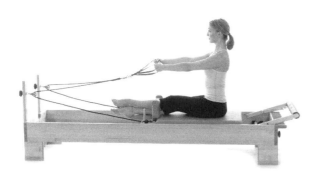

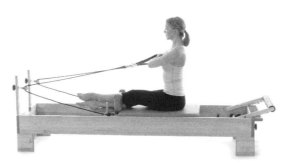

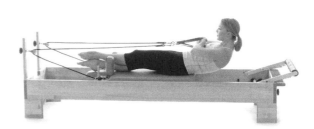

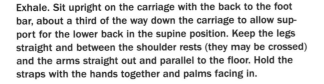

Exhale. Sit upright on the carriage with the back to the foot bar, about a third of the way down the carriage to allow support for the lower back in the supine position. Keep the legs straight and between the shoulder rests (they may be crossed) and the arms straight out and parallel to the floor. Hold the straps with the hands together and palms facing in.

Inhale. Bring the hands to the sternum, with the elbows wide.

Exhale. Roll down into a supine position, keeping the hands in front of the sternum and maintaining flexion of the trunk.

Imagery

Rowing a boat is a good visual image of the action in this exercise. I like to imagine a long, sleek boat gliding across smooth water as I use long, dynamic strokes to propel it.

☐ Place the foot bar in the down position before starting.

☐ Bring the hands to the chest before rolling down in the first phase of the exercise.

☐ Keep the carriage still when moving from the supine position to forward flexion and taking the arms from the side to the back.

☐ Take the arms out to the sides of the body and over as high as possible, as if swimming the butterfly, before rolling the spine up to a sitting position.

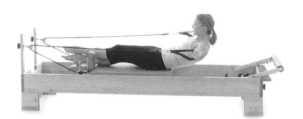

Inhale. Remaining in the supine position, internally rotate the shoulders and straighten the arms out to the sides to attain a T position with the arms. Pause.

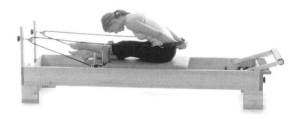

Exhale. Transfer the trunk into forward flexion over the legs while reaching the arms behind the body and touching the hands together. Keep the carriage still and maintain tension on the straps throughout this phase.

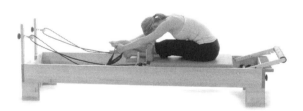

Inhale. Remain in forward flexion, stretching the hamstrings. Bring the arms through the sides of the body and over, as if swimming the butterfly, to the front alongside the legs. Exhale. Roll up to the starting position.

Rowing Back II

Muscle Focus

- Biceps

Objectives

- To strengthen the elbow flexors
- To develop abdominal and back control

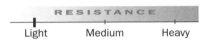

RESISTANCE		
Light	Medium	Heavy

The emphasis on full-body integration continues in this exercise. The focus is directed to the recruitment of the biceps, which are held in an isometric contraction at 90 degrees of elbow flexion for much of the exercise. Again, this exercise requires great control of the upper body.

Focus on the coordinated contraction of the abdominal muscles and the back extensors, particularly when lifting from supine into a sitting position. There is a tendency to throw the pelvis forward at this point, which results in an anterior tilt and hyperlordosis, placing excessive strain on the lower back. In the classic form of this exercise the trunk was held in extension throughout the movement. I prefer to roll down, reinforcing the familiar pattern of spinal articulation and reducing the chance of hyperextending the lower back. Throughout the movement, the arm motion should feel like an extension of the movement of the trunk.

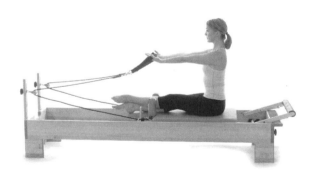

Exhale. Sit upright on the carriage with your back to the foot bar, approximately one-third of the way down the carriage (to allow support for the lower back when in the supine position) and with the legs straight and between the shoulder rests (they may be crossed). Hold the straps in the hands, with the arms straight out in front and parallel to the floor, hands facing upward.

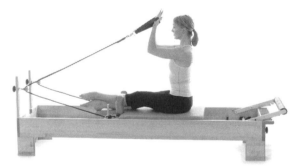

Inhale. Bend the elbows to 90 degrees.

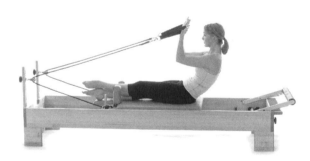

Exhale. Roll down into a supine position, maintaining flexion of the trunk and lowering the elbows to the sides of the body, holding the 90-degree angle in the elbows.

Imagery

I enjoy feeling the undulating, circular motion of the entire trunk as it rolls down and then unwinds to roll up; coordinating the arm movement with that of the trunk accentuates the rolling sensation. Visualizing this flowing, rhythmic motion will assist in giving the desired dynamic to this exercise.

☐ Place the foot bar in the down position before starting.

☐ Keep the elbows at a 90-degree angle when rolling down to the supine position.

☐ Hold the elbows firmly by the sides of the body when supine.

☐ Begin the lift with slight lumbar flexion before transitioning into trunk extension.

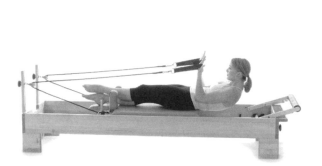

Inhale. Pause in the supine position, maintaining a stable trunk and arm position.

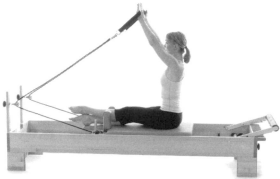

Exhale. Lift the body by drawing in the abdominal muscles and deepening the spinal flexion. Articulate through the spine to reach the upright sitting position. Simultaneously bring the arms up and forward to the starting position.

Rowing Front I

Muscle Focus

- Deltoids
- Lower trapezius

Objectives

- To strengthen the shoulder flexors and scapulae stabilizers
- To develop trunk stabilization

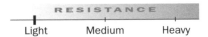

RESISTANCE

Light   Medium   Heavy

In this exercise the trunk should be upright, facing the foot bar, and should feel as sturdy as the trunk of a huge tree. This feeling is achieved by co-contracting the abdominal muscles and the back extensors. The focus is on stillness of the trunk and mobility of the shoulders. Having the resistance pulling from behind makes the movement more challenging and gives the sensation that the body is being pulled backward. If the hamstrings are tight or the back muscles are weak, sitting on a pad or small box to elevate the body is advisable; this takes the strain off the hamstrings and back extensors. Avoid leaning back and prevent the arms from going behind the body, keeping them in your peripheral vision as they circle around.

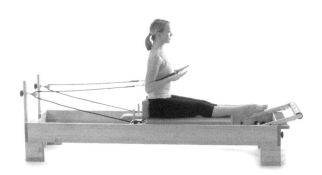

Inhale. Sit upright facing the foot bar with the back of the pelvis against the shoulder rests. Straighten the legs forward and bend the arms with the hands touching the sides of the chest, palms facing down and elbows reaching out to the sides. Place the thumbs in the straps with the rope running under the armpits.

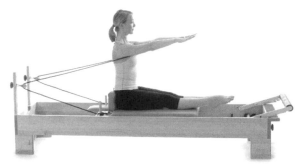

Exhale. Straighten the arms forward on a slight upward diagonal.

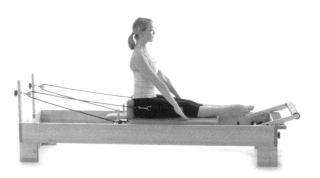

Inhale. Lower the arms to the carriage, reaching as far forward as possible, and touch the carriage with the fingertips.

Imagery

Visualize laser beams shooting out from the fingertips as you take the arms through this multidirectional movement, maximizing the range in all directions.

☐ Stabilize the trunk and maintain an upright position throughout the movement.

☐ Depress the scapulae prior to the movement.

☐ Reach as far forward as possible on the carriage while lowering the arms after the elbow extension.

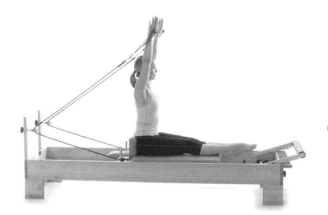

Exhale. Lift the arms overhead, internally rotating the shoulder so that the ropes pass the arms unobstructed.

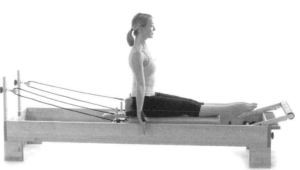

Circle the arms around and down to the sides, palms facing forward.

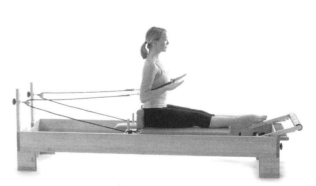

Inhale. Bend the arms and lift them up to the starting position.

187

Rowing Front II

Muscle Focus

- Back extensors
- Deltoids

Objective

- To strengthen the back extensors, elbow extensors, and shoulder flexors

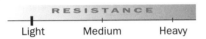

RESISTANCE

Light   Medium   Heavy

Proper execution of this exercise requires not only trunk strength and stability but also hamstring flexibility. The transition from flexion to extension of the trunk should be initiated from the lower back, with the energy flowing up through the trunk toward the arms and then the fingers. By focusing on extending the spine and achieving a straight diagonal line with the body and then with the arms, you avoid common mistakes such as shoulder elevation and inadequate extension of the trunk.

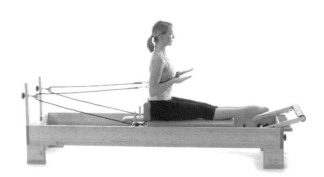

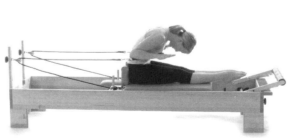

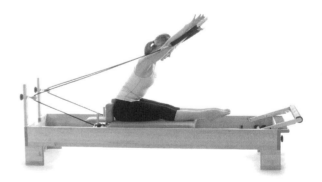

Inhale. Sit upright, facing the springs, with the back of the pelvis against the shoulder rests. Straighten the legs forward and bend the arms, with the hands touching the sides of the chest, palms facing down, and elbows reaching out to the sides. Place the thumbs in the straps with the rope under the armpits.

Exhale. Round the trunk into forward flexion over the thighs, keeping the arms close to the sides of the body and the hands directly under the shoulders.

Inhale. Extend the back into a flat diagonal position. Follow this by straightening the arms on the same diagonal line, internally rotating the shoulders so that the ropes pass the arms unobstructed.

Imagery

Imagine a wave of energy, like an electrical current, moving up the back through the arms and fingers. Or think of a color rising up the back, like litmus paper changing color.

☐ Initiate the extension from the lumbar spine before transitioning into the arm movement.

☐ Pause in the diagonal straight back position before lifting to sitting upright.

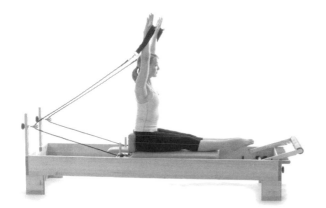

Continue to inhale. After a momentary pause, lift the body to the upright position, keeping the shoulders internally rotated.

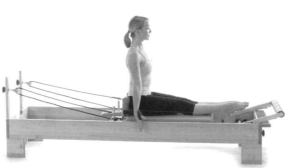

Exhale. Circle the arms around and down to the sides, palms facing forward.

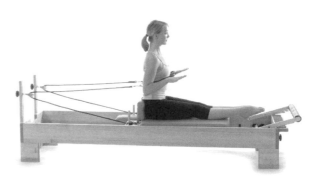

Inhale. Bend the arms to the starting position.

Leg Work

This block of exercises supplements the foot work block. It provides a space in the session for work on the legs (in addition to the foot work) but allows the instructor or practitioner to decide how to fill that space to meet individual goals, whether the goals are those of a professional football player, runner, cyclist, gymnast, dancer, or someone who just wants to maintain good general fitness.

Typically we use this block to work the hip adductors and abductors, which tend to be weak in relation to the larger muscles of the leg. The exercises chosen can be performed on the mat or the appratatus and may involve resistance, balance, specific skills, or a combination of all three.

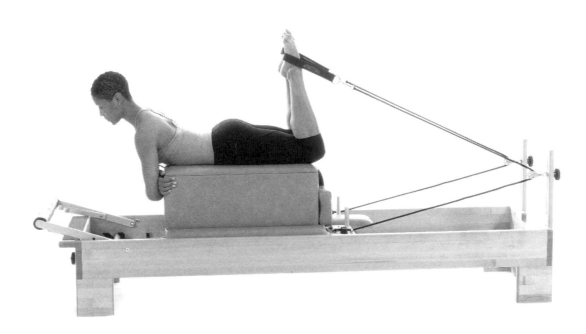

Side Split

Perhaps no other exercise so clearly demonstrates the concept of functional range of motion better than this one does. In essence, it coordinates strength and flexibility in a controlled split, striving for maximum range of motion.

The "down and out" phase involves an eccentric contraction of the adductors, and the "up and in" phase involves a concentric contraction of the adductors. Both phases require coordinated muscle activation of the hip adductors, abdominals, and back extensors. Focus on the pelvic floor as part of the ISS is ever present, yet here it seems especially pertinent in protecting the internal viscera and supporting the body from the base as it is "opened up" as wide as possible. The abdominal engagement prevents hyperlordosis and anterior pelvic tilting, which otherwise often occur at the point where the hips are in maximum abduction and the concentric phase begins. Avoid leaning the trunk forward during the movement.

Note that the resistance must be light or the abductors begin working instead of the adductors. Initially it is best to be safe and place the foot in the middle of the carriage rather than against the shoulder rest in order to limit the range of motion.

Imagery

I like the image of a string puppet being lifted from a string running from the base of the pelvis through the body and out the top of the head. There should be a sense of suction as the legs come together.

☐ Slightly tilt the pelvis posteriorly until you can maintain a neutral pelvic position.

☐ Keep the trunk upright throughout the movement.

☐ Use an arm position that allows the arms and shoulders to relax.

Muscle Focus

▪ Hip adductors

Objectives

▪ To strengthen the hip adductors
▪ To develop pelvic–lumbar stabilization

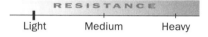

RESISTANCE		
Light	Medium	Heavy

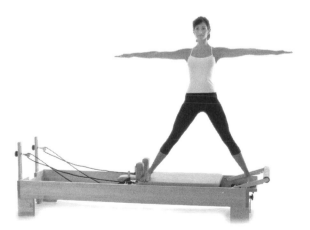

Exhale. Stand on the foot platform. Place one foot as far out as possible on the carriage (against shoulder rest if possible). Hold the arms in a T position.

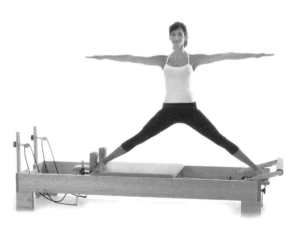

Inhale. Allow the carriage to move outward, controlling the movement with the adductors. Pause at the end of the range of motion.

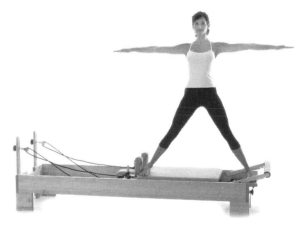

Exhale. Draw carriage back to the starting position.

Single-Leg Skating

Muscle Focus

- Gluteus medius
- Quadriceps

Objectives

- To strengthen the hip abductors
- To develop pelvic–lumbar stabilization

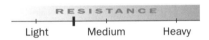

RESISTANCE

Light   Medium   Heavy

This exercise is a strong hip abductor exercise with a specific focus on the gluteus medius, a muscle quite important for healthy hip function and seen in everyday movements such as the gait cycle.

It is important to distinguish between the standing leg and the working leg, as they perform very different functions. The standing leg creates a solid foundation from which to work. The moving leg performs the action, relying on a stable pelvis to push off. Although the motion is created in the working leg, an equal amount of attention must be paid to the standing leg, which remains stable. Avoid the common mistake of pushing with the standing leg rather than the working leg. This often indicates that the resistance is too heavy. Another indication that resistance is too heavy is the body lifting as the working leg straightens.

Imagery

I like to use the image of a sidekick in karate, powerful and directed. The image of the fluid lateral force of speed skating may be useful in this exercise as well.

- ☐ Keep the weight on the standing leg, and avoid pushing it out.
- ☐ Maintain a level pelvis throughout.
- ☐ Straighten the working leg completely and control its return from the straight position.

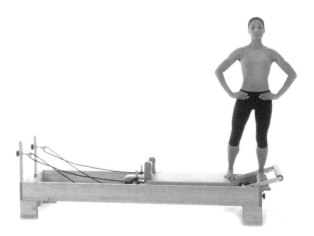

Inhale. Stand on the foot platform, then place one foot on the front edge of the carriage, keeping the weight entirely on the standing leg. Place the hands on the hips, and keep the trunk upright. Squat deeply with the standing leg, still keeping weight off the nonstanding leg at this point.

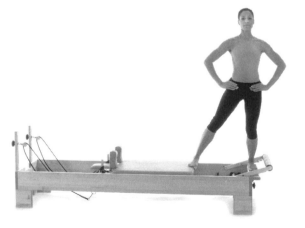

Exhale. Straighten the working leg completely, pushing the carriage outward.

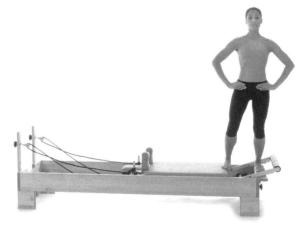

Inhale. Return to the starting position.

Hamstring Curl

As its name implies, this exercise focuses primarily on knee flexion. We add to this action hip extension, which again involves the hamstrings. Engaging the hip extensors prior to flexing the knee will enable stronger work by the hamstrings. Also, using the hip extensor component of the hamstring contraction will inhibit the use of the hip flexors, which often become involved when the knee bends, in turn pulling the pelvis into anterior tilt and creating hyperlordosis. This should be avoided at all costs. Once again, engagement of the abdominals and the back extensors stabilizes both the lumbar spine and the mid- and upper back, helping to prevent hyperlordosis and rounding of the thoracic spine. Hugging the front of the box offers additional support for the upper body.

Imagery

The image of the body being like an archer's bow is a powerful one. This is the position the body should assume prior to the actual curl (knee bend). The bending of the knee can then be viewed as pulling the string and placing tension on the bow. However, this image should not encourage excessive extension of the back, particularly the lower back.

☐ Maintain hip extension throughout the exercise.

☐ Keep the upper back slightly extended.

☐ Use the abdominals throughout the exercise to protect the lower back and prevent hyperlordosis.

Muscle Focus

▪ Hamstrings

Objective

▪ To strengthen the knee flexors and hip extensors

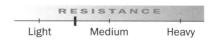

RESISTANCE		
Light	Medium	Heavy

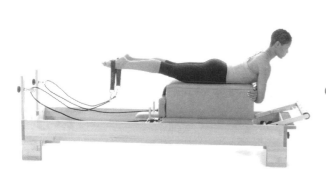

Inhale. Lie prone on the long box, facing the foot bar. Extend the upper back and engage the abdominals. Place the feet in the straps, extend the hips, and lift the legs straight so that they are slightly off the box. Hug the front of the box with the arms.

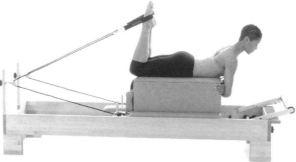

Exhale. Bend the knees and press the pubic symphysis into the box, keeping the hips extended.

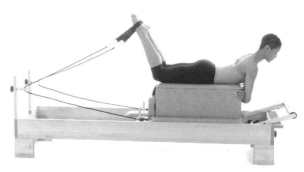

Inhale. Partially straighten the knees, maintaining tension in the straps. Do 5 to 10 repetitions. Return to the starting position.

Lateral Flexion and Rotation

Lateral flexion and rotation are important in both everyday activities and in athletic pursuits. Yet in many fitness programs they are severely neglected. For instance, when it comes to training the abdominals, the action predominantly if not exclusively used is forward flexion. This is only a small part of the whole. Without spinal lateral flexion and rotation, the abdominals are not being trained to their full capacity. This will result in less than optimal performance and may eventually lead to ailments and injury. Training the abdominals fully contributes significantly to engaging the spinal stabilization mechanism, which protects the spine.

Every program should have within it some lateral flexion and rotation movements, at whatever level is appropriate. Approximately 25 percent of the trunk work should be alloated to this category. The muscles must be addressed in terms of both strength and flexibility. Often in rotational activities the arms and shoulders compensate for lack of rotation in the trunk; this results in compromised performance and excessive wear and tear on the body. When the power emanates from the trunk, utilizing the strong abdominal muscles, the power of the movement is infinitely greater. This is the *powerhouse*!

Circular and spiral energy form the basis of the imagery for lateral flexion and rotation. These types of energy promote smooth and flowing movement. I like to visualize a circle or spiral, and, as I go through the range of motion, I try to touch every point on the circle or spiral.

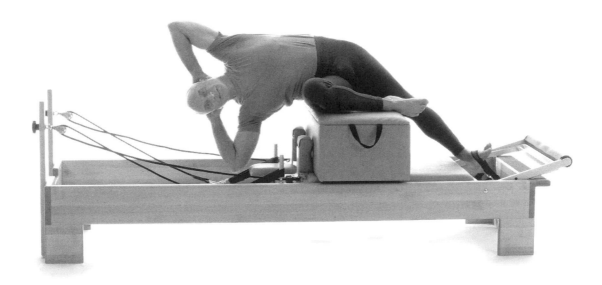

Although the tilt is not a particularly challenging exercise, it teaches correct alignment and muscle recruitment for lateral flexion that is then used in more difficult exercises. An important aspect of this exercise is initiating the lateral motion from the region of the waist as the pelvis remains stable with equal weight on the sit bones.

The movement works its way up through the spine, keeping the head aligned with the spine. The motion should never start from the shoulders or elbows. Aim to achieve maximum range of motion, moving as far as possible with the pelvis anchored on the box. The lower body provides the foundation for this exercise and remains still throughout.

Imagery

The image of a young, green tree trunk being pulled over and springing back to an upright position illustrates the elongated, gentle curve that is desired. The movement occurs in the saggital plane and as such the image of moving between two panes of glass is also helpful.

☐ Co-contract the abdominals and back extensors.

☐ Keep both sit bones in contact with the box throughout.

☐ Avoid thrusting the ribs forward and arching the back.

Muscle Focus

- Oblique abdominals

Objectives

- To stretch the oblique abdominal muscles
- To develop control of the oblique abdominal muscles

RESISTANCE		
Light	Medium	Heavy

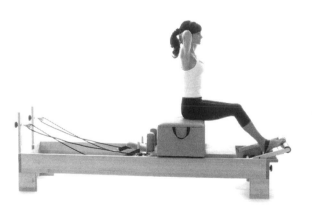

Exhale. Sit upright on the box close to the front. Place the feet under the foot strap, bend the knees, and interlace the fingers behind the head.

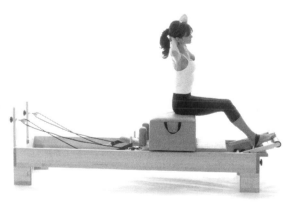

Inhale. Reach the trunk over to one side, keeping the pelvis stable and moving from the waist.

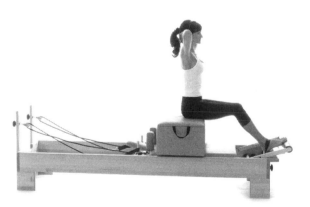

Exhale. Return to the starting position. Alternate sides.

Twist

Muscle Focus

- Oblique abdominals

Objectives

- To strengthen the abdominal muscles, especially the obliques
- To develop trunk stabilization

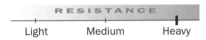

RESISTANCE

Light   Medium   Heavy

This exercise has two distinct phases: the trunk rotating around the longitudinal axis, followed by the trunk gliding diagonally back as one unit, hinging from the hips. This sequence is repeated in reverse as you return to the starting position.

During the second phase, focus on a coordinated contraction of the abdominal muscles and the back extensors in order to prevent the common error of hyperextending the back. As in the Reformer: Tilt (page 195), the range of motion is dictated by the ability to keep the pelvis anchored on the box.

Imagery

Rotation around the longitudinal axis—in the initial and final phases—is key to executing this exercise correctly. I use the image of a revolving door. When the body is then taken into a diagonal position, I visualize the entire door being tilted on its side.

- ☐ Co-contract the abdominals and back extensors.
- ☐ Rotate around the longitudinal axis prior to gliding backward.
- ☐ Lift the trunk back onto the longitudinal axis prior to returning to the starting position.

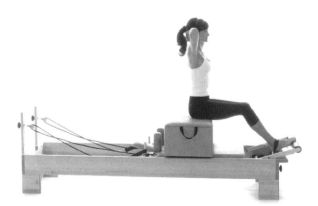

Exhale. Sit upright on the box, close to the front. Place the feet under the foot strap, bend the knees, and interlace the fingers behind the head.

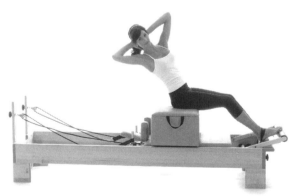

Inhale. Rotate around the longitudinal axis, focusing on elongation of the spine; then hinge from the hip joints, gliding the trunk backward on a slight diagonal.

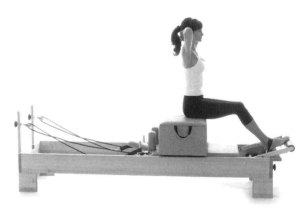

Exhale. Return to the upright position, maintaining the rotation, and then face forward. Alternate sides.

Side Over

I consider this to be the bread and butter of lateral flexion exercises—it is my favorite! The idea of an energy line that stretches from the feet through the leg and then the spine and out the top of the head is particularly pertinent in this movement. With the body in the straight diagonal starting position, the movement is initiated in the region of the waist. As the trunk reaches out and over, the energy line begins to arch as the pelvis and lower body remain stable.

Be mindful that the head is a continuation of the spine and extends the body line. When the body is in lateral flexion, avoid lifting back up with the head, which creates tension in the neck. Similarly avoid pulling on the leg to lift. The lift must come from the lateral flexors of the trunk. As in many of the lateral flexion exercises, co-contracting the abdominals and back extensors helps maintain the body line and keeps the movement in the saggital plane, preventing hyperextension or trunk flexion and encouraging

activation of the correct muscles. Keep the pelvis anchored and as still as possible. However, tipping the pelvis slightly forward or back may be necessary to achieve optimal activation of the oblique abdominals. In addition, maintaining activation of the obliques on the underside of the body is important in achieving the elongated alignment of the spine.

Imagery

The two Reformer: Tilt (page 195) images work well—a young tree trunk being pulled over and then allowed to return to its upright position, and a sense of moving between two panes of glass.

☐ Co-contract the abdominal muscles and the back extensors.

☐ Avoid lifting the trunk higher than the diagonal line created with the straight leg.

☐ Distribute the lateral flexion through the entire spine, creating an arch with the body.

Muscle Focus

▪ Oblique abdominals

Objectives

▪ To strengthen the abdominal muscles, especially the obliques
▪ To develop trunk stabilization

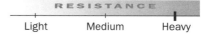

RESISTANCE

Light   Medium   Heavy

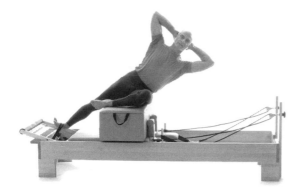

Exhale. Sit sideways on the short box. Place one foot, dorsiflexed, under the foot strap with a straight leg, and bend the other leg on top of the box. Interlace the fingers behind the head. The body should be on a straight diagonal line running from the foot that is under the strap to the head.

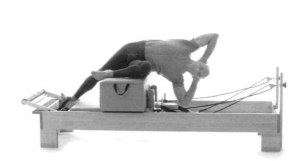

Inhale. Arch the body over the box, keeping the pelvis and leg still.

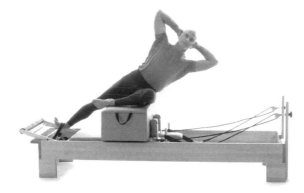

Exhale. Lift up to the starting position, forming a straight diagonal line.

Mermaid

The mermaid has a beautiful flow and exemplifies the choreographic skills involved in Pilates. It can be viewed as a movement sequence with three positions or parts. One, a stable position of the trunk is established. Two, the carriage is pushed out as far as possible and the trunk sinks toward the floor. The movement should feel as if it is emanating from under the arm but also as if you were moving the trunk as one unit, maintaining stable alignment. Three, the body rotates. During this phase the back extensors should *not* be released; instead there should be a feeling of disassociating the trunk from the pelvis and rotating the trunk around a pole. Although we attempt to keep the pelvis still with both sit bones connected to the carriage, the pelvis will move and one side will lift slightly, depending on the body's flexibility. At this point, the shoulders are square, in line with each other and parallel to the floor.

Muscle Focus

- Oblique abdominals

Objectives

- To increase spinal mobility
- To develop oblique abdominal and shoulder control

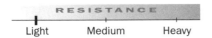

RESISTANCE

Light   Medium   Heavy

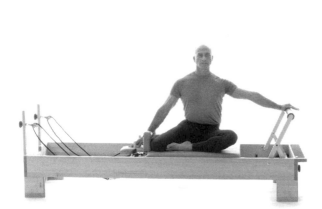

Exhale. Sit sideways on the carriage with one leg bent in front of the pelvis and the other leg bent to the side with the shin against the shoulder rests. Place the hand of the arm closest to the foot bar on the foot bar opposite the shoulder, and straighten the arm. Place the other arm down by the side with the fingers reaching toward the headrest.

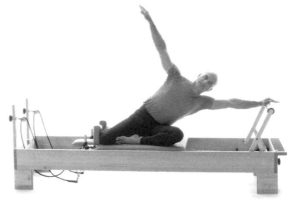

Inhale. Push the carriage away from the foot bar until the pushing arm is parallel to the floor. The trunk sinks down as one unit toward the carriage. Keep the head aligned with the spine. Simultaneously lift the breathing arm and reach out and up on a diagonal.

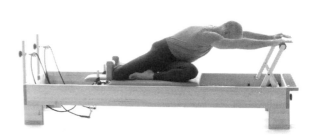

Exhale. Rotate the trunk, drawing in the abdominal muscles and pivoting around the shoulder. Bring the free arm around to touch the foot bar. Do not move the carriage during this transition. The trunk and shoulder girdle should now be square and parallel to the floor.

The return from the third part to position two should be precise and clear, pivoting around the shoulder joint. Finally the return to the starting position should be gradual without allowing the supporting arm to bend or the shoulder to elevate. (The carriage does not need to reach the stopper.) The transition between each position should display clarity and control. Avoid excessive movement with the free arm. I call it the *breathing arm*—it should float weightlessly, responding to the breath and the movement of the trunk.

Imagery

I like to think of the body as a spring being wound up, and then unwinding with control and precision.

☐ Keep the supporting arm straight throughout.
☐ Pivot around the supporting shoulder during the rotation.
☐ Allow the breathing arm to move weightlessly with the movement of the trunk.

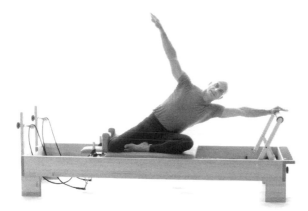

Inhale. Return to the previous position, again pivoting around the shoulder.

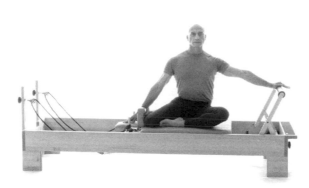

Exhale. Return to the starting position, keeping the supporting arm straight. (It is not necessary to reach the stopper.)

Back Extension

I suppose I might be regarded as a back extension fanatic. There are many reasons I qualify for this title, the most apparent being that I virtually never forgo back extension in a session. Also I am now over 50 years old, and I realize more every day that as we get older we do not gain more extension; instead our modern lifestyle coupled with gravitational pull and the natural inclination of the spine to fold forward predispose us to a forward-leaning posture and can lead to a loss of this range of motion (spinal extension).

So much focus is placed on the abdominals and hence on spinal flexion, often at the expense of back extension; at the very least, the ratio of abdominal work to back extension work is disproportionate. We must not forget that it is the extensors that hold us up; although the abdominals are certainly important in offering additional support, it is the extensors that do the primary work.

It is also important to recognize that there are distinct regions in the back and that different exercises target different regions and different muscles. Typically when teaching fundamental level movements, I focus on bracing and stabilizing the lumbar region and creating the movement in the mid- and upper back. The main reason for this is that most people are inclined to immediately move from their lumbar spines and the natural inclination of this region is in the direction of extension, which can lead to a weakening in the mid- and upper back. This is exacerbated by a modern lifestyle that encourages round shoulders and kyphotic posture. It takes time to become reacquainted with neglected mid- and upper back muscles while learning to stabilize the lumbar region.

Often, in order to facilitate activation of the mid- and upper back, the program needs to be augmented by exercises to stretch the muscles of the chest, which, if tight, restrict thoracic extension.

Once students of Pilates become accomplished in doing movements featuring back extension, they can move on to exercises with more extreme ranges of motion that require the participation of the lumbar extensors and focus on these muscles.

There are three distinct images that relate to extension exercises, each resulting in a different outcome and the recruitment of different muscles. The first is the concept of elongation. In this case the goal is typically to emphasize the mid- and upper back, with the height of the extension being somewhat limited. Reaching out from the top of the head and relaxing the legs and gluteal muscles will help achieve this goal.

The second image is used when proper extension has been accomplished and one of the goals is height. In this case I use the image of an archer's bow ready to unleash its power. This image works well for exercises that move in and out of extension as well as those in which holding an arched, stable position is important, such as the Mat Work: Swan Dive (page 104).

The third image requires very intricate execution. It uses the concept of spinal articulation, but in reverse direction. Starting from the very tip of the head, the spine is articulated into extension. This is much more challenging than spinal articulation in flexion, such as in the pelvic curl. The goal is seamless movement that utilizes the deep intervertebral muscles that are crucial to the integrity of the movement and stabilization of the spine.

Breaststroke Prep

This exercise is an excellent back extensor exercise for people of all age groups and every fitness level. It uses relatively low resistance and has a large base of support, making it safe and user-friendly. It works the arms and shoulders together with the back extensors, and the degree of extension can be easily moderated.

Once you have achieved good muscle activation and correct form in the basic version, add extension, lifting the body into an arch as the arms straighten. This increases the range of motion of the movement, stretches the abdominal muscles, and activates the lower back muscles more strongly.

Imagery

The image of effortlessly gliding across a smooth surface as you push away from the foot bar gives a flowing quality to the exercise. When doing the variation with added extension, the same gliding quality should be achieved; however as the body arches, the energy lines will move both horizontally and vertically.

☐ Engage the back extensors prior to moving the carriage.

☐ Keep the wrists firm and the fingers pointing forward.

☐ Keep the head aligned with the spine.

Muscle Focus

▪ Back extensors

Objectives

▪ To strengthen the back extensors

▪ To develop scapular stabilization

▪ To develop abdominal control

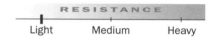

	RESISTANCE	
Light	Medium	Heavy

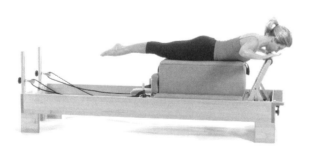

Inhale. Lie prone on the long box, facing the foot bar, with the sternum at the front edge. Place the hands on the foot bar, shoulder-width apart. Direct the elbows out toward the sides as if the arms were on a flat surface, and keep the body horizontal (parallel to the floor) with the back extensors and hip extensors engaged.

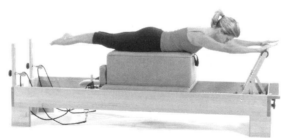

Exhale. Straighten the arms while elongating the entire body, moving horizontally.

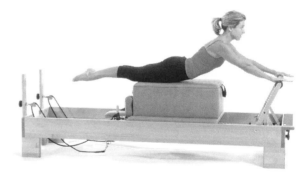

Alternatively, you can extend the trunk into a moderate arch before inhaling and returning to the starting position.

Muscle Focus

- Back extensors

Objective

- To strengthen the back extensors, shoulder abductors, and elbow extensors

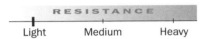

RESISTANCE		
Light	Medium	Heavy

Breaststroke

This exercise emphasizes coordinated movement of the shoulders and arms with the back extensors. The arms should always follow, rather than lead, the action of the back extensors and scapulae stabilizers. As in Reformer: Rowing Front II (page 188), the movement is initiated from the base of the spine and flows up the spine. The degree of extension should be moderate initially and evenly distributed throughout the back.

Following the extension of the back and straightening of the arms, the arms remain straight until they have circled around; avoid bending the elbows too soon. At the point that they do bend, having reached the sides of the body, keep the upper arms still and maximize shoulder external rotation. It should appear as if the forearms are moving on a horizontal surface.

Everyone can benefit from this exercise. The height of the back extension should be determined by the muscle focus and objectives. Keeping the position of the trunk lower, with the movement having a horizontal orientation, works the mid- and upper back extensors more. Lifting into a high arch activates the lower back more.

Imagery

I encourage the use of the image of swimming the breaststroke on the surface of the water or in a 1-inch-deep pool of water, keeping the movement almost two-dimensional. This exercise (as well as Reformer: Pulling Straps I and II, pages 203 and 204) promotes the concept of a strong horizontal component in back extension work.

- ☐ Move the arms as extensions of the trunk.
- ☐ Maintain external rotation of the shoulder as the elbows bend in the final phase.
- ☐ Focus on back extension without excessive hip extension, keeping the legs parallel to the floor.

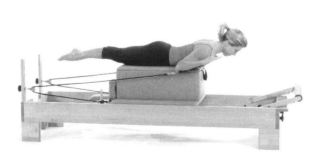

Exhale. Lie prone on the long box, facing the foot bar, with the sternum at the front edge. Place the thumbs in the straps so that the ropes run under the arms with the elbows bent by the sides and the shoulders biased toward external rotation. Face the fingers forward with the hands higher than the elbows.

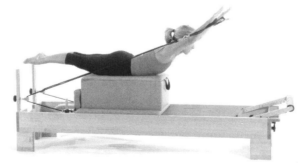

Inhale. Extend the trunk followed immediately by straightening the arms forward.

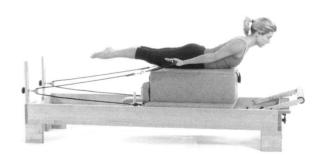

Still inhaling, circle the arms around to the sides of the body while holding the trunk stable in extension. Then exhale and bend the elbows, keeping them close by the sides and the hands lower than the elbows. Maintain external rotation of the shoulders. Simultaneously lower the body to the starting position.

The pulling straps exercises emphasize the importance of the back extensor complex and highlight correct muscle activation: Starting from the top of the head, the muscles are sequentially recruited toward the lower back. The back extension is accompanied by extension of the shoulders as the straps are pulled back—a powerful combination. As the extension occurs, the legs remain in a stable position parallel to the floor. The degree of extension depends on which area of the back you wish to target. The higher the arch, the more the lower back extensors will be activated. Keep the palms facing the reformer throughout, avoiding internal rotation of the shoulders and the temptation to round the chest. Focus on arching the thoracic spine and opening the chest as the arms pull back.

Imagery

Being a surfer, I find it difficult to resist using the image of paddling a surfboard during this exercise, which combines back, shoulder, and arm strength in a coordinated pattern. No exercise will better prepare surfers for that elusive perfect wave!

☐ Engage the back extensors from the outset.

☐ Keep the elbows straight.

☐ Press the hands against the thighs at the conclusion of the shoulder extension.

Muscle Focus

- Back extensors

Objective

- To strengthen the back and shoulder extensors

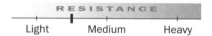

RESISTANCE

Light   Medium   Heavy

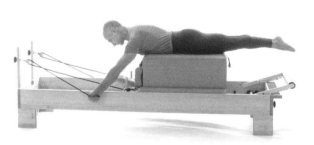

Inhale. Lie prone on the box, facing away from the foot bar with the sternum at the edge of the box. Hold the ropes with the arms straight and approximately 20 degrees forward of the perpendicular line of the shoulders.

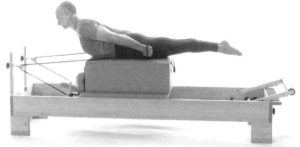

Exhale. Extend the trunk, arching the back and pulling the straps toward the sides of the thighs, with the palms facing the body.

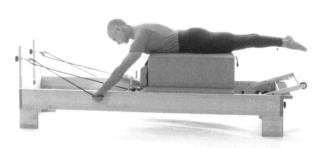

Inhale. Return to the starting position.

Pulling Straps II

Muscle Focus

- Back extensors

Objectives

- To strengthen the back extensors and shoulder adductors

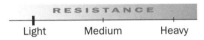

RESISTANCE

Light   Medium   Heavy

Like the Reformer: Pulling Straps I (page 203), this exercise emphasizes the importance of the back extensor complex and focuses on muscle activation patterning. However in this case back extension is accompanied by shoulder adduction rather than shoulder extension. This is a more complex and difficult movement that demands tremendous strength of the back extensors, which serve as a platform for the arms to move on.

Both pulling straps exercises demand strong recruitment of the latissimus dorsi, which extends the shoulders in the first one and adducts the shoulders in the second one. The action of the latissimus dorsi that is neutralized is internal rotation. The shoulder external rotators function as synergists in both these exercises, countering the temptation to internally rotate the shoulders. The close relationship of the shoulder external rotators and the back extensors is exemplified in this exercise. Keeping the palms facing the floor and the shoulders externally rotated encourages extension of the upper trunk.

Imagery

Imagine pulling the body forward along two rails, one on either side of the body, with the arms never rising above shoulder level. Although the motion is primarily horizontal and the horizontal energy line is very powerful, a vertical energy line appears as the trunk lifts into hyperextension.

- ☐ Keep the shoulders externally rotated.
- ☐ Hold the arms at the same height as the body throughout the exercise.
- ☐ Pause with the arms in the T position after each repetition.

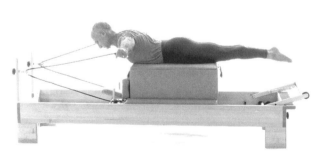

Inhale. Lie prone on the box, facing away from the foot bar with the sternum at the edge of the box. Hold the ropes with the arms in a T position, parallel to the floor, and with the palms facing down.

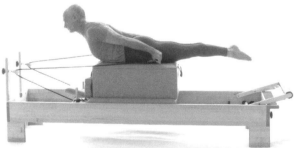

Exhale. Extend the back and pull the arms to the sides of the thighs, with the palms facing the floor. Lead the movement with the small finger.

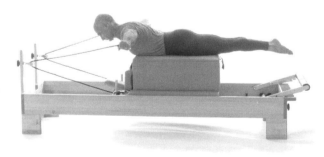

Inhale. Return to the starting position, moving the arms along a horizontal line parallel to the floor.

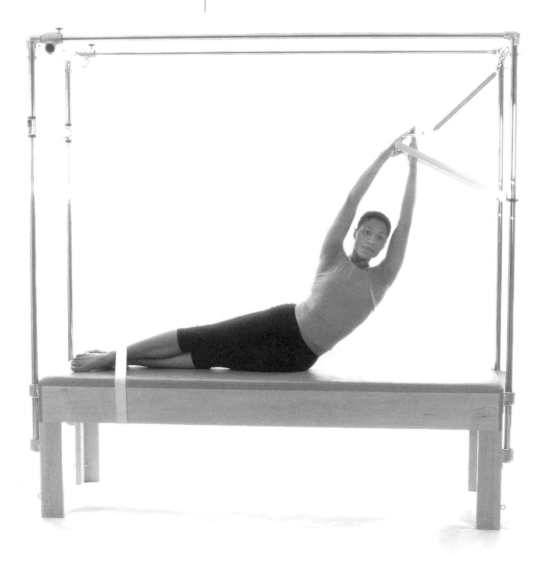

CHAPTER 6

Cadillac

Much has been written about Joseph Pilates' work with the ill, the sickly, and the injured. He helped rehabilitate them and in turn was inspired by them. When viewing the cadillac (also called the *trap* or *trap table*) it is clear that the inspiration for this piece of apparatus was a hospital bed.

Like all the Pilates apparatus, the cadillac is unique and versatile, with infinite applications. It differs from the reformer in that, during the foot work, it highlights the hamstrings in terms of both flexibility and strength. This is advantageous; as long as you are flexible enough to maintain the correct position (or close to it), the hamstrings are in a state of stretch, and the stretch increases as the work commences.

The cadillac's structure also permits hanging exercises, opening up tremendous possibilities for the upper and lower body. These exercises develop balance, coordination, and strength through acrobatic-type movements, which are very beneficial as well as a lot of fun.

The fact that the cadillac does not move, providing a stable base of support, is an advantage for people who lack balance and stability, such as the elderly or injured. In addition, because it sits high off the ground it is easier for those with limited mobility to mount and dismount. These advantages also make it comfortable for the teacher to teach and provide physical support.

The cadillac facilitates ranges of motion that surpass even those of the reformer, particularly in the leg spring work, which can be performed supine, side-lying, prone, and standing, facing all directions. The cadillac is a three-dimensional piece of apparatus in every sense of the word.

Finally, just as the reformer offers stretches for the legs that cannot be duplicated on the other apparatus, the cadillac offers unique stretches for the upper body that can only be performed on the cadillac. Enjoy this intriguing piece of equipment—it always makes me feel like a kid again, spending hours on my favorite jungle gym!

The foot work on the cadillac (pages 207 to 209) duplicates much of that done on the reformer (see pages 112 to 121) and all the same cues and directives apply. Although the foot positions are identical, the positioning of the legs is different: On the cadillac the legs move on a vertical line perpendicular to the trunk; on the reformer they move horizontally, on the same plane as the trunk. This translates to approximately 90 degrees of hip flexion on the cadillac when the legs are straight.

People with tight hamstrings who are unable to maintain the recommended position may lie with the head facing the opposite direction to decrease the stretch on the hamstrings and allow correct alignment; they will still reap the same benefits. A great advantage of the cadillac is that the position for foot work, while engaging the internal support system (ISS), minimizes the possibility of hyperlordosis and, in fact, stretches the lower back. However, you must avoid the common mistake of allowing the pelvis to curl up (tilt posteriorly), lifting the sacrum from the mat. The sacrum should serve as an anchor.

Double-Foot Positions

The double-foot positions on the Cadillac include the parallel and wide V positions for the heels and toes and the small V position for the toes (see pages 112 to 117). Note that on the cadillac, the range of knee flexion is not as great as on the reformer. Although it can be increased slightly in the V positions, particularly the open V, which allows deep flexion of the knees and hip joints, an effort must be made to maintain good form and to keep the sacrum anchored.

The toe positions generate greater resistance, and maintaining plantarflexion in the feet is important in order to keep the resistance constant. Although the stretch on the hamstrings is not as prominent in these positions as in the heel positions, you can clearly feel the sense of elongation up the back of the legs.

Imagery

Imagine that the legs are like pillars, holding up the ceiling of a large building. You lift the ceiling a little higher with each extension of the knees and then lower it as the knees bend. You should feel tremendous power in the legs.

☐ Bend the knees as far as possible without tucking the pelvis.

☐ Keep the hip extensors engaged throughout the movement.

☐ Straighten the legs with each repetition, fully extending the knees.

Muscle Focus

- Hip extensors and knee extensors

Objectives

- To strengthen the hip extensors and knee extensors
- To improve hamstring flexibility
- To develop pelvic–lumbar stabilization

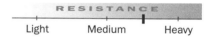

RESISTANCE

Light   Medium   Heavy

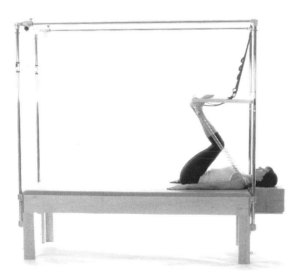

Inhale. Lie supine, knees bent, with the feet on the foot bar in one of the following positions: heels parallel, toes parallel, toes in small V position, heels in wide V position, toes in wide V position (see pages 112 to 116).

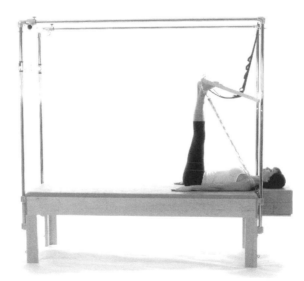

Exhale. Straighten the knees and extend the hips.

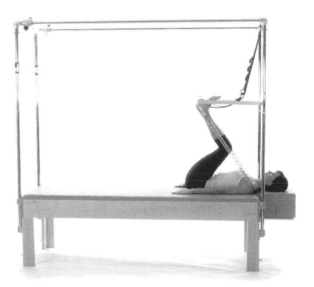

Inhale. Bend the knees and flex the hips.

Calves and Prances

Muscle Focus

- Foot plantarflexors

Objectives

- To strengthen the foot stabilizers and plantarflexors
- To stretch the foot plantarflexors and hamstrings

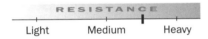

RESISTANCE

Light   Medium   Heavy

The calf exercises take advantage of a full stretch down the back of the legs that can often be felt all the way up the trunk. The stretch on the cadillac is more intense than on the reformer because of the upright position of the legs. Another advantage of being in this position is the opportunity to actually look at the alignment of the feet during the exercise. The visual feedback assists in correcting alignment.

During the prances on the cadillac, the same flow and smooth transitions that are required on the reformer should prevail. The anchored position of the pelvis helps stabilize it, avoiding the tendency to tilt from side to side during the prances.

Imagery

I try to imagine lightness in the feet, as if I were tossing a ball into the air with the feet, first together and then one at a time.

- ☐ Use the full range of motion of the ankle and foot.
- ☐ Keep the knees straight during the calf exercises.
- ☐ Transition through full plantarflexion after each repetition.

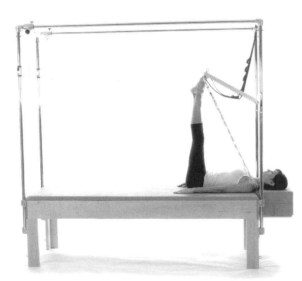

Exhale. Lie supine with the toes on the bar, the legs parallel and hip-width apart, and the feet plantarflexed. This position applies to both the calves and the prances exercises.

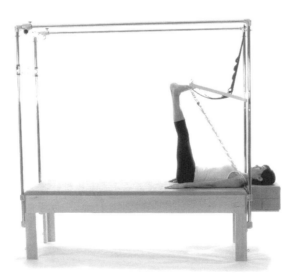

Inhale. Dorsiflex both feet. Then exhale and return to the plantarflexed position.

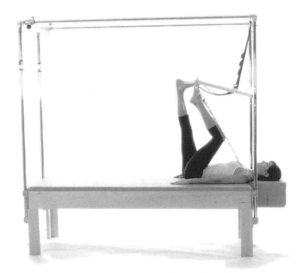

For prances, while one foot plantarflexes, the other knee bends and the foot dorsiflexes. Straighten the bent leg and plantarflex the foot so that both legs are straight and both feet plantarflexed before transitioning to the other leg to repeat the cycle and continue alternating.

Single-Foot Positions

The single-leg positions place the body in optimal alignment to stretch the hamstrings of the working leg and to stretch the hip flexors of the supporting leg. This interplay between strength and flexibility of the working leg fortifies the principle of *balance* in Pilates.

Similar benefits are reaped from the heel and toe positions. When on the heel, you can more readily feel the stretch and the work in the back of the leg. In the toe position, the resistance increases slightly because the springs are being stretched more, and the muscles that control the foot and ankle play a more prominent role.

Imagery

Energy lines offer a profound image for this position, with one line shooting upward vertically from the hip joint of the working leg. The other shoots horizontally through the supporting leg and out through the toes, and in the opposite direction through the trunk and out through the head. This image helps keep the alignment true.

☐ Bend the knee of the exercising leg as far as possible without allowing the pelvis to tuck.

☐ Bend the supporting leg if the hamstrings are tight.

☐ Keep the pelvis stable.

Muscle Focus

- Hip extensors and knee extensors

Objectives

- To strengthen the hip extensors and knee extensors
- To improve flexibility of the hamstrings
- To develop pelvic–lumbar stabilization

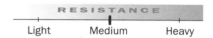

RESISTANCE

Light　　Medium　　Heavy

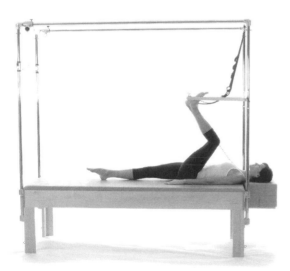

Inhale. Lie supine, working knee bent with the foot on the bar in either the single-leg heel or single-leg toes position (see pages 119 and 120). Keep the supporting leg straight and anchored on the bed.

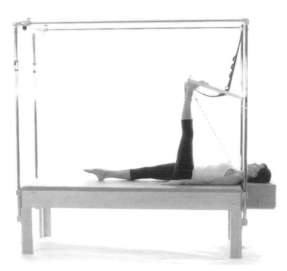

Exhale. Straighten the knee and extend the hip.

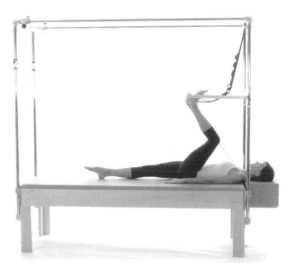

Inhale. Bend the knee and flex the hip.

Roll-Up

This is a spring-assisted roll-up, identical to the Mat Work: Roll-Up (page 52). This exercise assists people who are experiencing difficulty performing the roll-up correctly. The springs help the abdominal muscles maintain good form and facilitate the recruitment of the correct muscles in the correct sequence. They also help release other muscles that may be hampering good execution of this exercise, in particular the hip flexors and the muscles of the lower back.

Muscle Focus

- Abdominal muscles

Objectives

- To strengthen the abdominal muscles
- To stretch the back muscles
- To develop trunk stabilization

Imagery

As with most of the spring-assisted exercises, work with the springs as if they were an integral part of the body and musculature, not an external force. In this case they become an extension of the abdominal muscles.

- ☐ Simulate the exact positions and muscle recruitment of the Mat Work: Roll-Up (page 52).
- ☐ Keep the knees soft while lengthening the legs.
- ☐ Engage the adductors throughout the exercise.

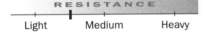

RESISTANCE

Light   Medium   Heavy

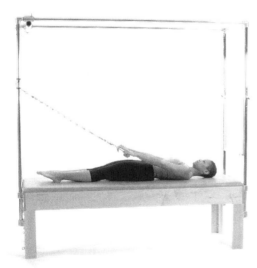

Exhale. Lie supine with the legs straight. Hold the roll-up bar with the hands shoulder-width apart, placing the body far enough back on the mat that there is tension in the springs.

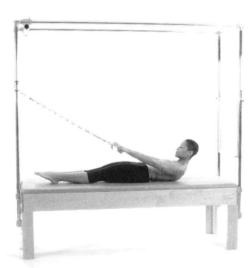

Inhale. Lift the head and shoulder girdle into spinal flexion.

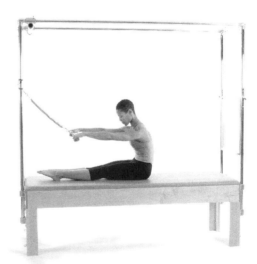

Exhale. Slowly roll up, maintaining the C curve in the trunk. Inhale and pause at the point where the shoulders are above the hip joints. Still exhaling, roll back down through each vertebra to the starting position.

This exercise is in essence a spring-assisted Mat Work: Chest Lift (see page 48). I view the springs as an extension of the abdominal muscles, supplementing their strength. The springs assist the abdominals in performing their function, helping you to overcome compensations and achieve perfect form. The assistance in this case relates largely to the release of the lower back extensors, which often prevent the trunk from achieving adequate forward flexion and the abdominals from fully contracting. Note that the trunk should remain in forward flexion throughout, and the feeling should be similar to that of the Mat Work: Rolling Like a Ball exercise (page 54). The movement occurs between the base of the scapulae and the sacrum, peeling the spine vertebra by vertebra off the mat and then placing it back down.

Imagery

Think of a wheel or ball rolling backward and forward in a small arc. Focus on deepening the hollow abdominal bowl with each roll (see also page 54).

☐ Focus on maintaining spinal flexion.
☐ Keep the shoulders relaxed.
☐ Maintain a neutral pelvis throughout the exercise if possible.

Muscle Focus

▪ Abdominals

Objective

▪ To strengthen the abdominal muscles
▪ To stretch the muscles of the lower back
▪ To teach the use of a neutral pelvis during abdominal work

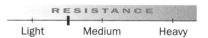

RESISTANCE

Light   Medium   Heavy

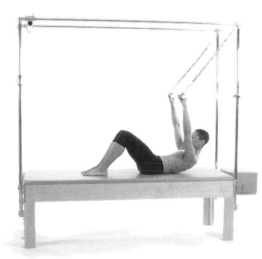

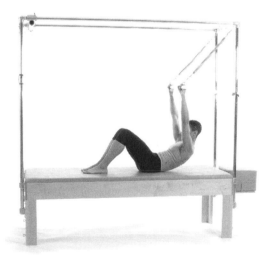

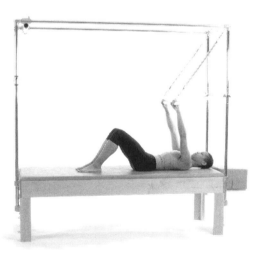

Inhale. Lie in a supine position with the knees bent and the feet anchored on the mat hip-width apart. Hold the push-through bar with an overhand grip, hands placed in line with the shoulders. Raise the head and shoulder girdle into trunk flexion. The arms should be directly under the push-through bar at this point.

Exhale. Slowly roll up, maintaining the C curve of the trunk.

Inhale. Lower to the starting position. Repeat 5 to 10 times before lowering to the starting position.

Roll-Up Top Loaded

The sequence of this exercise is similar to the spring-assisted Cadillac: Roll-Up (page 210). However, in this variation, there is a transition through trunk extension into an upright sitting position. An arm and shoulder movement is then added to stretch the shoulders and challenge the upright alignment of the trunk. (There is a tendency to thrust the ribs forward at this point, which should be avoided.) During the flexion of the elbows, accentuate shoulder external rotation and abduction of the scapulae. An alternate form of this exercise can be done by loading the springs from the bottom rather than the top, in which case the springs resist rather than assist the motion, generating an increased challenge for the abdominals, back extensors, arms, and shoulders. The exercise is then called the roll-up bottom loaded.

Muscle Focus

- Abdominals

Objectives

- To strengthen the abdominal muscles
- To stretch the shoulders

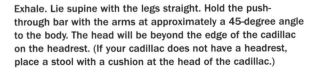

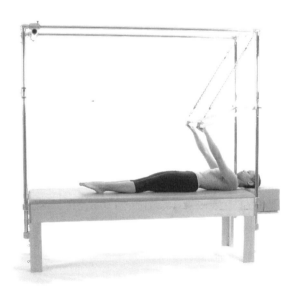

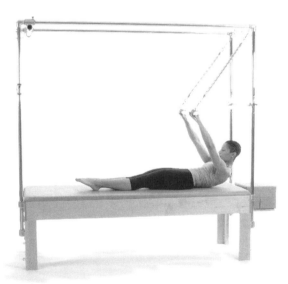

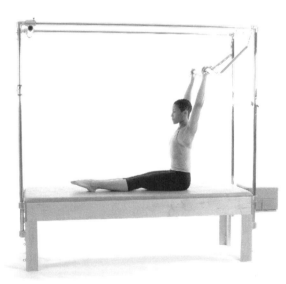

Exhale. Lie supine with the legs straight. Hold the push-through bar with the arms at approximately a 45-degree angle to the body. The head will be beyond the edge of the cadillac on the headrest. (If your cadillac does not have a headrest, place a stool with a cushion at the head of the cadillac.)

Inhale. Raise the head and shoulder girdle into trunk flexion.

Exhale. Slowly roll up by articulating the spine. Extend the trunk to a perpendicular sitting position with the arms straight overhead, pushing the push-through bar up.

Imagery

I always feel a sense of pushing the ceiling up and supporting it with my arms, like pillars holding up a building. When the elbows bend it should feel as if they were being pulled out to the sides with a spring attached to each side; they then draw back in, against the pull of the imaginary side springs, as the arms straighten.

☐ Position the body at the start of the exercise so that the trunk will be at a 90-degree angle in the final sitting position.

☐ Co-contract the abdominals and back extensors to stabilize the trunk when sitting upright.

☐ Maintain slight shoulder external rotation while bending the elbows.

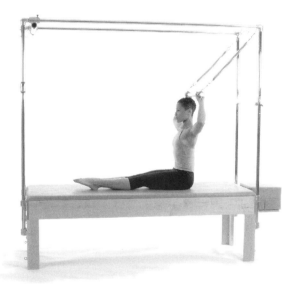

Inhale. Bend the elbows out to the sides and slightly forward (external shoulder rotation), abducting the scapulae, then straighten the elbows.

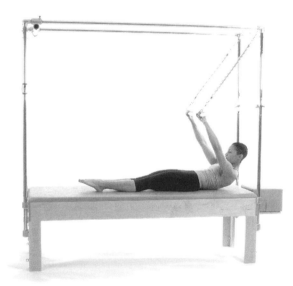

Exhale. Roll down to the starting position.

Oblique Mini Roll-Up

Muscle Focus

- Oblique abdominals

Objectives

- To strengthen the abdominal muscles, emphasizing the oblique abdominals
- To stretch the muscles of the lumbar region
- To establish the use of a neutral pelvis during abdominal work

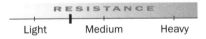

RESISTANCE

Light   Medium   Heavy

This exercise uses the same form and positioning as the Cadillac: Mini Roll-Up (page 211), but it is made more challenging by adding a rotational component. During the rotation the pelvis is inclined to tilt laterally and lift on one side; resist this by activating the abdominals in a balanced manner and keeping the feet evenly weighted. Also, the shoulders tend to elevate. Switching to an underhand grip assists in maintaining scapular depression and relaxed shoulders. Avoid allowing the ribs to flare on one side of the trunk (typically the side you are rotating to) by drawing the ribs in on the side you are rotating toward. Finally, avoid the temptation to pull up with the arm; it should remain straight and function simply as a connecting rod between the trunk and the push-through bar.

Imagery

Imagine a perpetual spiraling added to the rolling action of a ball, so that it spins slowly and rolls back and forth at the same time. Generate the movement from the abdominal region rather than from the arms or feet. Another good image to assist in the rotation is keeping the distance between the lower rib and the pelvic crest on both sides equal.

- ☐ Engage the internal and external oblique abdominals on both sides of the body.
- ☐ Maintain flexion of the spine.
- ☐ Keep the holding arm straight and relax the shoulders.

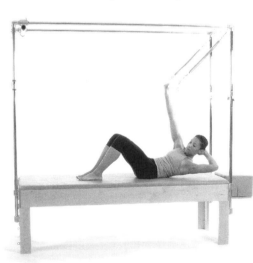

Inhale. Lie supine with the knees bent and the feet anchored on the mat hip-width apart. Hold the push-through bar with an underhand grip and the hands shoulder-width apart. Place one hand behind the head, raise the head and shoulder girdle into trunk flexion, and rotate the trunk away from the arm holding the push-through bar.

Exhale. Roll back up, keeping the C-curve position and maintaining rotation of the trunk.

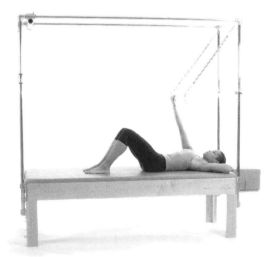

Inhale. Lower to the starting position, maintaining rotation of the trunk. Repeat 5 to 10 times before returning to center and lowering to the starting position.

The support provided by the springs supplements the abdominal muscles, diminishing the chance of lumbar strain and allowing refinement of the movement and muscle recruitment in this very demanding exercise, which is performed in various forms on the mat, reformer, barrel, and of course the cadillac. The push-through bar on the cadillac can be used to assist in all the variations of the teaser, from the most basic to the most advanced. Note that the starting position should be calculated so that in the final teaser position, the arms are aligned with the trunk to form a straight diagonal line. Bend the knees if any stress is felt in the back.

Imagery

The fact that you are hanging from a spring-loaded bar allows the feeling of weightlessness, of floating up and slowly rolling down. We strive for this quality of movement in the teaser and teaser prep, whether it is performed on the mat (page 101), the reformer, the step barrel (page 284), or the cadillac.

☐ Articulate through the spine during the roll-up and roll-down phases.

☐ Extend the back fully in the final V position.

☐ Keep the legs as high and as still as possible throughout.

Muscle Focus

- Abdominals
- Back extensors

Objectives:

- To strengthen the abdominals and back extensors
- To develop hip flexor control
- To develop trunk stabilization

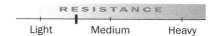

RESISTANCE

Light   Medium   Heavy

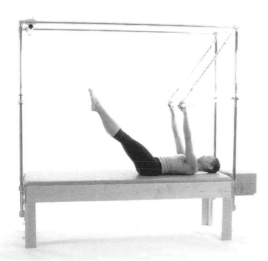

Exhale. Lie supine, holding the push-through bar. Position the shoulders directly below the hands. Keep the legs straight at an approximately 45-degree angle to the mat.

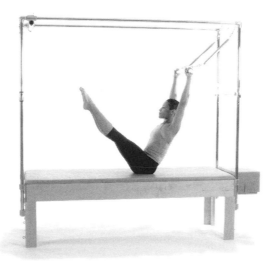

Inhale. Roll up from the head through the spine. Transition from spinal flexion to extension, creating a V position with the body, the arms overhead in a straight diagonal line with the trunk.

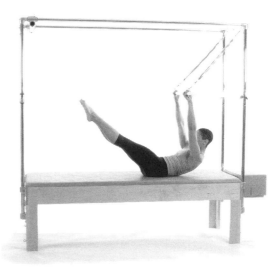

Exhale. Roll down through the spine to the starting position, keeping the legs still.

Frog

Muscle Focus

- Hip adductors

Objective

- To strengthen the hip adductors and extensors
- To develop pelvic–lumbar stabilization

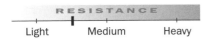

RESISTANCE

Light   Medium   Heavy

Hip exercises performed on the cadillac have several advantages over the same exercises done on the reformer. First, lying on the cadillac promotes a feeling of stability. Second, the height of the cadillac mat makes mounting and dismounting easier than on the reformer. Finally, with the cadillac each leg uses a separate spring, which translates to individual work on each leg. This is an advantage as it addresses directly any imbalances that may exist in the legs.

This exercise is similar to the same exercise done on the reformer (page 135); however, because of the angle of resistance, it places a greater load on the hip extensors. Think of the movement as following a horizontal path rather than the diagonal one used on the reformer.

Imagery

The Reformer: Frog (page 135) is a good reference, but the frog on the cadillac has a distinctly different feel. I visualize pushing away from a wall, with the feet remaining in one place while the body moves. This translates into the feet remaining on a consistent horizontal plane and creates the feeling of internal resistance.

- ☐ Maintain a neutral spine throughout the movement.
- ☐ Keep the feet traveling along a consistent horizontal plane.
- ☐ Initiate the movement with the hamstrings and adductors.

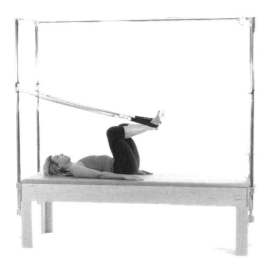

Inhale. Lie supine with the feet in the straps in a V position and dorsiflexed. Press the heels together and bend the knees. Place the arms by the sides or hold the poles, and relax the shoulders.

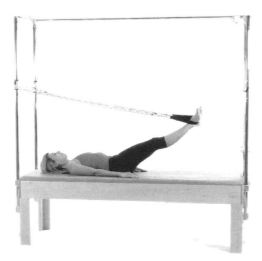

Exhale. Straighten the knees, squeezing the heels together as the feet move forward.

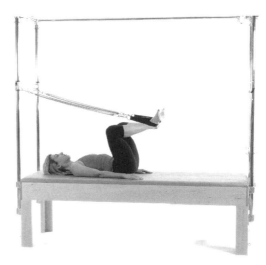

Inhale. Bend the knees, returning to the starting position.

Hip Circles

Like the Reformer: Down Circles and Up Circles (pages 136 and 137), this exercise highlights the principles of hip disassociation and hip joint mobility. Doing this series on the cadillac, however, shifts the emphasis from the adductors to the hamstrings, primarily because of the angle of resistance. In addition, on the cadillac, each leg has an individual spring and therefore works independently; this prevents a dominant side from overpowering the weaker side and doing more of the work.

Imagery

The Reformer: Down Circles and Up Circles (pages 136 and 137) is a good reference, yet this exercise has a distinctly different feel. As on the reformer, initially you should work on drawing two back-to-back D shapes in the air, increasing the size as your control improves. On the cadillac, when moving down the centerline, imagine the legs not only squeezing together to highlight the adductor work but also pressing down, as if against a big balloon.

☐ Maximize hip disassociation.

☐ Maintain external rotation of the hip joints.

☐ Keep the size of the circles within a range that can be comfortably controlled.

Muscle Focus

- Hamstrings
- Hip adductors

Objectives

- To strengthen the hip extensors
- To develop adductor control
- To improve hip disassociation

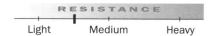

RESISTANCE

Light   Medium   Heavy

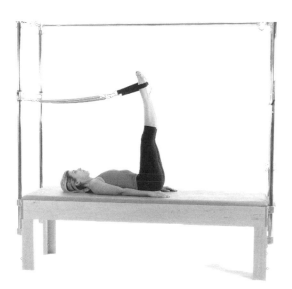

Inhale. Lie supine with the feet in the straps and the legs straight at an approximately 90-degree angle to the mat. Hips are externally rotated and feet are plantarflexed. Place the arms by the sides or hold the poles, relaxing the shoulders.

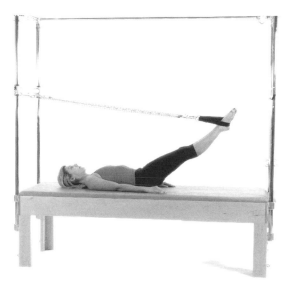

Exhale. Extend the hips, pressing the legs down the centerline squeezing them together.

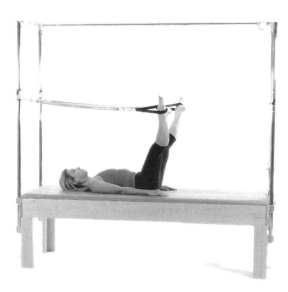

Inhale. Circle the legs around to the sides and back up to the starting position. Repeat 5 to 10 times and then reverse the direction.

Walking

Muscle Focus

- Hamstrings

Objectives

- To strengthen the hamstrings
- To develop hip disassociation
- To develop pelvic–lumbar stabilization

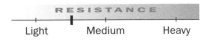

RESISTANCE

Light   Medium   Heavy

This exercise shifts the emphasis, after the Cadillac: Frog (page 216) and Cadillac: Hip Circles (page 217), from the hip extensors and adductors to the hip extensors only. Since the action of the hamstrings becomes the primary focus, the legs change from an externally rotated position to a parallel one.

Because two movements are occurring at the same time, the legs continuously switching as they move down toward the mat and then up again to a 90-degree angle in the hip joints, coordination becomes challenging. The small, vigorous scissoring movement of the legs continues throughout the exercise.

Imagery

Rather than thinking of this as walking, I prefer to imagine flutter kicks as in swimming. The movement should be small and contained, as opposed to the larger movement of the Cadillac: Bicycle (page 219) or actual walking.

- ☐ Keep the leg switches small.
- ☐ Keep tension in the springs throughout the exercise.
- ☐ Maintain a stable pelvis.

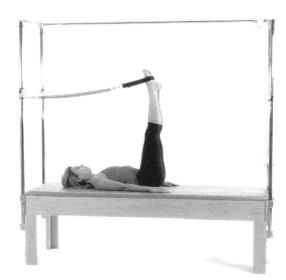

Inhale. Lie supine with the feet in the straps. Keep the legs straight and together in a parallel position at an approximately 90-degree angle to the mat. Place the arms by the sides of the body or hold the poles with the shoulders relaxed.

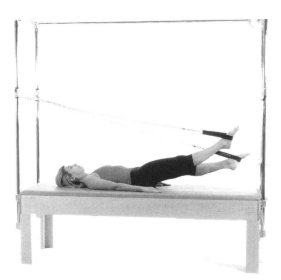

Exhale. Alternate legs with a small scissorlike motion while simultaneously extending the hips and pressing the legs down toward the mat for five counts.

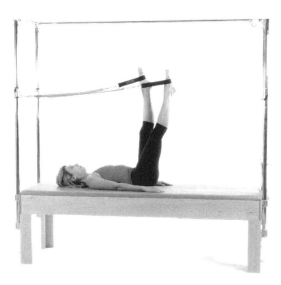

Inhale. Using the same scissoring motion, raise the legs while resisting the springs, moving upward for five counts. Return to the starting position.

The coordination required for this exercise can be challenging. Focus on making a large cycling motion with the legs while maintaining tension in both springs throughout. The movement should be fluid, with a sense of elongation, at all times keeping the hip extensors recruited. Keeping the legs in a parallel (neutral) position helps fully engage the hamstrings. Also keep the knee of the leg that is pressing down toward the bed slightly bent and stable, which helps promote strong contraction of the hamstrings, both as knee flexors and hip extensors.

During this large movement of the hip and knee joints, the pelvis must remain anchored and provide a stable platform for the legs. Once you have gained proficiency in the initial movement pattern you can reverse the direction, which changes the muscle action and coordination substantially, producing a feeling of stretching the hip extensors more than strengthening them.

Imagery

The image I often use is of a penny-farthing bicycle, one of those old-fashioned bikes with a large front wheel and a small back one. The small wheel (the pelvis) stabilizes the bicycle while the big wheel (the legs) provides the movement.

☐ Straighten both legs, establishing an L position before switching.
☐ Maintain pelvic stabilization and spring tension throughout the exercise.

Muscle Focus

- Hamstrings

Objectives

- To strengthen the hip extensors
- To develop hip disassociation
- To develop pelvic–lumbar stabilization

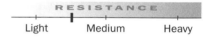

RESISTANCE

Light   Medium   Heavy

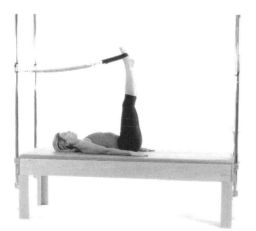

Inhale. Lie supine with the feet in the straps and the legs straight and together in a parallel position at an approximately 90-degree angle to the mat. Place the arms by the sides of the body or hold the poles with the shoulders relaxed.

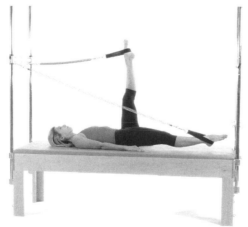

Exhale. Extend one leg, pressing it straight down toward the bed.

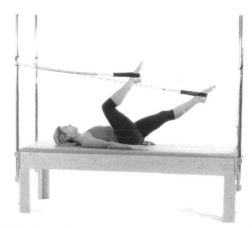

Inhale. Bend the extended leg in toward the chest, sliding the toes on or slightly above the bed and then straighten the leg toward the ceiling. Simultaneously extend the other leg straight down toward the mat, keeping tension in both springs throughout. After 10 repetitions, reverse the direction.

Muscle Focus

- Abdominals
- Hamstrings

Objectives

- To develop abdominal control
- To increase spinal mobility
- To improve flexibility of the hamstrings and calves

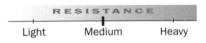

RESISTANCE

Light   Medium   Heavy

Monkey

This exercise, which focuses on spinal articulation and hamstring flexibility, serves as an excellent preparation for the next exercise in the series (Cadillac: Tower, page 222). It also introduces the deep pike position, which is used in many of the flexion exercises, particularly on the wunda chair (pages 250 to 252). Use the abdominals, followed by the back extensors, to reach the deep pike position: the arms are used only for support, like rods connecting the trunk and the push-through bar.

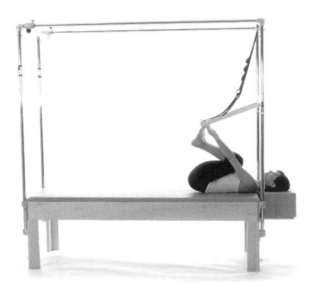

Inhale. Lie supine with the head facing the push-through bar. Place the toes on the bar with the hips directly under the feet. Hold the bar with the hands slightly wider apart than the feet. Strive to anchor the sacrum.

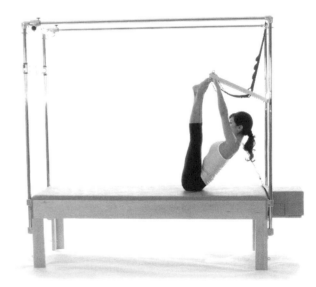

Exhale. Roll up through the spine into a pike position while straightening the knees and maintaining plantarflexion of the feet.

Imagery

The top phase of this exercise is reminiscent of a springboard diver's body folding into a tight pike position in the air. This powerful image will encourage the correct muscle recruitment and dynamic of this exercise and lay a solid foundation for all the exercises that use a similar position.

- ☐ Engage the abdominal muscles prior to the movement.
- ☐ Maintain plantarflexion while articulating up and down through the spine.
- ☐ Deepen the pike position when dorsiflexing.
- ☐ Keep the shoulders relaxed and the scapulae stabilized.

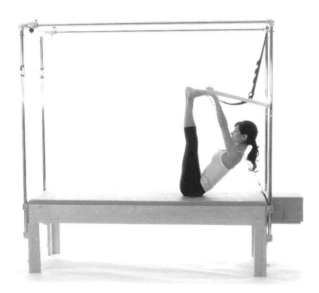

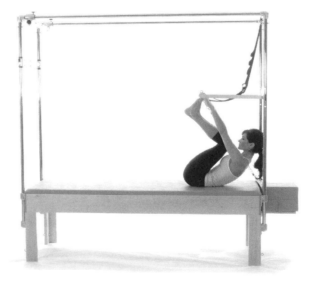

Inhale. Dorsiflex and plantarflex the feet, maintaining the deep pike position and keeping the shoulders relaxed.

Exhale. Roll down to the starting position, bending the knees.

Tower

Muscle Focus

- Abdominals
- Hamstrings

Objectives

- To develop spinal articulation
- To improve flexibility of the hamstrings and lower back muscles

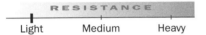

This exercise addresses spinal articulation as well as back and hamstring flexibility. It is a wonderfully satisfying and enjoyable exercise, however it must be approached with caution because of the loading of weight on the spine. To protect the spine, emphasize pushing away from the poles with straight arms. This alleviates excessive pressure on the spine, particularly the neck.

In addition, activate the back extensors together with the abdominals to support the trunk, especially when rolling up on the shoulders. This will help avoid sinking into the back and neck. When rolling down, focus on the eccentric contraction of the back extensors and maximize the stretch of the hamstrings and calves, particularly when the feet are dorsiflexed during the final phase. At this point the sacrum must be firmly anchored.

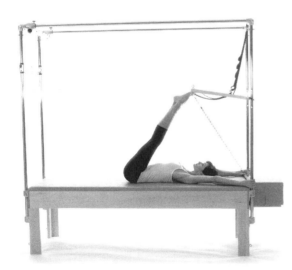

Exhale. Lie supine with the head facing the push-through bar. Reach the arms straight overhead to hold the poles. Place the toes on the push-through bar in a parallel position with the legs straight.

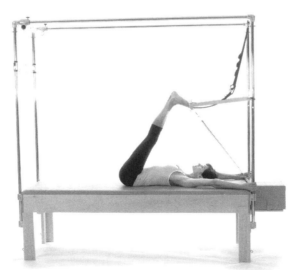

Inhale. Dorsiflex and plantarflex the feet.

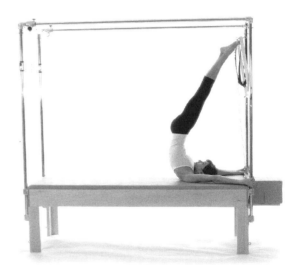

Exhale. Roll up, articulating the spine, onto the shoulder girdle.

Imagery

The image of an accordion opening and closing illustrates the opening, folding, and reopening of the body. This image relates more to the sensation of the movement than the physical positions of the exercise.

- ☐ Initiate the spinal articulation with activation of the abdominals and deep lumbar flexion.
- ☐ Engage the hip extensors and back extensors when up on the shoulders.
- ☐ Bend the knees moderately at the top without sinking into the spine and shoulders.

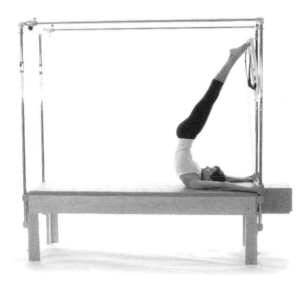

Inhale. Bend and straighten the knees, keeping the hip extensors engaged.

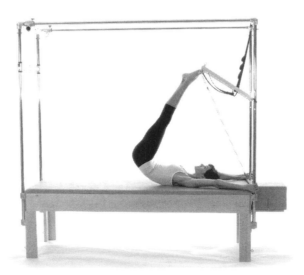

Exhale. Roll down through the spine to the starting position, anchoring the sacrum in the final phase.

Push-Through Sitting Forward

Push-through sitting forward nicely demonstrates the transition of the trunk from spinal flexion to spinal extension and vice versa. It also includes extension of the shoulders and their relationship to spinal flexion, a muscle recruitment pattern that appears in many Pilates exercises, particularly the abdominal ones. Along with the trunk work is the added benefit of a hamstring stretch, which is maximized by efficient, effective spinal extension. It truly is a full body integration exercise in every sense.

Muscle Focus

- Abdominal muscles
- Back extensors

Objectives

- To strengthen the abdominal muscles
- To develop back and shoulder extensor control
- To improve flexibility of the hamstrings

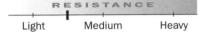

RESISTANCE

Light   Medium   Heavy

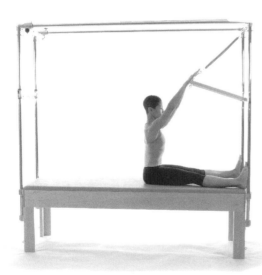

Inhale. Sit upright, facing the push-through bar, and press the feet against the poles. Hold the bar with the arms straight and shoulder-width apart.

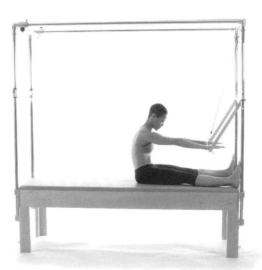

Exhale. Round the trunk, and then press the push-through bar down and through, leaning the body forward over the legs.

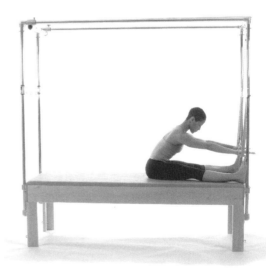

Inhale. Flatten the back on a diagonal, extending the spine.

Imagery

The backward and forward motion of the trunk and the control of the push-through bar always remind me of rowing a boat.

☐ Keep the arms straight throughout the exercise.

☐ Differentiate between the movement of the trunk and that of the arms.

☐ Press the heels against the upright poles of the cadillac throughout the exercise.

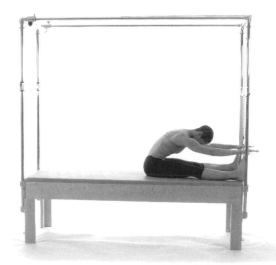

Exhale. Draw the trunk back into spinal flexion. Control the push-through bar while bringing it though and up, and maintaining the flexion of the trunk.

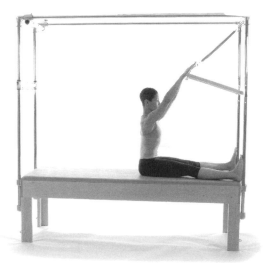

Inhale. Then extend the spine to the starting upright sitting position.

Cat Stretch

Muscle Focus

- Abdominal muscles
- Back extensors

Objectives

- To improve spinal articulation
- To improve shoulder flexibility
- To develop trunk stabilization

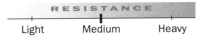

RESISTANCE

Light   Medium   Heavy

I perform this exercise when I want to spoil myself because it feels so good! The cat stretch fortifies the neutral alignment of the spine, both in an upright position and then in the more demanding forward-leaning position. The exercise requires both shoulder stability and flexibility. The shoulder-stretch position is challenging, and the stretch should be limited to the range in which you can comfortably maintain stability of the shoulders and trunk. Be careful not to hyperextend the back and place stress on the lumbar spine and the shoulders.

During the articulation of the spine when rolling down (at the beginning of the exercise) and rolling up (at the end), keep the body as close to the plumb line as possible.

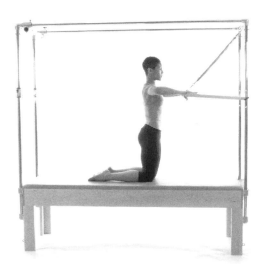

Inhale. Kneel facing the push-through bar. Hold the bar with hands shoulder-width apart and the arms bent, elbows reaching out to the sides.

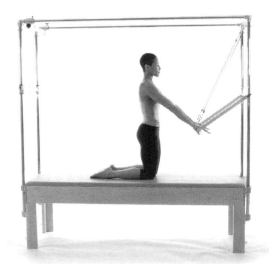

Exhale. Press the arms down, straightening the elbows.

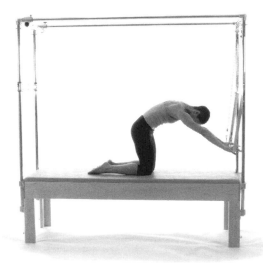

Continue exhaling, and roll down, articulating through the spine. Extend the trunk forward into a neutral spine position, parallel to the floor.

Imagery

The name says it all—stretch like a cat! The cat exemplifies immaculate spinal articulation and the quality of stretching out. Of course, it is important to establish control before you try to reach the more extreme ranges of catlike movement, but the image helps.

☐ Maintain abdominal support throughout the movement.

☐ Avoid thrusting the ribs forward during the shoulder stretch.

☐ Maintain scapular stability during the shoulder stretch.

☐ Align the spine in a neutral position in the initial phase and during the shoulder stretch.

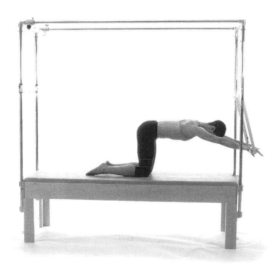

Inhale. Extend the trunk forward into a neutral spine position, parallel to the floor. Optional (if you feel secure and stable): Press the trunk down toward the bed, stretching the shoulders further toward shoulder flexion.

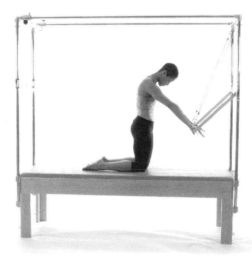

Exhale. Draw back into spinal flexion, articulating the spine as you return to the upright position. Bend the elbows and lift the arms to the starting position.

Standing Chest Expansion

Muscle Focus

- Latissimus dorsi

Objectives

- To strengthen shoulder extensors and elbow extensors
- To develop trunk stabilization

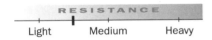

RESISTANCE

Light   Medium   Heavy

Relatively few exercises from the classic repertoire are performed in a standing upright position; therefore the ones that are should be fully utilized and integrated into a comprehensive program. They are very valuable, and I regard them as gems of the Pilates repertoire. The standing series not only develops arm and shoulder strength, flexibility, and control but also demands core strength and good posture and alignment. To intensify this exercise, develop balance, and increase the challenge, it can be performed on an unstable surface, such as a balance board or rotating disk, or while standing on one leg or standing farther away from the cadillac (increasing the resistance).

Imagery

This exercise is performed in different positions on various apparatus. Each position offers unique ben-efits and lends itself to different imagery, although the imagery from one can be used for any of the others. I like to visualize the body as a statue (think of Michelangelo's *David,* although he too has some alignment issues!) with one moving part, the glenohumeral joint. Feel the solidity of the structure and the intricate, controlled movement of the shoulder.

- ☐ Reach the arms down as if touching the fingertips to the floor.
- ☐ Minimize scapular movement.
- ☐ Engage the stabilizers of the trunk, maintaining correct alignment.
- ☐ Increase upper back extensor activation as the shoulders extend.

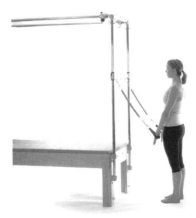

Inhale. Stand approximately 24 inches (60 centimeters) away from the cadillac, facing the apparatus, with the crossbar a little above shoulder height. Hold the handles with the palms facing back and slight tension in the springs. The farther away from the cadillac you stand, the more tension there is.

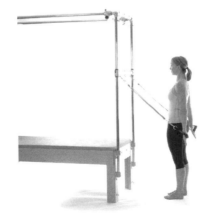

Exhale. Extend the shoulders, pressing the arms back while maintaining the upright alignment of the body.

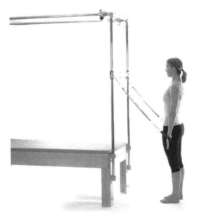

Inhale. Slowly return the arms to the starting position, keeping tension in the springs.

This exercise is similar to the reformer (page 175) and arm chair (page 296) versions and as with each variation, trunk stabilization is crucial. However, when standing the stabilization is taken a step further with the integration of the element of balance, and this makes the entire arms standing series particularly fascinating. Few exercises are better for discovering your *center*.

Lean forward just enough to counteract the pull of the springs backward, but not enough to rely on the springs for support or deviate from ideal alignment. Recruiting the ISS, particularly the abdominals, is vital in maintaining ideal alignment and is the essence of successful execution of this exercise.

Imagery

The image I offer here is a large bird spreading its wings. The arms spread like wings with the largest span possible, moving in and out. There are few sensations as wonderful as feeling centered, stable, and that you are soaring like an eagle.

- [ ] Keep the back broad and the scapulae stabilized.
- [ ] Lean slightly forward throughout the series while maintaining ideal posture and alignment.
- [ ] Keep the arms elongated with the elbows soft and the fingers reaching out.

Muscle Focus

- Pectoralis major

Objectives

- To strengthen and increase flexibility in the shoulder horizontal adductors
- To develop trunk and scapular stabilization

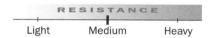

RESISTANCE

Light   Medium   Heavy

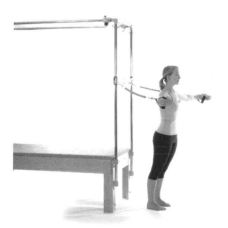

Inhale. Stand approximately 12 inches (30 centimeters) away from the cadillac, with the back to the apparatus and the crossbar a little above shoulder height. The farther away from the cadillac you stand, the greater the resistance; adjust accordingly. Lean slightly forward with the body and engage the abdominal muscles. Reach the arms out to the sides, holding the handles, with the hands either open or in a fist position. The elbows should be soft and the hands facing forward, with slight tension in the springs.

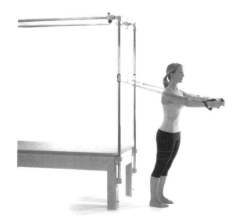

Exhale. Bring the arms toward each other until they are parallel and in line with the shoulders.

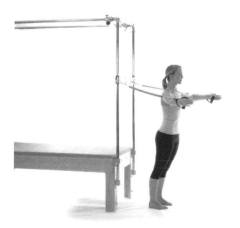

Inhale. Return to the starting position, maintaining some tension in the springs. Utilize the eccentric contraction of the horizontal adductors of the shoulders, keeping the scapulae still and maximizing the stretch across the front of the chest.

Standing Arm Circles

Muscle Focus

- Shoulder extensors
- Shoulder horizontal adductors

Objectives

- To develop control of the scapulae
- To strengthen the shoulders
- To increase the range of motion of the shoulders
- To develop trunk stabilization

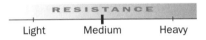

RESISTANCE

Light   Medium   Heavy

The arm circles highlight control and range of motion of the shoulder complex. It is an extension of the hug-a-tree exercise (page 229), performed in the same unique balanced position, but rather than executing only horizontal adduction before returning to the starting position, the arms circle overhead and back around to the T position and then circle in the opposite direction. The standing arm circles resemble the Arm Chair: Circles (page 297), which I recommend learning as a preparation for this exercise, but the arm chair provides support for the body while the cadillac relies on the body's ability to support itself. This is the essence of progression in many Pilates exercises: The movements become more challenging as a higher level of stabilization and internal support is required.

Imagery

Imagine the arms moving through a thick gel—not thick enough to create tension, but sufficient to provide a sense of equal resistance at every point of the circle.

- ☐ Face the palms toward the floor as the arms move from directly in front to overhead.
- ☐ Keep the circles within peripheral vision.
- ☐ Avoid elevating the scapulae as the arms rise above shoulder height.

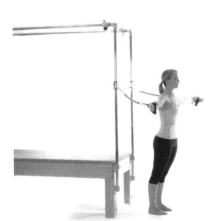

Inhale. Stand approximately 12 inches (30 centimeters) away from the cadillac, with the back to the apparatus and the crossbar a little above shoulder height. Step farther away or closer in to adjust the resistance according to your need. Lean slightly forward and engage the abdominals. Reach the arms out to the sides at shoulder height, with the palms facing forward, elbows soft, and slight tension in the springs.

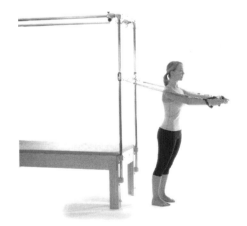

Exhale. Bring the arms toward each other, stopping when they are in line with the shoulders, with palms facing each other, as in the hug-a-tree (page 229).

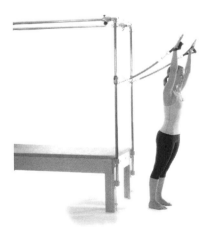

Inhale. Rotate the arms so that the palms face the floor, and lift the arms overhead. Keeping the scapulae stable, circle the arms out to the sides to the T position, with the palms facing forward (starting position). After 5 to 10 repetitions reverse the direction.

Standing Arm Punches

Besides the obvious element of developing arm strength, this movement demands tremendous trunk stabilization because of the tendency to rotate with each punch. Once a high degree of stabilization has been achieved, you can add trunk rotation to the punches, rotating with the straightening of each arm.

Imagery

As the name indicates, this movement should feel like punching. Imagine a precise point in front of you, in line with the shoulder; the hand reaches this same point with each punch.

☐ Start with tension in the springs.

☐ Focus the movement in the arms while the trunk and shoulder girdle remain still.

☐ Face the fingers toward the direction of the movement throughout the exercise.

☐ Move the arms on a horizontal line.

Muscle Focus

▪ Triceps
▪ Pectoralis major

Objectives

▪ To strengthen the elbow extensors and shoulder horizontal adductors
▪ To develop core strength

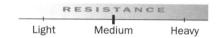

RESISTANCE

Light   Medium   Heavy

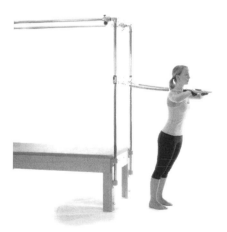

Inhale. Stand approximately 12 inches (30 centimeters) away from the cadillac, with the back to the apparatus and the crossbar a little above shoulder height. Lean slightly forward, placing the hands directly in front of the shoulders. Bend the elbows out to the sides while holding the handles with the palms facing downward and the fingers forward.

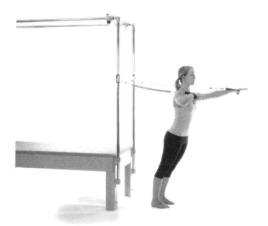

Exhale. Straighten one arm in a forward direction, then bend it as the other arm simultaneously straightens; the change should occur midway through the movement.

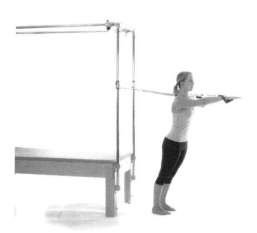

Inhale. Repeat the cycle, performing two to four punches with each breath.

231

Standing Biceps

Muscle Focus

- Biceps

Objectives

- To strengthen the elbow flexors
- To stretch the anterior aspect of the chest and shoulder

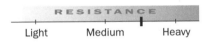

RESISTANCE

Light   Medium   Heavy

Although this movement is essentially a typical biceps curl, the position of the arms and trunk offer certain advantages. A significant stretch can be felt across the chest, a benefit after all of the work of the shoulder horizontal adductor that preceded it (hug-a-tree, arm circles, and punches, pages 229-231). In addition, the long head of the biceps is held in a fully stretched position, which enhances flexibility and provides a unique angle for developing strength. Step forward, if necessary, to increase the resistance and keep tension in the springs.

Imagery

The position of the body can be likened to the figure-head of an old ship. With each bend of the arms, the chest should open more. The feeling should be one of reaching the chest forward (without thrusting the ribs and hyperextending the back).

- ☐ Maintain constant and consistent shoulder extension.
- ☐ Keep the upper arms still and the scapulae stable throughout the movement.
- ☐ Keep the elbows parallel to each other.

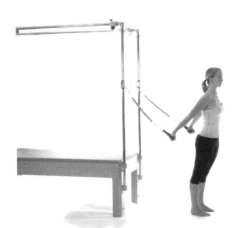

Inhale. Stand approximately 48 inches (120 centimeters) away from the cadillac, with the back to the apparatus and the crossbar a little above shoulder height. Lean slightly forward and reach the arms behind the body, parallel to each other. Hold the handles firmly.

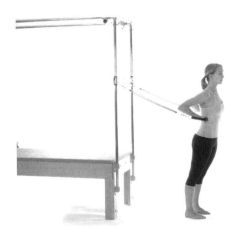

Exhale. Bend the elbows, keeping the upper arms still and the elbows at the same height as in the starting position.

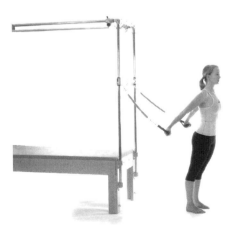

Inhale. Straighten the arms and return to the starting position.

Although this squat does challenge the legs, it presents even more challenge for the upper body. Also, the trunk is held in an upright position, rather than the typical forward tilt, throughout the movement, encouraging neutral alignment and making it more functional. The conventional squat position can place an excessive load on the lower back.

Adding the isometric contraction of the biceps to the squat action of the legs not only develops biceps strength but also core strength, particularly of the back extensors. While I've included this exercise in arm work as it addresses many areas of the body, it is a valuable addition to any program and can comfortably fit into the leg work, hip work, or full-body integration blocks.

Imagery

Maintain a good position of the trunk by imagining that you are leaning against a wall as the body slides up and down. Track the legs by picturing each one gliding between two panes of glass, making sure they are properly aligned to accommodate a smooth gliding movement.

☐ Keep the trunk upright in a neutral spine position.

☐ Hold the arms parallel to each other with the palms facing toward the ceiling (or toward the face when the elbows are in flexion).

☐ Maintain correct tracking of the legs as they bend and straighten.

Muscle Focus

- Biceps
- Quadriceps

Objective

- To strengthen the biceps and quadriceps
- To develop stability in the knees
- To align and stabilize the trunk

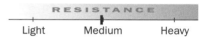

RESISTANCE

Light   Medium   Heavy

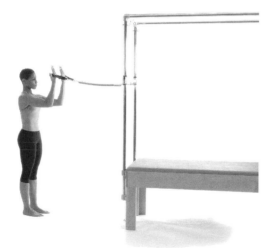

Exhale. Stand facing the cadillac with the legs parallel. Bend the elbows to a 90-degree angle, holding the straps in a biceps-curl position with slight tension in the springs.

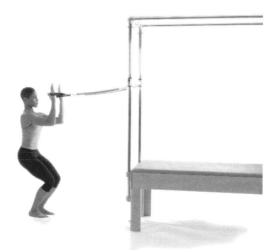

Inhale. Bend the knees into a deep squat, keeping the heels on the ground and maintaining a stable arm and trunk position.

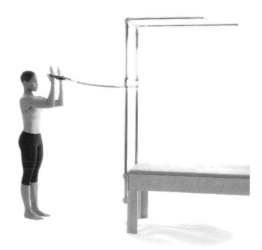

Exhale. Straighten the knees, returning to the starting position. Perform 5-10 squats and straighten the arms only after the final repetition.

Butterfly

Muscle Focus

- Oblique abdominal muscles

Objectives

- To stretch the oblique abdominals and lower and mid-back muscles
- To develop control of the oblique abdominals

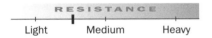

This complex movement with a beautiful name is a combination of lateral flexion and rotation that also makes use of the resistance of springs and the element of balance. The movement should be viewed in two distinct phases: lateral flexion, followed by rotation. This pattern can be found in several advanced Pilates exercises such as Mat Work: Twist (page 98), as well as in many sports, such as golf, volleyball, and baseball.

In the first phase, the movement is pure lateral flexion of the trunk with no arm movement. The arms maintain an exact T position, resisting the backward pull of the springs. This is followed by the rotation of the trunk, and only at the point of maximum rotation do the arms circle around to reach the T position facing the cadillac. The movement is then reversed to return to the starting position.

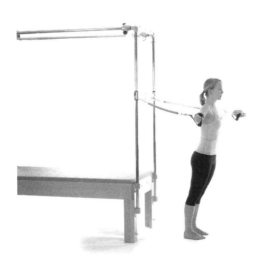

Exhale. Stand approximately 12 inches (30 centimeters) away from the cadillac, with the back to the apparatus and the crossbar a little above shoulder height. Lean forward with the hands in the straps, the arms in a T position, and the palms facing forward with slight tension in the springs.

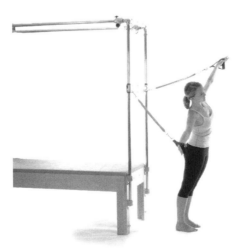

Inhale. Reach over to one side, laterally flexing the trunk.

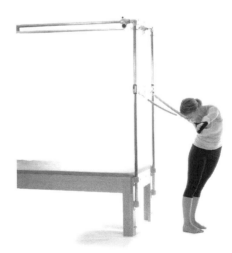

Exhale. Rotate and round the upper body to face the cadillac, bringing the top arm up and over and the other arm down and across, striving to create a T position while now facing the cadillac. The arms continue pulling the springs out to the sides and back.

Imagery

The feeling of this movement is like a spring being wound up and then carefully unwound, similar to the dynamic of the Reformer: Mermaid (page 198). These two exercises are closely related; finding the connection between them may prove valuable in mastering both of these challenging exercises. Another image I like to use is that of the exercise name, the butterfly. As the arms reach out to the sides throughout the exercise, they should feel like wings.

☐ Keep the pelvis facing forward as long as possible before allowing it to adapt to the rotation.

☐ Maintain constant tension in the springs.

☐ Keep the arms as wide as possible throughout.

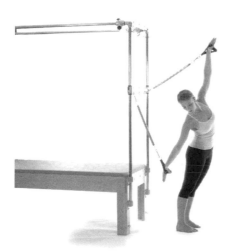

Inhale. Return to lateral flexion, following the exact path of the body and arms in reverse.

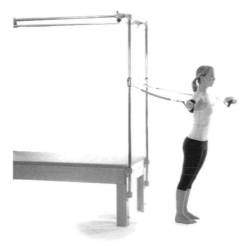

Exhale. Return to the starting position.

Side Lift

This exercise is not from the classic Pilates repertoire, but it has evolved from the traditional work. It has a wonderful flow, and besides being a valuable exercise for developing the lateral flexors of the trunk, it is beautiful to watch and wonderful to perform.

Although ideally the body is in a straight line, it may be necessary to place the legs slightly forward of the centerline, which in turn emphasizes activation of the oblique abdominal muscles. This is helpful when the back extensors, particularly the quadratus lumborum, tend to overpower the other muscles. The same result can be achieved by tipping the upper side of the pelvis slightly back.

People tend to try to lift the body by pulling on the push-through bar with the arm. Avoid this by keeping the arm straight and focusing on lifting from the waist. Complete the movement by lifting the bottom arm to the push-through bar (or as close to it as possible) and touching it. This provides a dramatic stretch to the underside of the body and works the lateral flexors on the upper side intensely. The lateral flexors on the underside should remain contracted throughout the exercise to provide stability.

Muscle Focus

- Oblique abdominal muscles

Objectives

- To strengthen the lateral flexors (upper side)
- To stretch the lateral flexors (lower side)

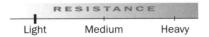

RESISTANCE

Light   Medium   Heavy

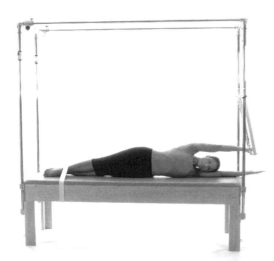

Exhale. Lie on one side with the legs straight and the top leg in front of the bottom leg. Place the feet under the foot strap. The bottom arm is straight overhead with the head resting on the shoulder. The top arm is also straight overhead, holding the push-through bar.

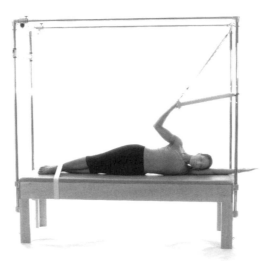

Inhale. Bend the top arm, bringing the push-through bar through to the inside of the cadillac.

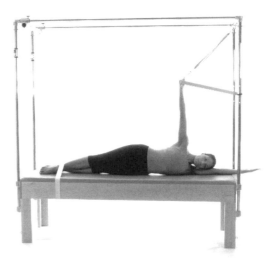

Still inhaling, straighten the top arm upward.

Imagery

This movement always reminds me of dance choreography. I like to imagine flying through the air after a leap, reaching up or out, depending on the phase of the exercise. If only we could fly!

☐ Keep the arm holding the push-through bar straight when lifting into lateral flexion.

☐ Engage the abdominal muscles throughout the exercise.

☐ Move up and down in the coronal plane as if between two panes of glass.

Maintain as close to a straight line as can be achieved without compromising balanced muscle activation.

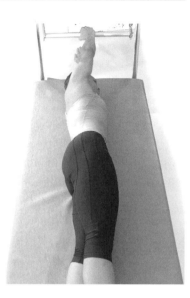

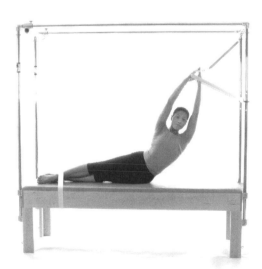

Exhale. Lift the trunk into lateral flexion. Then lift the bottom arm to touch, or to come as close as possible to touching, the push-through bar.

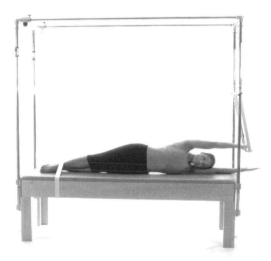

Inhale. Lower the body, then exhale as you bend the upper arm, bringing the push-through bar through to the outside of cadillac, and straighten it overhead. Return to the starting position.

Side Reach

Muscle Focus

- Oblique abdominal muscles

Objectives

- To develop abdominal control
- To improve oblique flexibility
- To stretch the shoulder adductors

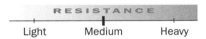

RESISTANCE

Light　　Medium　　Heavy

Few exercises feel as good as this one. It provides a focused stretch to one side of the trunk and the underarm. Maintaining a good anchor with the legs and pelvis in order to maximize the stretch is vital. This is a unique position because the pelvic–lumbar region remains in flexion to reinforce the anchoring of the pelvis, while the upper trunk stretches laterally and extends, displaying the control we strive for in each segment of the spine and the body as a whole.

Imagery

The movement should be a sweeping action out to the side and back as the body opens like a large fan. Or think of the body as a rubber band that is being stretched by an external force pulling on the arm; when the force is removed, it is pulled back to the center.

- ☐ Maintain pelvic–lumbar stabilization when reaching the arm back.
- ☐ Press both heels against the upright poles, particularly the one on the reaching side.
- ☐ Turn the palm of the free hand toward the ceiling while reaching back.

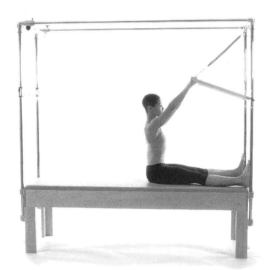

Inhale. Sit upright, facing the push-through bar. Place your feet against the upright poles and the hands on the push-through bar, shoulder-width apart. Keep the arms straight.

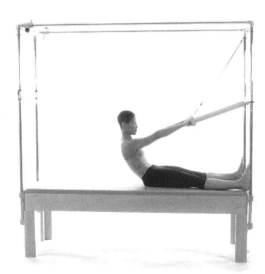

Exhale. Round the trunk, hanging back on the push-through bar and pressing the feet into the upright poles.

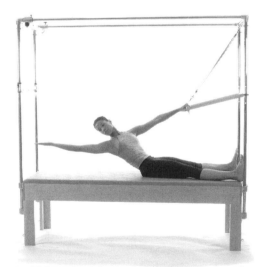

Inhale. While maintaining lumbar flexion, sweep one hand, palm up, out to the side and back, reaching as far from the feet as possible and maximizing the stretch. Exhale and return to the previous position, deepening the flexion and placing the hand back on the bar. Inhale and extend the spine to the upright sitting position.

Prone I is the foundation of a wonderful series of back extension exercises on the cadillac. This exercise teaches the fundamentals of distributing the extension throughout the spine by recruiting the spinal extensors together with the abdominals, which assists in protecting the lower back from excessive pressure. It also teaches coordination of scapular stabilization and shoulder mechanics along with spinal extension.

Imagery

The image of an archer's bow being stretched and then released works well to create the powerful, arching shape of the body. The energy is never completely released; the power is held within the musculature at all times, available on demand.

☐ Glide the scapulae down the back prior to the movement.

☐ Engage the abdominal muscles throughout the movement.

☐ Keep the hands pressing down on the push-through bar, with the arms straight.

Muscle Focus

▪ Back extensors

Objectives:

▪ To strengthen the back extensors
▪ To develop control of the shoulder girdle and abdominal muscles

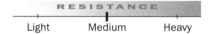

RESISTANCE

Light   Medium   Heavy

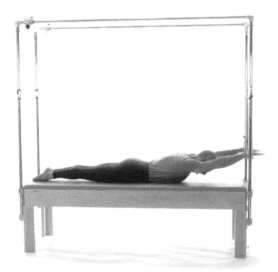

Exhale. Lie prone, holding the push-through bar with the arms straight overhead.

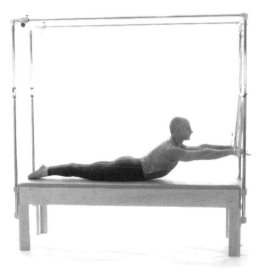

Inhale. Lift the trunk into spinal extension, pressing the arms down gently on the push-through bar.

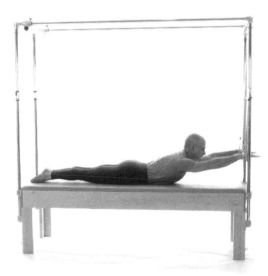

Exhale. Lower the trunk to the starting position without releasing the supporting musculature between repetitions.

Prone II

Muscle Focus

- Back extensors

Objectives

- To strengthen the back extensors
- To develop control of the shoulder and abdominal muscles
- To improve flexibility in the shoulder region

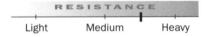

RESISTANCE

Light   Medium   Heavy

Few exercises combine spinal extension as beautifully and intricately with the strength and flexibility of the shoulder girdle. Stretching the shoulders as much as possible before extending the back is important; although the shoulder stretch and the back extension are linked, they should be regarded as two separate movements. When the trunk reaches full hyperextension, the effort is transferred largely to the back exten-sors, not relying on the arms and the push-through bar to maintain the elevation of the trunk.

When you reverse the movement, again maximize the stretch of the shoulders (you should feel like you are hanging from the arms) before lowering the body completely and bringing the push-through bar down to the starting position.

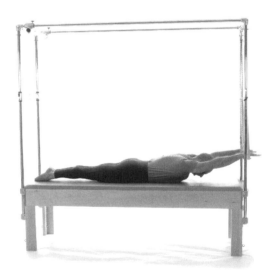

Exhale. Lie prone holding the push-through bar with the arms straight overhead.

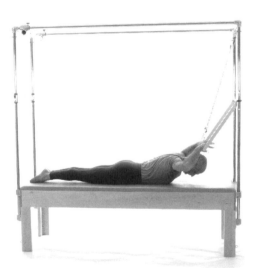

Inhale. Bend the elbows out to the sides, bringing the arms back and behind the head.

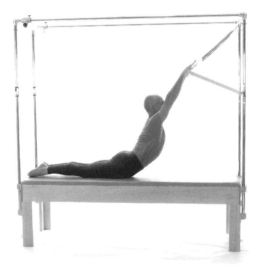

Exhale. When the arms can move no further, start lifting the trunk and continue by straightening the arms upward until the elbows and back are fully extended.

Imagery

The image of stretching a bow (see Cadillac: Prone I) serves well in this variation as the body reaches a higher, more extreme bow shape.

☐ Achieve maximum stretch of the shoulders before lifting the trunk into extension.

☐ In the second part of the exercise, lower the trunk as far as possible, stretching the shoulders, before bringing the arms through to complete the movement.

☐ Engage the abdominal muscles throughout the movement.

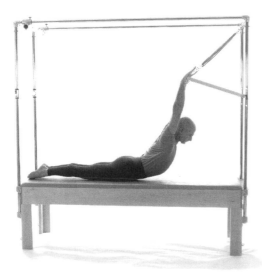

Inhale. Lower the trunk, keeping the arms straight and reaching up.

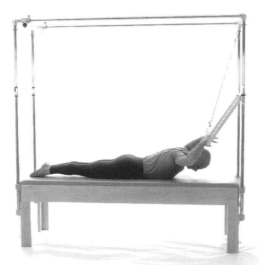

Exhale. Bend the elbows and lower the trunk, bringing the push-through bar down, then straighten the arms directly overhead to return to the starting position.

Muscle Focus

- Back extensors

Objectives

- To strengthen the back extensors
- To stretch the chest muscles
- To develop hip extensor control

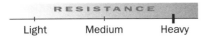

RESISTANCE

Light   Medium   Heavy

Hanging Back

This exercise is impressive to watch and fun to do. Although categorized as an advanced exercise, it is within the reach of many people, even those who may not believe they can perform such a challenging movement. It encapsulates fundamental concepts such as spinal articulation, well-distributed back extension, scapular stabilization, abdominal support, and the relationship between back extension and hip extension.

I like to focus this movement in the mid-back, just below and between the scapulae. You should stabilize the pelvic–lumbar region until you have achieved maximum thoracic extension and only then add lumbar extension and further hip extension to provide the finishing touches to the movement.

The arms serve as levers; they simply connect the body to the crossbars. The shoulders, however, fulfill an important role; good shoulder mechanics are critical to successful execution of this exercise.

The position of the head follows the line of the spine. Avoid the tendency to throw the head back too far when in the hanging-back position, which results in neck tension. Instead, you should feel like the crown of the head is reaching down toward the mat, completing the smooth, arcing shape.

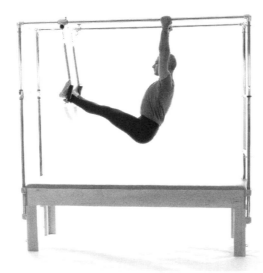

Inhale. Hold onto the crossbars of the cadillac with straight arms. Place the feet on the trapeze swing in a turned-out, dorsiflexed position so that they wrap around the springs (for safety). Hold the spine in as close to a neutral position as possible while hanging.

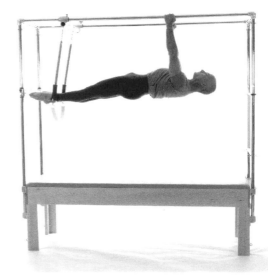

Exhale. Roll up, articulating through the spine, into a plank position so that the body hangs parallel to the mat in neutral alignment. Plantarflexing the feet is optional.

Imagery

Visualizing energy lines works well for this exercise. In the cradle-hanging position, one energy line runs down through the legs and the other through the trunk, both meeting in the pelvis, creating a V shape. In the hanging-back position, the energy line runs from the feet to the pelvis, then arcs through the trunk and head, reinforcing the arc shape of the body.

☐ Reach the tailbone toward the mat when hanging in the starting position.

☐ Depress the scapulae in the hanging position prior to starting the movement.

☐ Draw in the abdominals, creating deep spinal flexion, to initiate the movement.

☐ Achieve maximum extension in the mid- and upper back before using lumbar and hip extension to complete the movement.

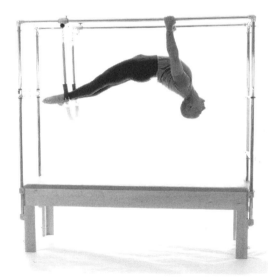

Inhale. Extend the spine further, maximizing the arch of the thoracic region. Add lumbar and hip extension, pivoting at the shoulders and keeping the arms straight.

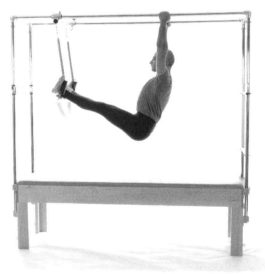

Exhale. Return to the plank position, and then articulate the spine down to the V shape starting position.

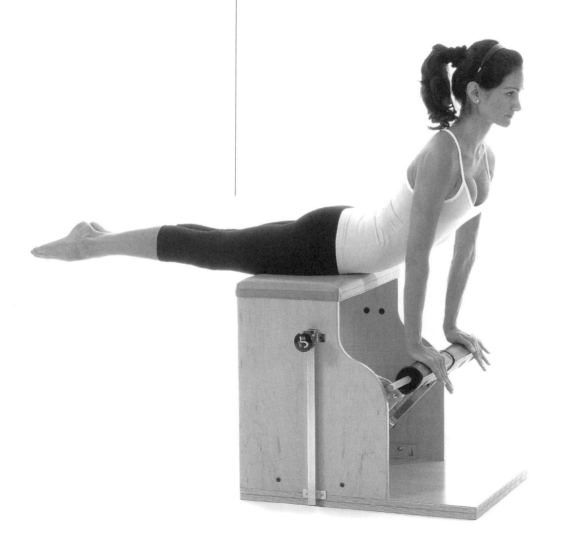

CHAPTER 7

Wunda Chair

I must admit, I have special feelings for the wunda chair (also known simply as *the chair*)—if I do have a favorite piece of Pilates equipment, this is it. The genius of its design never ceases to amaze me. This unassuming box with four springs offers infinite possibilities. It was arguably the first piece of home gym equipment, displayed proudly by Joseph Pilates in what looks like the first infomercial, yet even today there are few if any pieces of equipment that can rival the wunda chair's capacity: there are hundreds of exercises for every part of the body and every fitness level. And to cap it all, it can double as a piece of furniture (as the original design did).

The chair is not easy to use, and it often proves unforgiving. It highlights imbalances and weaknesses like no other piece of apparatus. At the same time it offers possibilities for dealing with these problems that are unique and specific to the chair only. It is also well suited for improving general fitness and enhancing athletic performance. In many ways it is more functional than other exercise equipment, even other pieces of Pilates apparatus. When doing the foot work on the chair, for instance, the body is in an upright position, demanding greater activation of the trunk stabilizers than the reformer or cadillac. Being upright also more closely simulates everyday movements, making the exercises more functional. It is extremely useful for pregnant women because it enables them to do the foot work in a sitting rather than supine position. (Lying supine for extended periods of time during pregnancy is not recommended.)

However, because of its design, the movements performed on the chair are typically short in range; it does not readily accommodate full ranges of motion. In some cases it may even prove advantageous to use pads or a small box to elevate the body and increase the range of motion. Also, the chair offers far fewer possibilities for developing flexion of the limbs than for extension. As long as you are aware of these possible shortcomings, the wunda chair is simply a must-have item.

I had the privilege of being introduced to the wonders of the chair by one of the greatest Pilates teachers to grace our community, Kathy Stanford Grant. She was among Mr. Pilates' early students, and one of only two people to receive a teacher's certification from him. (The other is Lolita San Miguel, also a teacher of great distinction and one I am honored to call a friend, who has the title of a Living Treasure of Puerto Rico.) Kathy may be singularly responsible for the rebirth of this apparatus, bringing it from obscurity to center stage in the early nineties.

I recall as if it were yesterday the day I met Kathy and I naively volunteered to perform several moves on the chair. I had some experience on this apparatus and had been doing Pilates for 12 years. Kathy, a woman small in stature and large in presence, honed in on every compensation, protection, tension, and imbalance in my body. If I have ever had an epiphany in my career, this was it. I recognized a depth of work that I had previously ignored. I had relied on a strong body to perform choreography well—but that was only the outside of the movement. My humbling experience on the chair taught me the meaning of moving from within and set my teaching on a new, exciting tangent. I had to go back to square one, learning and exploring every movement anew. It also taught me to see inside people with "MRI vision" (beyond X-ray vision!), to detect where the movement is coming from before it even happens. This awareness taught me to cue differently, to teach differently, and to anticipate more profound results. I have never looked back.

The double-leg foot work on the wunda chair, as on the cadillac, duplicates that on the reformer. The foot positions are identical (see Reformer: Parallel Heels, Parallel Toes, V-Position Toes, Open V-Position Heels, and Open V-Position Toes on pages 112 to 116) while the positions of the trunk and legs are quite different—the trunk is upright and the legs push down toward the floor on the wunda chair.

The dynamic of the leg movement on the chair is like a pumping action, with a relatively short range of motion compared to the full-range knee extension on the reformer and cadillac. On the wunda chair, feeling the quadriceps more prominently is common; I refer to this as having "wunda chair legs," a delightful, wobbly sensation on completion of the series.

Rather than detailing all the foot work positions, I describe only the double-foot positions, calf raises, and single-foot positions (see pages 248 to 249).

Many of the same cues and directives that are noted in the foot work on the reformer and cadillac apply to the chair.

Imagery

On the cadillac the feeling is like supporting the ceiling, with the legs as pillars; on the reformer it is propelling yourself on a horizontal line by pushing away a wall. On the wunda chair the feeling is like pressing against the floor, becoming taller with each leg extension, to the point of feeling levitated above the chair.

☐ Maintain a stable, upright trunk throughout the series.

☐ Push down through the heels when in the heel positions.

☐ Maintain plantarflexion when in the toe positions.

Muscle Focus

- Quadriceps
- Hamstrings

Objectives

- To strengthen the knee extensors
- To develop hip extensor control
- To develop trunk and pelvic stabilization

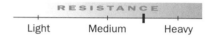

RESISTANCE

Light   Medium   Heavy

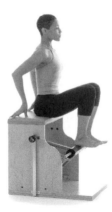 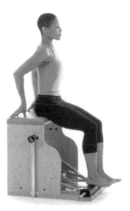 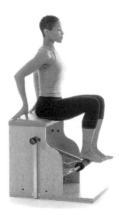

Inhale. Sit upright on the chair on the front part of the platform, hands near the rear of the platform resting on the fingertips, with elbows bent and reaching back. Place the feet on the pedal in one of the double-foot positions. Start the movement with the thighs parallel to the floor or slightly higher.

Exhale. Press down with the legs, lowering the pedal until it is about to touch the base.

Inhale. Lift the legs, raising the pedal to the starting position.

Calf Raises

Muscle Focus

- Foot plantarflexors (calves)

Objectives

- To strengthen the calves
- To stretch the calves and hip flexors

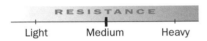

RESISTANCE

Light   Medium   Heavy

This position exemplifies the concept of multidimensional, full-body integration. Although the calf of the moving leg is the focus of the exercise, trunk stability is being challenged, the hip flexors and calf of the opposite leg are being stretched, and even the shoulder stabilizers are being activated. This position is exceptional for highlighting correct foot alignment.

Imagery

The diagonal position of the body in this exercise reminds me of a ski jumper flying down the ramp.

Add to this powerful image the completely isolated movement of the foot.

- ☐ Maintain a level pelvis.
- ☐ Keep the legs parallel rather than externally rotated, with the back heel pressing into the floor.
- ☐ Control the up-and-down movement of the foot through the full range of motion of the ankle.

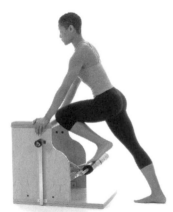

Inhale. Stand facing the chair with the trunk stable on a diagonal line, and place the hands firmly on the sides of the front section of the platform. Place the toes of one foot on the pedal, pressing the leg just below the knee into the front edge of the platform. The back leg is straight, creating a long diagonal line with the trunk, and the heel presses into the floor.

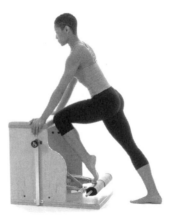

Exhale. Plantarflex the foot, lowering the pedal.

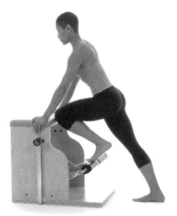

Inhale. Dorsiflex the foot, raising the pedal.

Single-Foot Positions

All of the advantages and benefits of doing single-leg work on the other apparatus apply to the wunda chair but are magnified. Stabilization is challenging in the sitting position, and every possible weakness, imbalance, and compensation is brought to the fore. Few pieces of apparatus, if any, are as valuable as the wunda chair for developing and improving leg function.

Imagery

See Reformer: Single-Leg Heel and Single-Leg Toes (pages 119 and 120). Also valuable is imagining a movement similar to kick-starting a motorcycle (something I have done many times, but you may need to be a little older to appreciate this image) while keeping the rest of the body stable.

☐ Maintain equal weight on both sit bones.
☐ Start with the thighs parallel to the floor or slightly higher, and press down until the pedal is about to touch the base.
☐ Keep the trunk stable, avoiding rotation as the leg presses down.

Muscle Focus

- Quadriceps
- Hamstrings

Objectives

- To strengthen the knee extensors
- To develop hip extensor control
- To develop trunk and pelvic stabilization

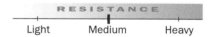

Light   Medium   Heavy

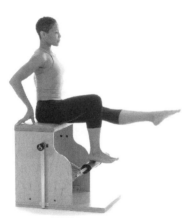

Inhale. Sit upright on the chair on the front part of the platform, with the hands placed near the rear of the platform, resting on the fingertips, and the elbows bent and reaching back. Place one foot on the pedal in either the single-leg heel or toes position. Hold the opposite leg directly forward, parallel to the floor. If this position proves too difficult, bend the knee or rest the leg on a large ball or box.

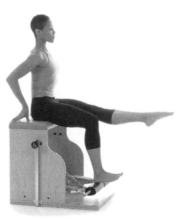

Exhale. Press down with the leg, lowering the pedal.

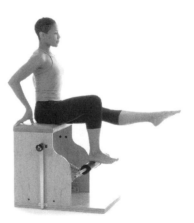

Inhale. Lift the leg, raising the pedal to the starting position.

Muscle Focus

- Abdominal muscles

Objectives

- To develop abdominal control
- To develop scapular stabilization
- To increase lumbar flexibility

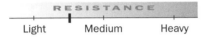

RESISTANCE

Light   Medium   Heavy

Standing Pike

The movement of this exercise is similar to the Mat Work: Roll-Down described on page 24, but it has the advantage of support provided by the spring. This alleviates potential strain on the spine during the roll-down, particularly when it is done with straight knees. This fundamental exercise lays the foundation for the abdominal exercises that follow, which are progressively more advanced and challenging. It teaches the pike position, which relies on deep flexion of the trunk and solid shoulder stabilization.

Imagery

All the spinal flexion pike exercises (and there are many, on all the apparatus) center on the image of folding the body in two, bringing the thighs and pelvis toward the trunk and vice versa. A diver in mid-flight, tucked into a pike position, is the perfect image.

- ☐ Aim for maximum lumbar flexion.
- ☐ Stabilize the scapulae.
- ☐ Keep the legs vertical and the knees soft.

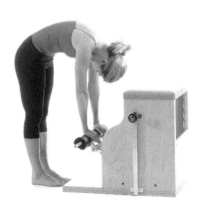

Exhale. Stand facing the chair, close to the front of it, with the legs parallel. Roll down, placing the hands on the pedal with the shoulders aligned over the hands.

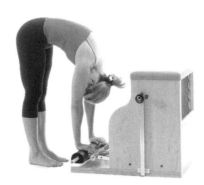

Inhale. Roll down, pressing the pedal toward the floor.

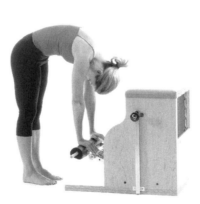

Exhale. Roll up, increasing the spinal flexion and raising the pedal. Repeat 5 to 10 times.

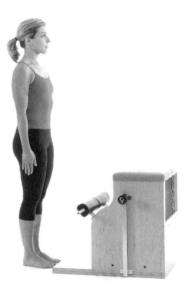

On the final exhalation, roll up all the way to the starting standing position.

Cat Stretch

The cat stretch is one of a series of exercises, including the Wunda Chair: Standing Pike (page 250) and the Wunda Chair: Full Pike (page 252), that focuses on deep spinal flexion. It also incorporates spinal extension and demonstrates the fine interplay between spinal flexion and extension. During the spinal extension, reach the head toward the floor and aim for 180-degree flexion of the shoulders, creating as close to a vertical line as possible with the trunk. At the same time, try to keep the hips over the knees so that the thighs remain vertical, which will help ensure that the movement occurs in the spine as opposed to rocking back and forth with the whole body. This will encourage the deep, hollow, round shape of the trunk as the pedal is lifted.

Imagery

The name says it all—the shape, the intricate articulation of the spine, the flexibility, the control—there is no better image to strive for than a cat stretching.

☐ Align the hips over the knees throughout the movement.

☐ Keep the head aligned with the spine.

☐ Reach the head down toward the pedal.

Muscle Focus

- Abdominal muscles
- Back extensors

Objectives

- To develop abdominal and back extensor control
- To stretch the lower back
- To develop scapular stabilization

RESISTANCE

Light　　Medium　　Heavy

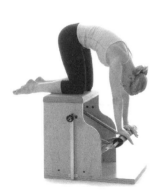

Exhale. Kneel on the chair close to the front edge facing the pedal, with the body upright and the hips over the knees. Roll down, placing the hands on the pedal, with the shoulders aligned over the hands.

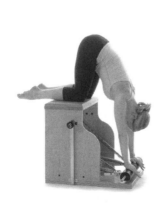

Inhale. Roll down, pressing the pedal toward the floor, extending the spine and keeping the head between the arms. Exhaling, roll up, rounding the trunk into deep spinal flexion, keeping the hips above the knees and raising the pedal (as shown in first photo in series). Repeat 5 to 10 times.

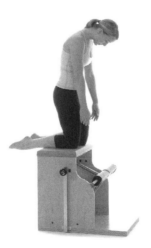

On a final exhale, roll up all the way to an upright kneeling position.

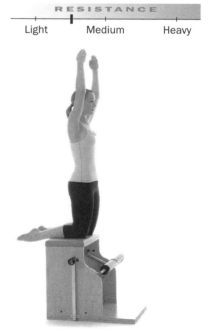

Circle the arms overhead and around to the sides of the body, returning to the starting position.

Full Pike

Muscle Focus

- Abdominal muscles
- Serratus anterior

Objectives

- To develop abdominal control
- To develop scapular stabilization
- To strengthen the shoulder girdle

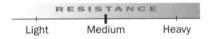

RESISTANCE

Light　　Medium　　Heavy

Few exercises exemplify masterful muscle coordination and integration better than the full pike. And few exercises can humble the fittest and strongest human specimens as the full pike can. You must perform it to understand how profound it is. Viewing from the sidelines simply does not impart full appreciation of its intensity, but those who attempt it will never look back. If one exercise can guide you to discover the sensation of working deep into the abdominals, this is it. The abdominal work is profound and often leads to a sensation of muscle activation never before experienced. Layered on top of the abdominal work is the intense shoulder work, which can be likened to performing a handstand. The influence gymnastics had on the development of the Pilates repertoire is evident in the full pike. This is a personal favorite!

Imagery

See the Wunda Chair: Standing Pike (page 250) for body-alignment information. In this exercise, the sensation should be of floating upward—levitating—a feeling that can be achieved only when all components, both mental and physical, are in place.

☐ Maximize lumbar flexion.
☐ Keep the shoulders over the hands and the head aligned with the spine.
☐ Maintain stable plantarflexion of the feet.

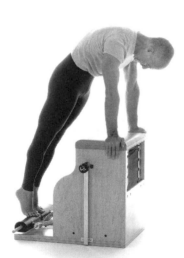

Inhale. Stand on the pedal, facing the chair. Place the hands on the back portion of the chair, holding it from the sides. Align the shoulders over the hands. Keep the scapulae stable and round the trunk, establishing a solid pike position.

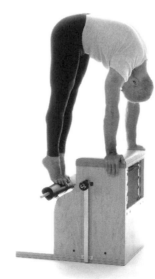

Exhale. Draw deeper into spinal flexion, raising the pedal to the top of its range.

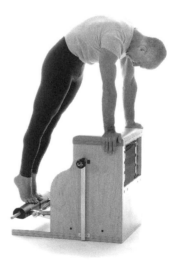

Inhale. Lower the pedal (not quite to the floor), maintaining the pike position.

Seated Torso Press

With the legs stable and still, and the trunk a solid integrated unit, the movement in this exercise occurs at the hip joint. Control of the hip flexors is important, but the focus of the effort should be on the abdominals and back extensors working in co-contraction to keep the trunk stable. This exercise demands a high level of precision and coordinated muscle activation. It also serves as a good preparation for advanced abdominal exercises, such as the Mat Work: Teaser (page 101), although some people find this exercise more demanding than the teaser. Because of the arm position, the torso press offers a significant stretch for the shoulders and the chest.

If you find that you are unable to maintain the neutral spine position of the trunk or keep the legs parallel to the floor, place a large ball or box under the feet and bend the knees slightly. This supports the legs and decreases the load on the hip flexors, making it easier for the abdominal muscles and back extensors to keep the trunk in alignment.

Imagery

I liken this position to a drawbridge, initially lying flat and then hinging as one segment lifts as a solid unit.

☐ Keep the legs stable and parallel to the floor.
☐ Maintain co-contraction of the abdominal muscles and back extensors throughout the movement.
☐ Align the head with the spine.

Muscle Focus

- Abdominal muscles
- Back extensors

Objectives

- To strengthen the abdominal muscles and back extensors
- To stretch the shoulders and chest
- To develop hip flexor control

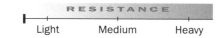
RESISTANCE
Light   Medium   Heavy

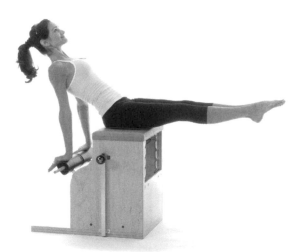

Exhale. Sit on the chair, facing away from the pedal. Place the hands on the pedal with the fingers facing backward and the shoulders aligned over the hands. Hold the legs directly forward, parallel to the floor, with the trunk in a neutral spine position on a diagonal line.

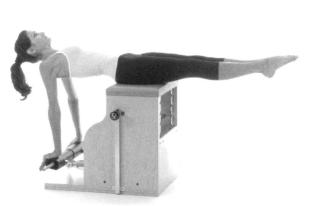

Inhale. Lower the trunk to a flat supine position parallel to the floor, pressing the pedal down.

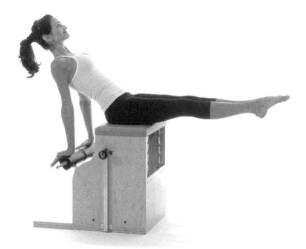

Exhale. Lift the trunk, raising the pedal to the starting position.

Seated Triceps

Muscle Focus

- Triceps
- Biceps

Objectives

- To strengthen the elbow extensors
- To develop trunk stabilization
- To emphasize scapular depression

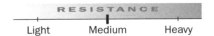

This exercise teaches the fundamentals of what are commonly called *dips.* I cannot overemphasize the importance of good trunk alignment and stability, in addition to excellent scapular stabilization. The movement is a combination of shoulder flexion, highlighting the long head of the biceps and the exterior deltoid, and elbow extension, focusing on the triceps.

I like to precede this exercise with shoulder shrugs, allowing the shoulders to lift toward the ears and then pressing them down to engage the scapular depressors, particularly the lower trapezius. (Note that in terms of muscle action this is the opposite of a typical shrug, in which the shoulders are actively lifted and the upper trapezius is engaged.) Once scapular stabiliza-tion has been established, setting the stage for the movement, the triceps exercise can commence.

Imagery

Visualize lifting the body off the ground rather than merely straightening the arms. The involvement of the back extensors and the image of the scapulae gliding down the back are vital to the success of this movement.

- ☐ Keep the elbows parallel to each other.
- ☐ Maintain scapular depression.
- ☐ Maintain an upright and stable trunk.

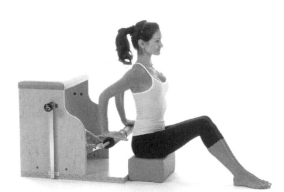

Inhale. Sit upright on a small box, facing away from the chair with the legs together, the knees bent, and the feet placed firmly on the floor. Place the hands on the pedal with the fingers facing the body and the elbows bent and reaching back.

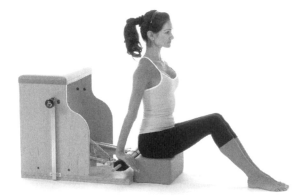

Exhale. Straighten the elbows, pushing the pedal down.

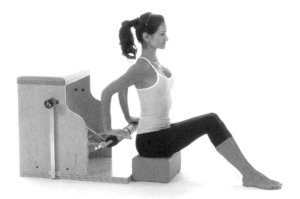

Inhale. Bend the elbows, raising the pedal.

This exercise resembles, and can teach correct and precise execution (seldom seen) of, the classic push-up. Two areas should be highlighted. The first is the pelvic–lumbar region, which is supported by the chair platform and is therefore less likely to collapse than during a push-up. The other area is the scapulae, which tend to adduct and elevate. Proper placement of the scapulae is often ignored in the push-up; it should not be neglected in any exercise. The trunk and scapulae must remain stable, requiring that the movement occur in the arms alone.

I recommend initially doing the prone triceps with the arms parallel and the elbows close to the sides.

This is equivalent to a triceps push-up. The exercise can also be performed with the elbows reaching out to the sides, in which case it is equivalent to a pectoral push-up. Another alternative is to perform it with one arm, reaching the other out to the side.

Imagery

Although it is the pedal that is lowered and lifted, the sense should be that the entire body is being lowered and lifted, as one integrated and stable unit.

☐ Keep the body stable and parallel to the floor.
☐ Avoid adducting and elevating the scapulae.

Muscle Focus

▪ Triceps

Objectives

▪ To strengthen the elbow extensors
▪ To develop trunk and scapular stabilization

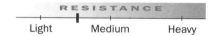

RESISTANCE		
Light	Medium	Heavy

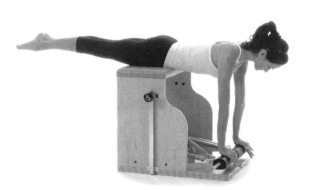

Exhale. Lie prone on the chair with the legs straight and together, and the hands on the pedal. Align the hands directly under the shoulders and straighten the arms.

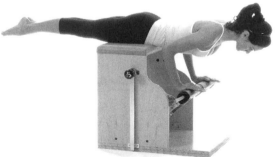

Inhale. Bend the elbows, raising the pedal.

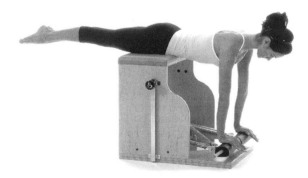

Exhale. Straighten the elbows, pressing the pedal down.

Backward-Facing Dips

Muscle Focus

- Triceps
- Biceps

Objectives

- To strengthen the elbow extensors and shoulder flexors
- To develop trunk and scapular stabilization

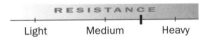

RESISTANCE

Light   Medium   Heavy

The similarity of these dips to the triceps dip commonly seen in a gym ends with the name. The placement of the body in these dips amplifies the intensity, requiring tremendous strength as well as body control, awareness, and muscle integration. As in the Wunda Chair: Seated Triceps (page 254; an excellent preparation for this exercise), good trunk alignment and stability and excellent scapular stabilization are important. The movement combines shoulder flexion and elbow extension, focusing on the triceps. Initiate the movement with the shoulder flexors and then follow with the elbow extensors.

The body should remain perpendicular to and in line with the pedal, holding true to the plumb line. Leaning back and bringing the shoulders over the handles makes it easier but is incorrect. When performed correctly, the exercise not only develops tremendous upper body strength but also improves trunk stabilization and back extensor control. Scapular depression should precede the actual movement. Set the height of the handles so that the upper arms are approximately parallel to the floor when starting. Some wunda chairs do not have side handles, in which case this particular exercise is not possible.

Imagery

See Wunda Chair: Seated Triceps (page 254). With the dips the image of the body levitating off the ground works well. It should appear and feel effortless, as if the force were being generated under the pedal.

- ☐ Keep the elbows facing back and parallel to each other.
- ☐ Maintain scapular depression.
- ☐ Maintain an upright, stable trunk.

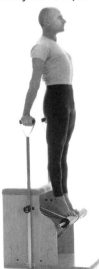

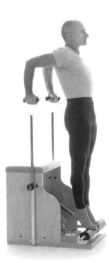

Inhale. Stand upright on the pedal facing away from the chair and place the hands on the handles with the elbows reaching back.

Exhale. Flex the shoulders and extend the elbows completely, pushing down into the handles and elevating the body.

Inhale. Bend the elbows, lowering the body and the pedal to the starting position (not quite touching the floor).

Hamstring Curl

This hamstring curl exercise is very focused and effective, with the body in a stable and comfortable position. The back is not in danger of being pulled into hyperextension, as is the case in other hamstring curl exercises performed in a prone position. Another advantage is the ability to perform this hamstring curl unilaterally, exercising each leg independently. This is of great benefit when a significant imbalance in the strength of the hamstrings is present.

The range of motion of this curl is limited; it works the flexors of the knee only from approximately 120 degrees to 90 degrees of knee flexion. Only the top section of the pedal's arc is utilized in this exercise as this entails pure knee flexion. The bottom part of the arc, in which the pedal would be pressed down to the base, requires hip extension, which is not the objective of this exercise and therefore is not used.

Imagery

Visualize pulling the heels toward the sit bones as if a rubber band connected each heel to the opposite sit bone. This image ensures the precise direction of pull. When you have maximized the knee flexion (before starting to extend the hips), straighten the knees and lift the pedal slowly, resisting the pull of the imaginary rubber band as you return to the starting position. Never fully release the tension.

☐ Maintain a neutral pelvis.
☐ Isolate the knee flexion.
☐ Keep the feet stable.

Muscle Focus

▪ Hamstrings

Objectives

▪ To develop knee flexor strength
▪ To develop pelvic–lumbar stabilization

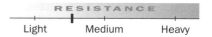

RESISTANCE

Light   Medium   Heavy

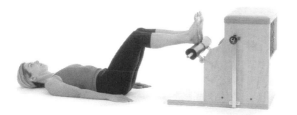

Inhale. Lie supine on the floor. Place the heels on the pedal, feet in a neutral position, with the legs parallel and the knees bent at approximately a 120-degree angle.

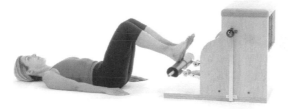

Exhale. Bend the knees, drawing the pedal halfway down.

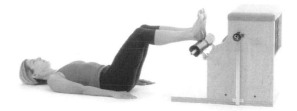

Inhale. Raise the pedal, returning to the starting position.

Standing Leg Press

Muscle Focus

- Hamstrings

Objectives

- To strengthen the hip extensors
- To develop knee extensor control
- To develop balance

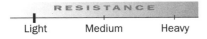

RESISTANCE

Light   Medium   Heavy

This exercise is important in teaching functional movement of the leg, improving balance, and perfecting muscle recruitment patterns pertaining to knee and hip extension. The combination of supporting with the standing leg, pelvis, and trunk and moving with the pressing leg enhances the ability to disassociate the action of the leg from the rest of the body and highlights the value of closed kinetic chain exercises (weight-bearing exercises in which the extremity, the distal point, is fixed). Balance is key.

The alignment of the body is key to activating the correct muscles and ensuring a successful outcome. In order to challenge the hip extensors, the standing leg must be sufficiently far back from the chair, and the initiation must occur in the hip extensors rather than in the knee extensors. Avoid the tendency to stand too close to the chair and lean forward; this transforms the movement, eliminating much of the challenge.

Imagery

Visualize climbing a vertical staircase while keeping the body perfectly upright. The sensation should be like doing the moonwalk, but moving in a vertical rather than horizontal direction.

- ☐ Initiate the movement with the hamstrings.
- ☐ Maintain plantarflexion with the pressing foot throughout the movement.
- ☐ Maintain upright posture; avoid leaning forward.

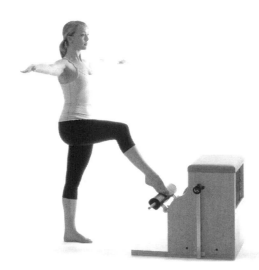

Inhale. Stand upright facing the front of the chair, 12 to 24 inches (30 to 60 centimeters) away from it. Place one foot on the pedal in a plantarflexed position. Hold the arms out to the sides in a T position.

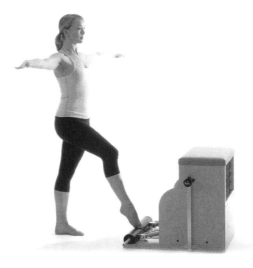

Exhale. Extend the hip, pressing the pedal down.

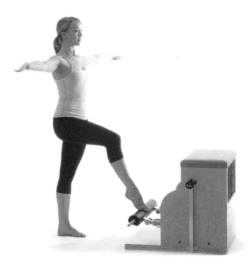

Inhale. Lift the leg, controlling the pedal as it returns to the starting position.

I have helped many athletes improve their running, leaping, jumping, and overall performance with this exercise. It is a great equalizer—no matter how strong the legs are, the exercise will not be successful without certain essentials in place: correct muscle activation patterns, pelvic–lumbar stabilization, balance, and full body integration, plus an optimal strength ratio between the hip extensors, hip abductors, and knee extensors.

Sequencing the muscle activation is key, starting with the hip extensors as the pedal lifts up, followed by the hip abductors as the back foot lifts off the pedal, and finally the quadriceps as the knee straightens completely. Also important is maintaining ideal vertical alignment. The tendency is to lean forward, using the strength of the quadriceps from the outset, which should be avoided.

Imagery

This exercise is about levitation. You should feel a sensation of rising from the starting position, as if a force under the pedal is propelling you upward or a string from the sky is lifting you up.

☐ Activate the muscles sequentially: hip extensors, hip abductors, then knee extensors.

☐ Maintain a stable, level pelvis throughout the exercise (particularly as the foot lifts off the pedal).

☐ Move on a vertical line, avoiding leaning forward.

Muscle Focus

▪ Hamstrings
▪ Gluteus medius
▪ Quadriceps

Objectives

▪ To strengthen the hip extensors, hip abductors, and the knee extensors

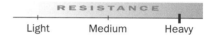

RESISTANCE

Light   Medium   Heavy

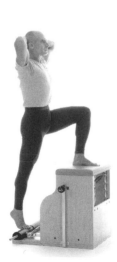

Inhale. Stand facing the chair. Place one foot on the pedal and press the pedal down. Place the other foot on the platform and align the knee above the ankle. Stand upright with the hips directly over the pedal and the hands behind the head or out to the sides.

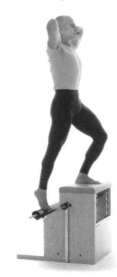

Exhale. Extend the hip, pressing down onto the platform of the chair and straightening the leg as the pedal rises.

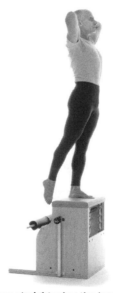

Continue straightening the leg and lift the back foot off the pedal, completing the knee extension.

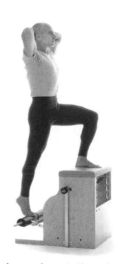

Inhale. Lower down to the point where the thigh is approximately parallel to the floor.

Side Over

This is an excellent exercise for teaching precise lateral flexion and correct alignment. By adding small increments of spring tension, the exercise can be made less challenging if necessary. By the same token, decreasing the spring tension will make the exercise more challenging. From a teacher's perspective, the student's body is in an ideal position for cueing and offering input and corrections.

Muscle Focus

- Oblique abdominals

Objectives

- To strengthen the abdominal muscles (particularly the obliques)
- To stretch the lateral flexors

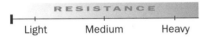

RESISTANCE

Light   Medium   Heavy

Imagery

Imagine the movement as two-dimensional, occurring between two panes of glass (i.e., do not lean forward or backward).

- ☐ Lift no higher than the diagonal line created by the straight leg and trunk.
- ☐ Keep the legs and pelvis stable with the foot of the straight leg anchored on the floor.
- ☐ Move from the waist area.

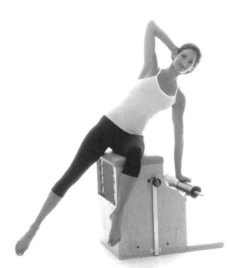

Exhale. Sit sideways on the chair, hooking one leg on the side and keeping the other leg straight and in line with the body, creating a long diagonal with the foot touching the floor. Place the lower hand on the pedal and the other hand behind the head (or reach the arm overhead).

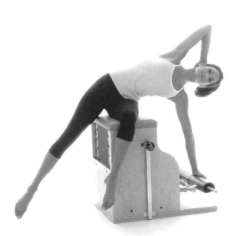

Inhale. Laterally flex the trunk, lowering it and pressing the pedal down.

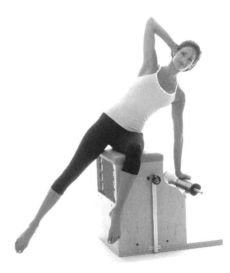

Exhale. Lift the trunk, raising the pedal and returning to the starting position.

Basic Swan

As in the Wunda Chair: Side Over (page 260), this exercise can be made easier by adding small increments of spring tension or more challenging by reducing the spring tension. This adjustability is valuable when dealing with back problems because it allows muscle activation to be regulated. The springs can move the body through a predetermined range of motion as neuromuscular patterns are reeducated, and then the muscles can be progressively challenged (by decreasing the tension) as improvement takes place.

This exercise is valuable for teaching the crucial role of the abdominal muscles in back extension work and how to recruit them correctly. Often, as soon as the abdominal muscles are activated, the trunk is drawn into flexion; then as the trunk is lifted all the extension occurs in the lumbar region. This is not the effect to strive for. Correct abdominal activation should provide support for the spine, assisting in the creation of a long, evenly distributed arc through the trunk.

Imagery

Visualize a reverse articulation of the spine, starting with the head and moving down the spine, drawing the trunk into extension. This tends to distribute the work through the entire back, creating a gentle arc rather than extreme hyperextension in the lumbar spine.

☐ Keep the abdominal muscles engaged.
☐ Maintain adduction of the legs.
☐ Press the hands back into the pedal, extending the shoulders, as the body lifts.

Muscle Focus

▪ Back extensors

Objectives

▪ To strengthen the back extensors
▪ To develop scapular stabilization
▪ To emphasize abdominal control

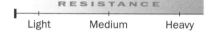

RESISTANCE
Light   Medium   Heavy

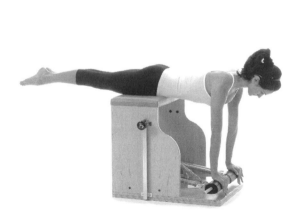

Exhale. Lie prone on the chair, with the legs straight and together, forming one long line with the trunk that is parallel to the floor. Place the hands on the pedal, aligning them directly under the shoulders, and straighten the arms. Lift the pedal slightly off the base.

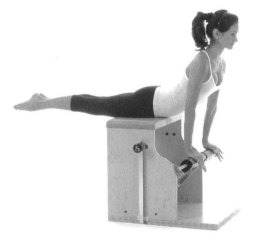

Inhale. Extend the back, lifting the pedal.

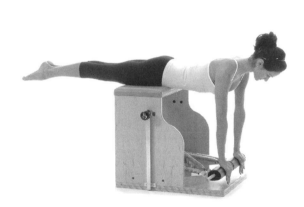

Exhale. Lower to the starting position.

CHAPTER 8

Barrels

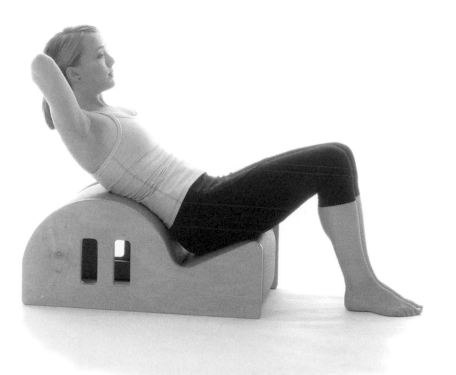

The barrels are as unique in their offerings as they are in appearance. They provide exceptional opportunities for both active and passive back extension at all ability levels. But of course they are not limited to back extension. Like the entire lineup of Pilates apparatus, the barrels have endless potential to work the body in every range of motion.

There are two kinds of barrels: the high, or ladder, barrel stands several feet off the ground and is attached to a ladder of the same height, and the step barrel sits on the floor. There are also variations of the step barrel such as the half barrel and baby arc.

As I have emphasized throughout this book, trunk extension is crucial to developing back strength and good posture; unfortunately it is often neglected. The barrels are exceptional tools for strengthening the back extensors and for passively relaxing in a position of spinal extension, thereby stretching the trunk flexors. During forward flexion abdominal exercises, the barrel supports the lower back in a neutral position; this is very important when flexion of the lumbar spine is contraindicated. The barrels also support the trunk during lateral flexion exercises from fundamental to advanced levels, facilitating the improvement of both strength and flexibility. Unique hip and arm work, full-body integration exercises, and stretches can be performed on the barrels, many of which cannot be easily duplicated on other apparatus.

The barrels utilize gravity rather than springs for resistance, a difference that is an important consideration in making exercises less or more difficult. I often add ankle weights or hand weights to the work on the barrels to increase the challenge when developing strength or to facilitate a deeper stretch when doing flexibility exercises.

I highly recommend ending a session by spending a few minutes in relaxation, lying supine over the step barrel with a cushion supporting the head. It leaves you stretched out, with a delightful *open* feeling.

The order of presentation of the following exercises is not necessarily the sequence in which they would be performed. Typically we would not do an entire session on the barrels but rather borrow exercises from the rich repertoire to fulfill certain blocks in a comprehensive session. I have placed certain categories of exercises together to make selection more convenient; for instance, the stretches are placed together, the lateral flexion exercises are together, and the back extension exercises are together. Students often wonder whether they should learn the ladder barrel before the step barrel or vice versa. In my opinion it does not matter; both have much to offer at every level of work.

Hamstring Stretch

This is a comfortable, relatively easy way to stretch the hamstrings. Although this exercise can be performed on a variety of apparatus (as can the Ladder Barrel: Gluteal Stretch, page 266), the ladder barrel helps keep the body in optimal alignment to achieve maximum stretch of the hamstrings.

Imagery

Visualize the body functioning like a hinge, with the trunk being the top part of the hinge and the pelvis and lower limbs the bottom section. One leg and the pelvis are attached to the ladder and remain stable. The other leg, placed on the barrel, is also part of the stable structure. The upper section of the hinge, the trunk, moves as one piece, closing over the stretching leg and then opening up again.

☐ Keep the back extensors engaged and tilt the pelvis in an anterior direction during the stretch.
☐ Dorsiflex the foot to intensify the stretch.

Muscle Focus

▪ Hamstrings

Objective

▪ To stretch the hamstrings

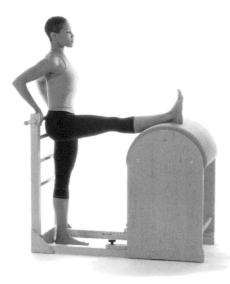

Inhale. Facing the barrel, stand on one leg, keeping it straight and against the ladder. Place the other leg on top of the barrel, keeping it as straight as possible (without hyperextending the knee). Hold the ladder with the hands, arms parallel and elbows facing backward.

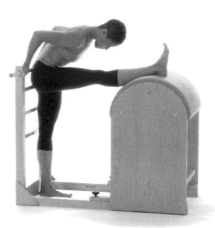

Exhale. Lean forward over the stretching leg, keeping the back as flat as possible. Extend the arms, pressing them against the ladder while reaching the trunk further over the leg and dorsiflexing the foot to intensify the stretch. Hold this position for three to five breaths.

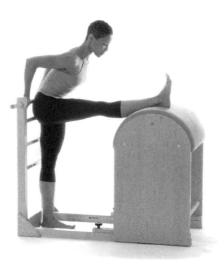

Inhale. Extend the back even further before returning to the starting position.

Gluteal Stretch

Muscle Focus

- Gluteal muscles

Objective

- To stretch the gluteal muscles

The gluteal muscles tend to get very tight. In addition there is often an imbalance in the relative strength of the muscles within this group, with the gluteus medius being weak and the gluteus maximus very strong. The strength factor should be addressed in a comprehensive program. However, a good stretch is always needed, and the ladder barrel is a comfortable location to perform it. It helps keep the body in good alignment to maximize the stretch. Note that this position potentially places a great deal of stress on the knee, particularly when the hip joint is tight and the knee compensates for this tightness. Move into the position with caution, and do not exceed the limits of your own structure. This stretch can be very intense, so remember to breathe!

Imagery

As with all stretches, stabilize the area above and below the region that is to be stretched, and then visualize the region being stretched becoming soft, like rubber, and elongating with each breath.

- ☐ Keep the back extensors engaged and tilt the pelvis in an anterior direction during the stretch.
- ☐ Stand closer to the barrel to intensify the stretch.

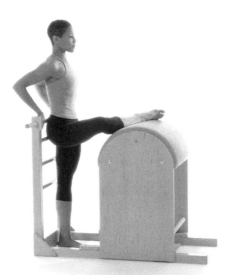

Inhale. Stand on one leg, keeping it straight and against the ladder. Place the lateral aspect of the other leg on the barrel, bend the knee, and externally rotate the hip. Hold the ladder, with the arms parallel and the elbows pointing backward.

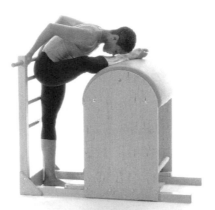

Exhale. Lean forward over the stretching leg and keep the back as flat as possible. Extend the arms, pressing them against the ladder while reaching the trunk farther over the leg to intensify the stretch. Hold for three to five breaths.

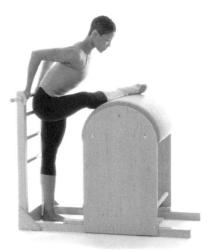

Inhale. Extend the back even farther before returning to the starting position.

Adductor Stretch

This stretch is similar to a ballet stretch at the barre. It is most effective when you turn out (externally rotate) the hip of the stretching leg as dancers often do. The rotation of the hip joint facilitates keeping the pelvis level, so that it doesn't hike up on the stretching side. If this position is not familiar to you, take particular care to achieve correct alignment of the pelvis so that undue stress is not placed on the joints, particularly the knee and hip. This exercise also stretches the lateral flexors of the trunk on the upper side and the shoulder adductors.

Imagery

I like to use the image of the body as a wishbone. This stretch creates a feeling of the body folding in two; the stretching leg and the trunk create the two sides of the wishbone. The foot of the stretching leg and the hand of the stretching arm elongate together. Visualize the area between the pelvic crest and the lower ribs opening and expanding. At the same time, the region under the armpit of the upper arm also opens, allowing the arm to reach further over the head. The breathing is important to facilitate the stretch of the trunk as well as the leg. Direct the breath into the upper lung, feeling the trunk expand without flaring the ribs.

☐ Keep the pelvis level.
☐ Dorsiflex the foot of the stretching leg to intensify the stretch.
☐ Prevent the ribs from flaring on the upper side of the trunk.

Muscle Focus

▪ Adductors

Objective

▪ To stretch the hip adductors, hamstrings, and lateral flexors of the trunk

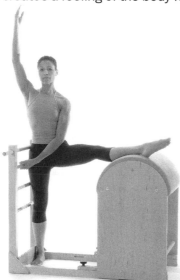

Inhale. Stand on one leg with your side to the barrel. Keep the standing leg straight, in a parallel position against the ladder. Place the stretching leg up on the barrel with the hip externally rotated, keeping the leg as straight as possible (without hyperextending the knee).

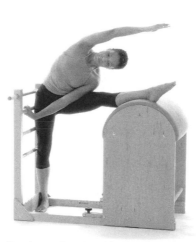

Exhale. Reach over the stretching leg, laterally flexing the trunk. Hold onto the ladder with the inside arm (the lower arm when stretching over) as the outside arm stretches overhead. Hold this position for three to five breaths.

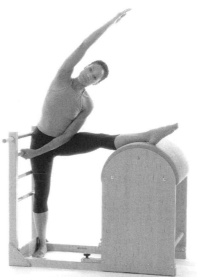

Inhale. Reach out further to the side before returning to the starting position.

Muscle Focus

- Oblique abdominals

Objectives

- To strengthen the oblique abdominals
- To develop trunk stabilization
- To stretch the lateral flexors

Side Over

This exercise resembles the Reformer: Side Over (page 197) and incorporates many of the same principles. However, performing the exercise on the barrel requires more balance, which demands deeper activation of the core muscles for stabilization. Also the shape of the barrel supports the body in perfect lateral alignment and facilitates a wonderful stretch for the upper side. As a preparation for the full side over, place the lower foot on the bottom rung and the other foot on the first or bottom rung, in front of or behind the first foot. This gives the trunk more support and shortens the lever arm, making the exercise less challenging.

Imagery

In the diagonal starting position, the energy line that runs up through the head and down through the body and the foot of the supporting leg gives the sense of directness and stability. The energy line that runs through the body during the lateral flexion is all about curve. The body is draped over the barrel like soft, cascading fabric. To help maintain correct alignment, imagine the movement occurring between two panes of glass.

- ☐ Keep the elbows wide and the fingers interlaced behind the head.
- ☐ Engage the internal support system (ISS) prior to the movement to stabilize the trunk.
- ☐ Keep the upper leg relaxed and avoid pulling up with the upper foot that is hooked under the ladder.

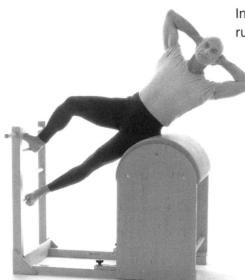

Exhale. Rest one side of the pelvis on the barrel. Place the bottom foot on the first rung of the ladder. Hook the top foot under the top rung with the hip externally rotated and the bent knee facing upward. Place the hands behind the head, creating a diagonal line from the supporting lower foot to the head.

Inhale. Lower the trunk over the barrel, maintaining correct alignment of the head with the spine.

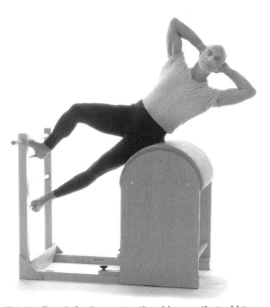

Exhale. Reach further out to the side, creating a big arc, before returning to the starting position.

Basic Back Extension

In all back extension exercises, keeping the abdominal muscles engaged throughout the movement is key. This protects the back and facilitates correct muscle recruitment and body alignment. When setting up the ladder barrel, be aware that the closer the barrel is to the ladder, the lower in the back the work will be focused. If the intention is to work the upper or mid-back, set the barrel farther away from the ladder. Also note that the closer the barrel is to the ladder, the greater the load will be on the back extensors because of the longer lever arm created by the trunk, and vice versa.

Imagery

I encourage visualizing a reverse spinal articulation, lifting the head and then continuing to articulate into spinal extension down through the spine to the mid-back. Emphasize elongation as opposed to height, reaching out from the tip of the head.

☐ Keep the abdominal muscles engaged and the pubic symphysis pressed forward.

☐ Keep the head in line with the spine.

☐ Create a straight line between the legs and the trunk when lifted in extension.

Muscle Focus

▪ Back extensors

Objectives

▪ To strengthen the back extensors

▪ To develop trunk stabilization

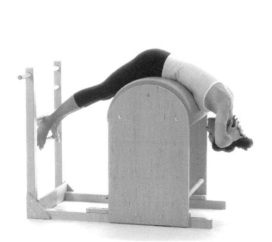

Exhale. Lie prone with the trunk draped over the barrel. Place the toes on the first rung of the ladder with the feet in a V position, heels together, and anchored under the second rung. Place the hands behind the head.

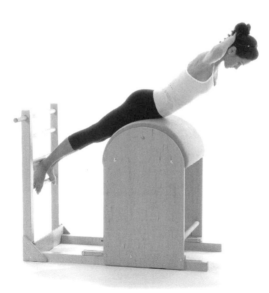

Inhale. Lift the trunk, extending the back.

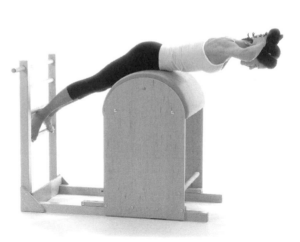

Exhale. Elongate further, lowering the trunk over the barrel to the starting position.

Swan

Muscle Focus

- Back extensors

Objectives

- To strengthen the back extensors
- To stretch the hip flexors
- To develop control of the hip extensors

The swan is one of the most aesthetically beautiful movements in the repertoire and very satisfying to perform. It is an advanced back extension exercise that demands strength, flexibility, and tremendous control. The key to success is integrated and organic movement throughout the body, utilizing the movement of the knees and hips in addition to the full range of motion of every vertebral joint. Many people focus only on the back, specifically the lower back. This results in shearing forces on the lower back, and the body folding over rather than arcing from the knees through the trunk to the fingertips.

Engaging the abdominals is critical in order to protect the back and achieve the desired shape. This exercise can help many gymnasts and dancers, who tend to rely almost entirely on flexibility when performing back extension, achieve a healthy balance of strength, flexibility, and control. Note that the barrel should be set relatively close to the ladder so that the thighs are pressing against the barrel.

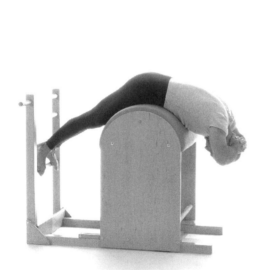

Exhale. Lie prone with the trunk draped over the barrel and the thighs pressing against it. Place the toes on the first rung of the ladder with the feet in a V position and the heels together, anchored under the second rung. Place the hands behind the head.

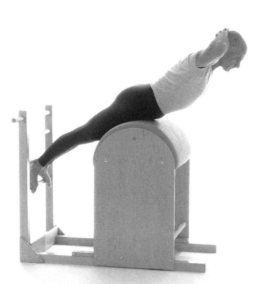

Inhale. Lift the trunk and extend the back, creating a diagonal line with the trunk and the legs.

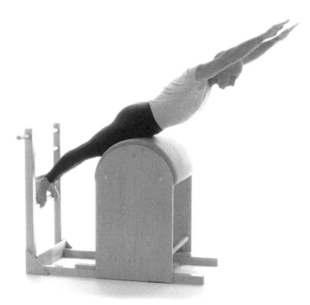

Exhale. Straighten the arms overhead in a V position in line with the ears, establishing a long, straight line from the fingers to the toes.

Imagery

The image of an arc when in full extension is so important in creating the correct movement pattern and muscle recruitment. Refer to the archer's bow mentioned in some of the previous exercises (see Mat Work: Rocking, page 80, which describes this powerful position well).

☐ Keep the abdominal muscles engaged and push the pubic symphysis forward.

☐ Bend the knees as the trunk arcs back and the hips extend.

☐ Distribute the extension of the back through the entire trunk and the hips.

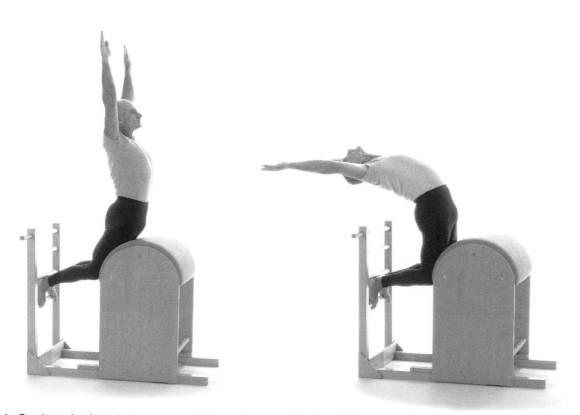

Inhale. Reach up, drawing a large arc, preparing for maximum extension of the body.

Continue inhaling as you bend the knees, pressing the thighs further against the barrel. Extend the hips to the point of maximum extension, and take the trunk as far back as possible into hyperextension.

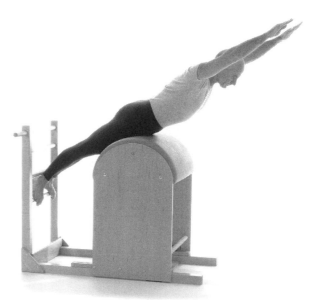

Exhale. Return to the long diagonal line, then inhale while placing the hands back behind the head. Then exhale and lower the body to the starting position.

Reach

This movement offers a wonderful interplay between deep spinal flexion and extension, with the added bonus of a shoulder stretch. The stretch for the back, particularly the lower back, should be maximized when in the C-curve position, as should the stretch for the shoulders when in the supine position.

In the supine position, the spine should be neutral, the legs straight, and the arms reaching overhead in a straight diagonal line, supported by the barrel. This is an ideal position in which to stretch the shoulders. However, be aware of the tendency to thrust the ribs forward in an endeavor to achieve more range in the shoulders; doing so results in hyperlordosis and possible stress on the lower back. Activate the ISS to help maintain a firm, elongated position when supine and to assist when transitioning from supine to sitting and vice versa.

Imagery

The visual of a green branch being pulled into an arc with twine tied to each side (like a bow) and then opening out to the straight position conjures up the perfect dynamic for this exercise.

☐ Maximize the C curve when in the sitting position.

☐ Maintain a straight line with the body when in the supine position.

☐ Keep the head aligned with the spine at all times.

Muscle Focus

- Abdominal muscles
- Shoulder extensors and flexors

Objectives

- To develop abdominal muscle control
- To stretch the abdominal and shoulder muscles

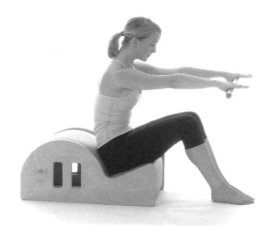

Inhale. Sit on the step of the barrel with the trunk in a C curve (deep spinal flexion). Hold a roll-up pole, approximately 36 inches (90 centimeters) in length, straight in front of you with the arms shoulder-width apart. Bend the knees, keeping the legs together and the feet firmly on the floor.

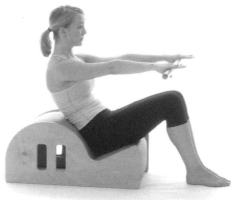

Exhale. Roll down onto the barrel, straightening the legs.

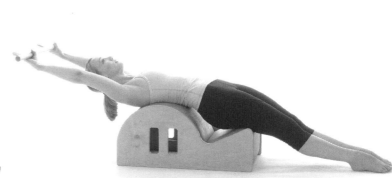

Inhale. Extend the trunk and reach the arms overhead to form a straight line with the legs, trunk, and arms. Inhale, further stretching the shoulders. Then exhale and draw the trunk back into the C curve, bending the legs in and bringing the arms forward to the starting position.

Overhead Stretch

This exercise resembles the Step Barrel: Reach (page 272) but offers a more intense stretch for the shoulders and chest. Whereas the reach calls for in a neutral position when supine, this stretch takes the trunk into hyperextension. The abdominal muscles must be activated to avoid excessive stress on the lower back. Although the apparatus itself offers some support, the role of the abdominal muscles in supporting and protecting the spine cannot be overemphasized.

This exercise challenges the mobility of the shoulder, so anyone with shoulder restrictions should approach it with caution. An important element of this exercise is the sequential movement that progresses through the body—starting at the core, the movement proceeds through the spine as you roll down, and then continues to the arms. The arms then circle around

and "pick up" the spine again to initiate the roll-up into a sitting C curve. The completion of the exercise is another sequential movement through the spine, transitioning from trunk flexion to sitting upright.

Imagery

The feeling should be one of a perpetual rolling wave permeating through the body as it goes through the full spectrum of movement: extension, hyperextension, and flexion.

☐ Lower the trunk onto the barrel before circling the arms.

☐ Keep the head aligned with the spine and the neck relaxed.

☐ Lift the head and spine sequentially as the arms circle around.

Muscle Focus

- Abdominal muscles
- Shoulder extensors and flexors

Objectives

- To increase shoulder mobility
- To stretch the thoracic region and shoulders
- To develop abdominal control

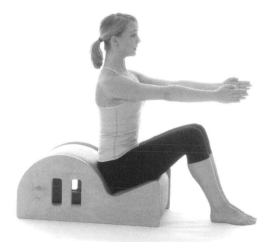

Inhale. Sit on the step of the barrel, holding the trunk upright and the arms straight out in front of the body at shoulder height, with the palms facing each other. Bend the knees, keeping the legs together and the feet firmly placed on the floor.

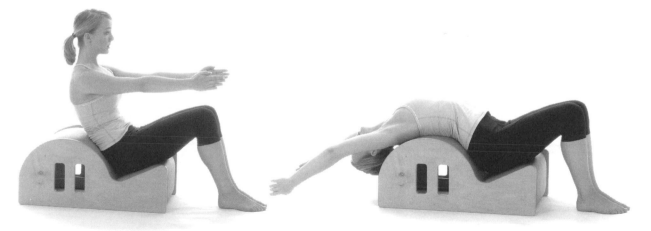

Exhale. Roll down onto the barrel.

Inhale. Reach the arms overhead and circle them around. Exhale. Roll up to the sitting C curve position, with the shoulders over the hips and the spine in deep flexion. Then extend the spine to the starting position.

Chest Lift

Muscle Focus

- Abdominal muscles

Objectives

- To strengthen and stretch the abdominal muscles
- To stretch the thoracic region

This exercise on the step barrel is similar to the Mat Work: Chest Lift (page 48) but with two fundamental differences. First, the range of motion achieved on the barrel is greater, spanning from spinal hyperextension to spinal flexion (as opposed to neutral spine to spinal flexion). This additional range of motion is very valuable because the abdominal muscles are seldom strengthened or stretched beyond a neutral position.

Second, the lumbar spine remains in a supported extended position throughout the exercise. This could be important in some cases; for example, if a medical practitioner requests that a patient with disc problems in the lower back improve abdominal strength but advises against flexion of the lumbar spine. The back is supported by the barrel, which protects the spine and minimizes the risk of tension buildup in the lower back. This exercise has the added benefit of a significant stretch for the chest, which most people desperately need, to help overcome or prevent round-shoulder syndrome and similar conditions.

Imagery

Although the "hollow bowl" concept still pertains in this chest lift to help engage the ISS (see Mat Work: Chest Lift, page 48), imagine the lumbar region remaining stable and the movement occurring from a hinge or pivot point directly under the sternum.

- ☐ Support the head with the hands. (Rest the head on a cushion when in the supine position if necessary.)
- ☐ Keep the elbows wide.
- ☐ Maintain contact between the lumbar spine and the barrel throughout.

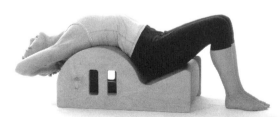

Inhale. Lie supine on the barrel with the pelvis anchored in the step. Interlace the fingers behind the head and stretch the thoracic spine over the barrel. Bend the knees, keeping the legs together and the feet firmly on the floor.

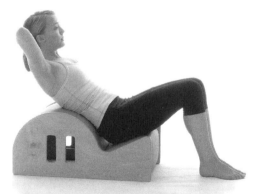

Exhale. Lift the head and chest into spinal flexion. Inhale, pausing in this position.

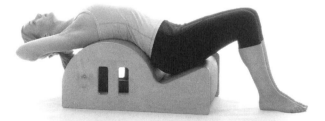

Exhale. Lower the head and chest to the starting position.

Scissors

The scissors provides a wonderful stretch for the hamstrings and hip flexors and develops control of both of these muscle groups, and in fact, of all the muscles surrounding the hip joint. Keeping the pelvis stable and maintaining abdominal activation throughout the movement are important. Without abdominal support, you are in danger of placing excessive pressure on the lower back. The spine is in a hyperextended position and the hip flexors are pulling on it with a very long lever, the legs.

Once immaculate control has been achieved, you can add ankle weights to this exercise to facilitate a deeper stretch and develop strength. Please employ extreme caution when using weights as they increase the potential danger of pressure on the lower back.

Imagery

The name says it all—visualize long scissors opening and closing. The movement is sharp, direct, and precise, just like that of scissors.

☐ Return the legs to the perpendicular position after each opening.

☐ Create a V shape with the legs, opening them equal distance to the back and front.

☐ Keep the trunk and pelvis adhered to the barrel throughout.

Muscle Focus

- Hamstrings
- Hip flexors

Objectives

- To increase hamstring and hip flexor flexibility
- To develop hamstring and hip flexor control
- To improve pelvic–lumbar stabilization

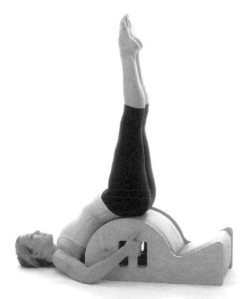

Inhale. Lie supine with the back and pelvis on the barrel, the legs perpendicular, and the shoulder girdle on the floor. Place a mat under the shoulder girdle and head to elevate the body in relation to the barrel if necessary.

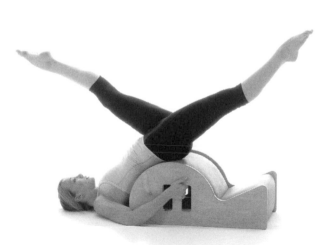

Exhale. Open the legs as wide as possible to the back and front in a scissorlike motion. Pulse twice.

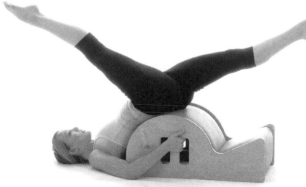

Inhale. Switch the legs, passing through the perpendicular position. Repeat 10 times on each leg, finishing in the perpendicular position.

Openings

Muscle Focus

- Hip adductors

Objectives

- To increase hip adductor flexibility
- To develop hip adductor control
- To improve pelvic–lumbar stabilization

The barrel is an excellent place to work the hip adductors, particularly for those with tight hamstrings. The position of the pelvis on the barrel places less stretch on the hamstrings than a supine position on the floor does. It requires less hip flexor activation to keep the legs lifted (a challenging feat in itself) and allows maximum focus on the hip adductors and on maintaining a stable trunk.

Once immaculate control has been achieved, add ankle weights for additional stretch and strength. (Use caution as the weights can load the hips excessively and cause pain or injury.)

Imagery

Whether using weights or not, imagine pressing against a huge spring or moving through a heavy gel, creating internal resistance as the legs open and close.

- ☐ Open the legs as wide as possible with control.
- ☐ Pause with the legs in the perpendicular position after each opening.
- ☐ Keep the hips externally rotated throughout the movement.

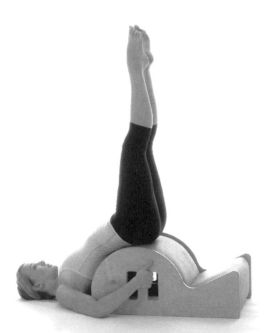

Exhale. Lie with the back and pelvis on the barrel, the legs perpendicular, the hips externally rotated, and the shoulder girdle on the floor. (Place a mat under the shoulder girdle and head to elevate the body in relation to the barrel if necessary.)

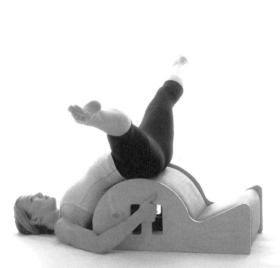

Inhale. Abduct the legs, opening them to a wide V position.

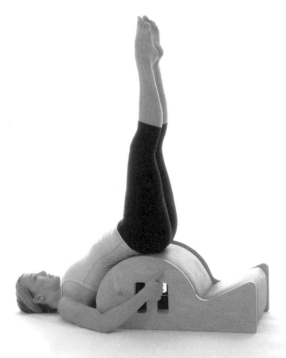

Exhale. Adduct the legs, closing them to the starting position. Repeat 10 times.

Helicopter

Coordination plays a vital role in this exercise. As the legs move in opposite directions, each leg must move at the same pace and the range of motion of each should be equal. This exercise combines the Step Barrel: Scissors (page 275) with Step Barrel: Openings (page 276), both being prerequisites. Adding ankle weights does help achieve a greater range of motion, but you must employ extreme caution as the hip joint is being challenged to the outer limits of its range.

Imagery

The name of this exercise serves the image well—visualize the blades of a helicopter circling around, preparing for takeoff. (Stay grounded!)

☐ Pass through the perpendicular position of the legs after each circle.

☐ Touch each point of the circle as the legs move around.

☐ Keep the pelvis stable.

Muscle Focus

- Hip flexors
- Hamstrings
- Adductors

Objectives

- To increase hip joint mobility
- To strengthen the muscles of the hip
- To develop pelvic–lumbar stabilization

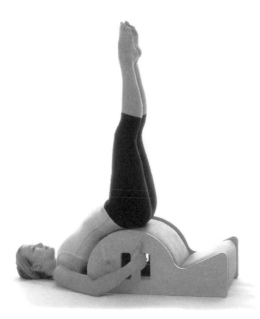

Exhale. Lie with the back and pelvis on the barrel, the legs perpendicular, hips externally rotated, and the shoulder girdle on the floor. (Place a mat under the shoulder girdle and head to elevate the body in relation to the barrel if necessary.)

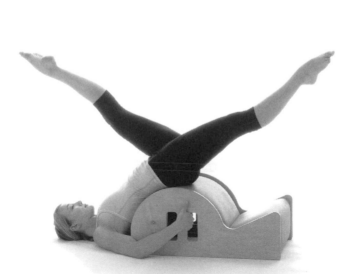

Inhale. Open the legs as wide as possible to the back and front in a scissoring motion.

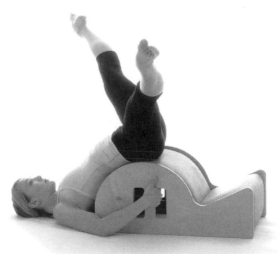

Exhale. Circle the legs around, moving them in opposite directions. (The front leg circles to the back; the back one circles to the front.) Return to the starting position. Repeat five times in the same direction before changing.

Bicycle

Muscle Focus

- Hip flexors
- Hamstrings

Objectives

- To stretch the hamstrings and hip flexors
- To develop hip flexor control

As with the Step Barrel: Helicopter (page 277), coordination is possibly the greatest challenge in this exercise. The legs move simultaneously, one bending while the other is straightening. The cycling movement should be as large and elongated as possible. The bicycle includes within it the Step Barrel: Scissors (page 275), and passing through this position is important because it will ensure that the circular motion remains very large and stretches the hip flexors and hamstrings. Adding ankle weights helps achieve a greater range of motion but requires caution since the weights load the hip flexors and challenge the hip joint to the outer limits of its range.

The legs are parallel, as opposed to externally rotated, and the path they follow should be close to the center line. This maximizes the stretch of the hip flexors and hamstrings. This version of the bicycle serves as an effective preparation for the Mat Work: Bicycle (page 91); in this case the body is supported by the barrel. As with the mat version, the movement pattern in this bicycle can be reversed.

Imagery

Imagine riding a bicycle with very large wheels and pedals. The movement should be circular, not linear, with each leg describing a large circle.

- ☐ Touch the step of the barrel with the foot as the back leg bends to come in.
- ☐ Maintain pelvic–lumbar stabilization throughout the exercise.
- ☐ Keep the legs parallel to each other; avoid splaying the knees as the legs bend.

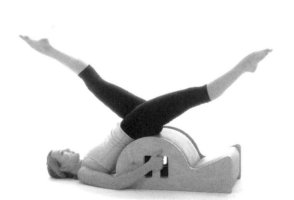

Inhale. Lie with the back and pelvis on the barrel, the legs in a scissors position, the hips in neutral, and the shoulder girdle on the floor. (Place a mat under the shoulder girdle and head to elevate them if necessary.)

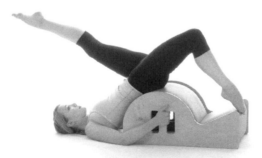

Exhale. Bend the front leg, touching the step with the foot. Simultaneously begin to extend the hip joint of the back leg, reaching the leg over the head.

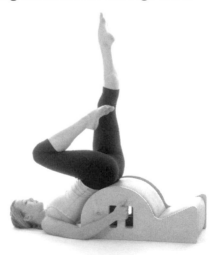

Still exhaling, draw the bent front leg toward the chest. It meets the other leg, now perpendicular, as it is being taken forward. Then inhale and open to the scissors position, straightening what is now the front leg near the face. Repeat five times in the same direction before reversing.

Side Over

The step barrel is exceptionally helpful in accomplishing correct alignment and muscle recruitment for lateral flexion. It supports the body and almost guides it in the desired direction. This lays a solid foundation for many similar and often more challenging lateral flexion exercises in the Pilates repertoire, such as the Reformer: Side Over (page 197) and the Ladder Barrel: Side Over (page 268). You can address both strength and flexibility of the lateral flexors with this exercise. Although I describe the movement sequence below as starting from the draped over the barrel position, I recommend building up strength to the point where you can begin in the diagonal position.

Keeping the head aligned with the spine and the neck uninvolved in this movement is important. There is a strong tendency to try to lift with the head; clearly this is not the goal. The spine supports this integrated movement, creating the shape of an elongated arc.

Imagery

Visualize tall grass being blown sideways in a soft breeze; then the breeze subsides and the grass lifts back up. I encourage you to strive for this effortless, soft quality.

- [ ] Lift the trunk only as high as the diagonal line created by the trunk and the top leg.
- [ ] Stabilize the core, engaging the abdominal muscles prior to the movement.
- [ ] Direct the movement up toward the ceiling rather than crunching sideways.

Muscle Focus

- Oblique abdominals

Objectives

- To strengthen the lateral flexors of the trunk
- To stretch the lateral flexors of the trunk

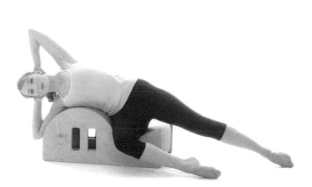

Inhale. Lie over the barrel on one side of the body. Bend the bottom leg to 90 degrees at the hip and knee joints, and rest it in the step of the barrel. Straighten the top leg, keeping the foot anchored on the floor. Interlace the fingers behind the head.

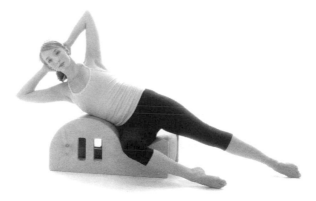

Inhale. Lift the trunk, creating a straight diagonal line with the trunk and the top leg.

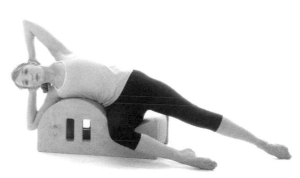

Exhale. Lower the trunk to the starting position. After 5 to 10 repetitions, complete the exercise by straightening the arms overhead and relaxing sideways over the barrel, stretching the lateral flexors.

Roll-Over

Muscle Focus

- Abdominal muscles
- Hamstrings

Objectives

- To develop abdominal muscle control
- To increase spinal articulation
- To stretch the hamstrings and back extensors

The roll-over on the barrel allows those who find the Mat Work: Roll-Over (page 64) difficult or impossible (because of tight hamstrings, a tight lower back, weak abdominal muscles, or other reasons) to successfully complete the exercise. The barrel elevates the pelvis, placing it in a position that alleviates the pull on the hamstrings and lower back. It also allows gravity to assist the abdominal muscles in the challenging roll-over phase of the exercise.

Once you have mastered this exercise on the barrel, it is easier to perform it on the mat. Be cautious when bringing the legs, which function as a long lever arm, back to the starting position because the pressure on the lower back can be excessive, particularly when abdominal support is lacking and hip flexors are tight. The lower back can easily be pulled into hyperextension because of the body's position on the barrel. The abdominal muscles must be firmly engaged throughout to counteract this danger.

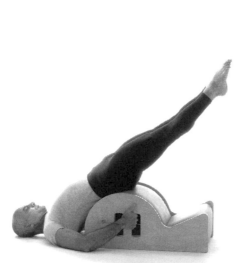

Exhale. Lie supine with the back and pelvis on the barrel, the shoulder girdle on the floor, and the legs straight on a diagonal line. (Place a mat under the shoulder girdle and head to elevate the body in relation to the barrel if necessary.)

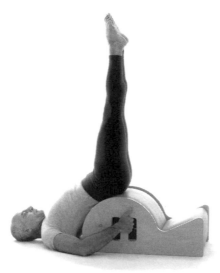

Inhale. Lift the legs to a perpendicular position.

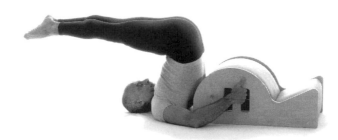

Exhale. Roll over, transferring the legs overhead. Pause with legs parallel to the floor.

Also of note is that this exercise can place pressure on the cervical spine and that it necessitates deep spinal flexion. Both aspects of the exercise may be contraindicated in certain situations. If in doubt, consult with a medical professional. Ideally minimal, if any, pressure should be placed on the cervical spine; after the roll-over the weight should fall on the shoulder girdle. Having the barrel behind the back also helps control the degree of spinal flexion.

Imagery

The visual of the vertebrae gently rolling back and forth like a necklace of pearls helps achieve the desired spinal articulation.

☐ Maintain abdominal support throughout the exercise.

☐ Keep the barrel connected to the back.

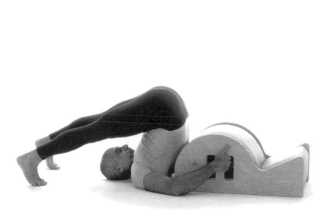

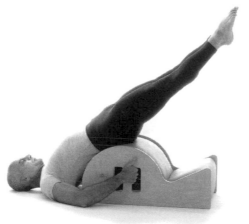

Inhale. Dorsiflex the feet, separate the legs to shoulder width, and lower the feet to the floor.

Exhale. Roll down through the spine, placing each vertebra on the barrel until the pelvis is anchored. Lower the legs and bring them back together to the starting position.

Swan

Muscle Focus

- Back extensors

Objectives

- To strengthen the back extensors
- To develop hip extensor control

Variations of the swan can be done on almost every piece of Pilates apparatus. The step barrel is an excellent place to teach the positioning, alignment, and muscle recruitment for this popular exercise. The support of the barrel alleviates some of the potential stress on the back and accommodates the perfect bow shape we work hard to achieve. The barrel sup-ports the trunk and the legs, thereby assisting the back extensors and hip extensors. Of course, this does not exempt the abdominal muscles from being active throughout the exercise. They are vital to sup-porting the movement, achieving the correct form, and protecting the back.

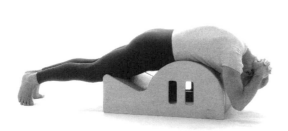

Exhale. Lie prone over the barrel with the knees slightly bent, the hips externally rotated, the feet in a small V position with the toes anchored on the floor, and the fingers interlaced behind the head.

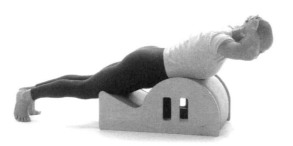

Inhale. Lift the trunk, extending the back.

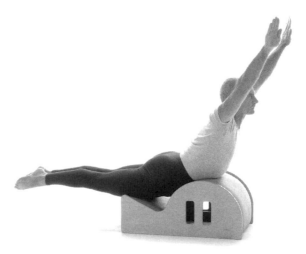

Exhale. Lift the trunk higher as the arms reach forward and up, slightly beyond shoulder-width. Simultaneously lift and straighten the legs while plantarflexing the feet.

Imagery

The image of a bow works well. This helps you visualize the position as well as integrate the important concept of keeping the work evenly distributed through the back .

☐ Glide the scapulae down the back prior to lifting the trunk.

☐ Engage the abdominal muscles throughout the exercise.

☐ Continue to adduct the legs as they lift into spinal extension.

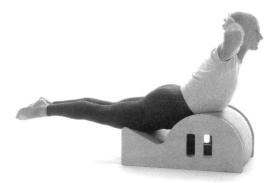

Inhale. Place the hands back behind the head.

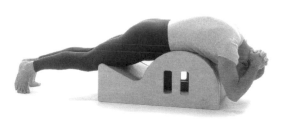

Exhale. Lower to the starting position.

Muscle Focus

- Abdominal muscles
- Hip flexors

Objectives

- To develop abdominal and hip flexor control
- To prepare for the teaser (pages 101 and 215)

Teaser Prep

The teaser prep assists in building a foundation for the many variations of the teaser (as well as any of the pike movements) performed on almost all the Pilates apparatus, including the step barrel. The barrel provides unique and welcome support for the body: behind the legs and upper back when the body is straight on a diagonal line, and behind the lower back, allowing the pelvis to sink into the step, when in the pike position.

Observing the intricate connections between the many exercises in the Pilates method, on all the different apparatus, is fascinating. These connections can be viewed as branches on a large family tree symbolizing close or more distant relationships. Understanding these multiple relationships helps immensely in preparing the body for the next level, whatever it may be. The teaser prep exercise has proven valuable for the athletes I have worked with over the years, particularly the divers and gymnasts.

Imagery

Imagine the body opening out and then closing like a switchblade; the action is sharp, precise, and controlled.

- ☐ Keep the head aligned with the spine.
- ☐ Activate the abdominal muscles prior to lifting the legs.
- ☐ Focus the eyes directly forward when in the pike position.

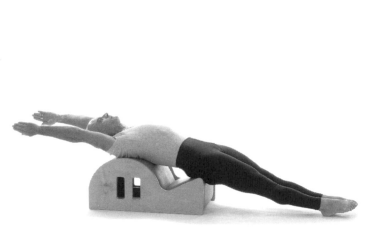

Inhale. Lie supine on the barrel with the coccyx (tailbone) on the edge of the step and the upper back resting on the barrel. Reach the arms overhead, creating a straight diagonal line from the fingertips to the tips of the toes.

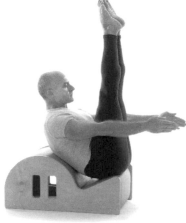

Exhale. Lift the arms and trunk forward and simultaneously lift the legs toward the ceiling, creating a deep pike position, with the legs perpendicular to the floor.

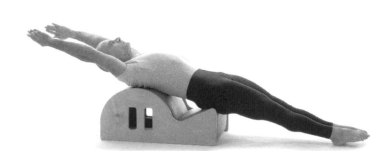

Inhale. Lower the trunk and legs to the starting position.

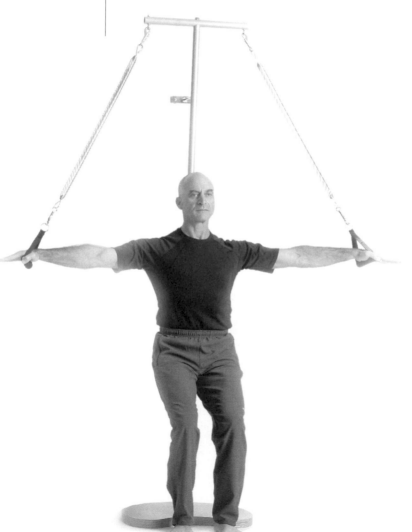

CHAPTER 9

Ped-a-Pul

The ped-a-pul is one of Joseph Pilates' original apparatus, but like the arm chair, it is not as commonly used as some of the other pieces such as the cadillac and the reformer. However, it has unique capabilities that cannot be easily duplicated on the other equipment. The ped-a-pul works the body in a standing position and is excellent for developing upright alignment and balance. In addition it focuses on the arms and shoulder complex, offering fundamental to advanced movements.

I have created a series of exercises on the ped-a-pul that works the shoulders below shoulder height. This is particularly advantageous when teaching scapular stabilization and working with shoulder ailments such as impingement syndrome. This series has proven to be invaluable when rehabilitating the shoulder and for general conditioning of the upper body.

Some ped-a-puls are adjustable, allowing you to vary the resistance to meet individual needs. When working with one that is not adjustable, you can increase the resistance by sitting on a stool or squatting lower. (The lower the body is in relation to the springs, the more resistance there will be.) Sitting on a stool offers more stability, which may be an advantage in certain situations.

Some ped-a-puls are attached to the wall and others are self-standing. I prefer to attach the equipment to the wall unless the base is extremely stable—it is safer and opens up more possibilities in terms of both repertoire and adding resistance.

Extension

This exercise focuses on shoulder extension from shoulder height and below, developing the shoulder extensors in this specific range of movement. It is an excellent preparation for a frequently recurring movement pattern in Pilates; shoulder extension together with trunk flexion, as found in much of the abdominal work (see Mat Work: Hundred, page 50 and Reformer: Coordination, page 125) or together with trunk extension (see Reformer: Pulling Straps I, page 203).

The series of arm exercises presented on the ped-a-pul duplicates the arms supine series on the reformer (pages 168 to 171), but it places the body in an upright position rather than a supine position, further challenging the postural muscles and making the exercises more functional.

Imagery

Visualize pressing the hands against a big inflated balloon. (See also Reformer: Supine Arm Extension, page 168.)

☐ Maintain scapular stabilization.

☐ Keep the arms straight.

☐ Move the arms in a straight line opposite the shoulders.

Muscle Focus

▪ Latissimus dorsi

Objectives

▪ To strengthen the shoulder extensors
▪ To develop scapular stabilization
▪ To improve trunk alignment

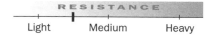

RESISTANCE

Light   Medium   Heavy

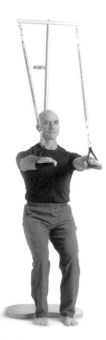

Inhale. Stand with the back against the pole and the feet 12 to 24 inches (30 to 60 centimeters) away from the base of the pole. Bend the knees, keeping the legs parallel to each other. Hold the handles; straighten the arms at shoulder height directly in front of the shoulders, palms facing down.

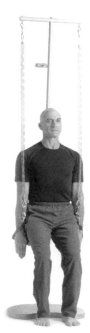

Exhale. Extend the shoulders, keeping the arms parallel to each other, and bring them down to the sides of the body.

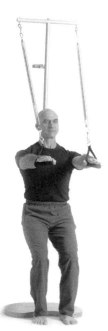

Inhale. Return to the starting position.

Adduction

Muscle Focus

- Latissimus dorsi

Objectives

- To strengthen the shoulder adductors
- To develop scapular stabilization
- To improve trunk alignment

This exercise focuses on shoulder adduction in this specific range of motion. Like shoulder extension, shoulder adduction is utilized in many Pilates exercises together with movement of the trunk. It is often accompanied by trunk flexion, as in the case of abdominal work, or back extension, as in the Reformer: Pulling Straps II (page 204).

Imagery

Imagine spreading your arms like the wings of an eagle as they move up and down. This is a powerful image; enjoy the sensation.

- ☐ Maintain scapular stabilization.
- ☐ Keep the arms straight and the palms facing the floor.
- ☐ Maintain a neutral spine position.

RESISTANCE

Light   Medium   Heavy

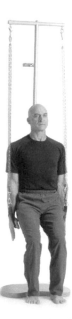

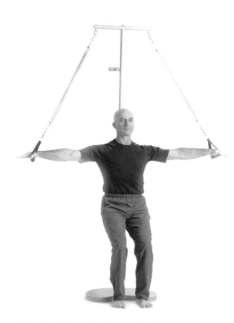

Inhale. Stand with the back against the pole and the feet 12 to 24 inches (30 to 60 centimeters) away from the base of the pole, knees bent and legs parallel to each other. Hold the handles and reach the arms straight out to the sides, establishing a T position, with the palms facing down.

Exhale. Adduct the arms, bringing them down to the sides of the body.

Inhale. Return to the starting position.

Triceps

This exercise offers extremely focused work of the triceps. Keeping the upper arms stable and close to the sides of the body is key to maximizing the work of the triceps and isolating the movement of the elbow. Not allowing the wrist to bend back (extend) is also important. When the wrist does bend back, it places excessive pressure on the joint and releases some of the tension from the springs. The lower arm should be viewed as one solid unit.

Imagery

Imagine the body levitating with each extension of the elbows. The trunk elongates and the scapulae glide even further down the back. The lower arm should feel like a mechanical lever attached at the elbow, and the joint like a well-lubricated hinge.

☐ Maintain scapular stabilization.
☐ Keep the upper arms close to the sides of the body.
☐ Isolate the movement of the lower arm.

Muscle Focus

▪ Triceps

Objective

▪ To strengthen the elbow extensors
▪ To develop scapular stabilization
▪ To improve trunk alignment

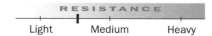

RESISTANCE

Light   Medium   Heavy

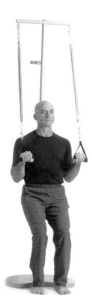

Inhale. Stand with the back against the pole and the feet 12 to 24 inches (30 to 60 centimeters) away from the base of the pole. Bend the knees and keep the legs parallel to each other. Hold the handles, either with a fist or fingers straight, and firmly anchor the arms by the sides of the body with the elbows at approximately a 45-degree angle.

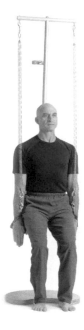

Exhale. Straighten the elbows. (Note alternative hand position.)

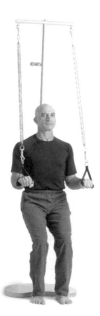

Inhale. Bend the elbows, returning to the starting position.

Circles

Muscle Focus

- Latissimus dorsi

Objectives

- To strengthen the shoulder adductors and extensors
- To improve shoulder joint mobility
- To improve trunk alignment

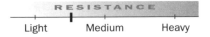

The circles combine shoulder adduction and shoulder flexion. There should be an almost indiscernible pause when the arms reach the sides of the body, the shoulders rotate, and the hands change from facing the body to facing back. Controlling the scapulohumeral rhythm (the relationship between the movement of the arm and the scapula) is a crucial aspect of this exercise and so important in establishing healthy shoulder mechanics. The feeling of the scapulae drawing down the back should always be present, even as they rotate in and out to accommodate the movement of the humerus.

Reversing the direction of the circles changes the type of contraction in each phase. The concentric phase of shoulder adduction becomes an eccentric contraction as the shoulders abduct. The same

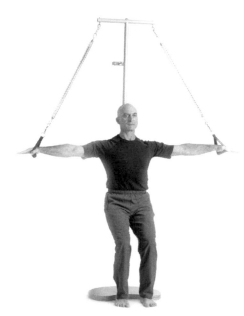

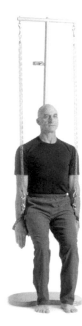

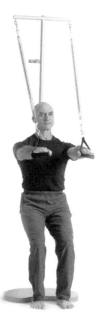

Inhale. Stand with the back against the pole and the feet 12 to 24 inches (30 to 60 centimeters) away from the base of the pole. Bend the knees and keep the legs parallel to each other. Hold the handles and reach the arms straight out to the sides, establishing a T position, with the palms facing down.

Exhale. Adduct the arms. When they are down at the sides of the body, rotate them so that the palms face backward.

Raise the arms in front of the body to shoulder height. Inhale. Horizontally abduct the arms, returning to the T position. After 10 repetitions, reverse the direction.

applies to the extensors, which work concentrically as opposed to eccentrically during the shoulder extension. I recommend working the shoulders and arms in both directions; the movement pattern feels different and the muscles work differently. In Pilates we always train the muscle in both concentric and eccentric modes, an approach that is widely supported in the world of exercise science.

Imagery

See Reformer: Kneeling Arm Circles, page 178.

☐ Maintain scapular stabilization.
☐ Allow the scapulae to glide and rotate according to the movement of the arm.
☐ Maintain a neutral position of the spine.

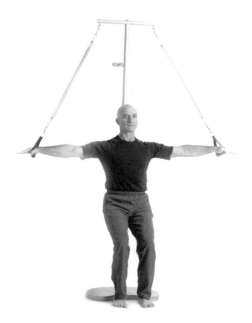

Exhale. Extend the shoulders. When the arms are down at the sides, rotate them so that the palms face the body. still exhaling abduct the arms to the T position.

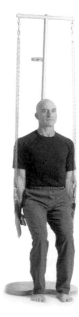

Inhale. Horizontally adduct the arms, returning to the starting position.

CHAPTER 10

Arm Chair

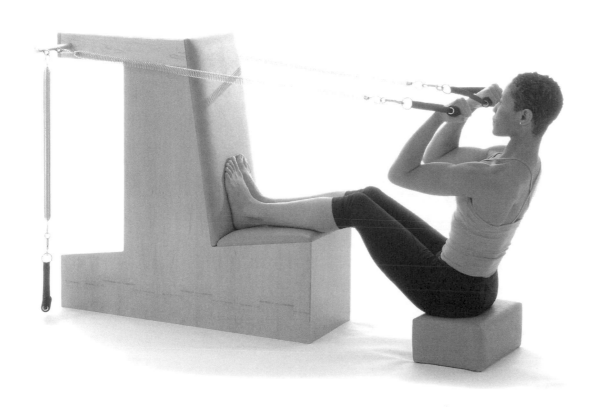

I would find it difficult to run a Pilates studio without the arm chair. Yet for some inexplicable reason this piece of equipment is not often used; many Pilates teachers are unaware that it even exists. The arm chair is comfortable and user-friendly, and it offers convenient access for tactile cueing by the teacher.

As the name implies, the arm chair is used primarily for the arms and shoulder complex. It is an excellent aid in teaching good shoulder mechanics and the concept of trunk stabilization during arm work. It also offers support, which is so important in the early stages of learning Pilates and a luxury later on.

Shoulder dysfunction is possibly the most common issue that Pilates teachers deal with. We give cues repeatedly to correct shoulder mechanics—to release tension, to lower them, or stabilize them. I ask teachers all over the world to name the most common correction they give students and clients, and invariably the answer is, "Relax the shoulders." Clearly we are dealing with a global epidemic of shoulder dysfunction! The arm chair is a user-friendly, versatile piece of apparatus for focusing on the shoulders and teaching good movement technique.

Because I believe that the arm chair has enormous untapped potential, I have designed a new chair (see www. Pilates.com for information on pieces of Pilates apparatus that I have designed), which promises to become a multifaceted piece of apparatus that addresses the entire body. I hope that it will become one of the central pieces of Pilates apparatus in the studio or the home. It is the simplicity of this apparatus, like the wunda chair (see chapter 7), that I find so appealing. The arm chair is relatively small and unassuming, yet packed with possibilities for developing the entire body.

Chest Expansion

The arm chair offers an excellent position for performing this exercise, particularly for those with tight hamstrings who find it difficult to sit upright on the reformer with the legs straight forward (see pages 172–176). The trunk must be in an optimum position in order to activate the correct muscles and benefit from the exercise. It is surprising how little resistance is required to work the shoulder extensors effectively when the body is in a good position.

The most typical compensations seen in this exercise are shoulder elevation, trunk flexion, and elbow flexion. These compensations occur when the resistance is too high or when body awareness and control are lacking. The arm chair can assist in overcoming these compensations and in laying the foundation for correct movement.

Imagery

The movement is similar to the Reformer: Seated Chest Expansion (page 172). The sitting position on the arm chair promotes the feeling of elongation. I also encourage a slight elevation of the chest, which in turn prompts deeper activation of the mid-back extensors. When I was a young dancer, I had a wonderful teacher who spoke about the feeling of having a fishhook placed through the sternum, with the fishing line pulling the body upward to the sky. The image, painful though it sounds, has always stuck with me; I think of it whenever I need to achieve a more upright position.

☐ Keep the range of movement relatively small (approximately 20 degrees forward of vertical to 5 to 10 degrees behind vertical).

☐ Maintain ideal upright alignment of the trunk.

☐ Reach down to the floor with the fingertips, keeping the elbows straight.

Muscle Focus

▪ Latissimus dorsi
▪ Triceps

Objectives

▪ To strengthen the shoulder and elbow extensors
▪ To develop trunk stabilzation

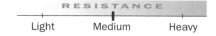

RESISTANCE

Light   Medium   Heavy

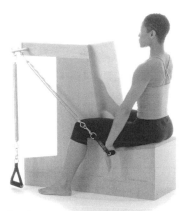

Inhale. Facing the back of the arm chair, straddle the chair and place the feet firmly on the ground. Hold the handles, with the arms straight down by the sides of the body and the palms facing back.

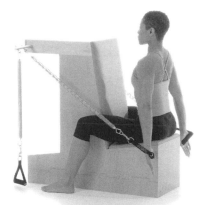

Exhale. Extend the shoulders, pulling the arms straight back.

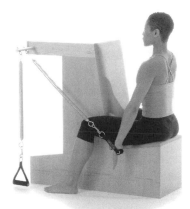

Inhale. Return to the starting position, maintaining tension in the springs.

Hug-a-Tree

Muscle Focus

- Pectoralis major

Objectives

- To strengthen and increase flexibility in the shoulder horizontal adductors
- To develop trunk stabilization

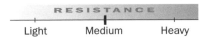

Having the back support from the chair while performing this series of exercises is invaluable. Not only does it support the trunk as you develop the strength to hold the body in good sitting alignment without external support, it also assists in maintaining good scapular positioning by providing a solid surface to press against. As with the reformer (see Reformer: Seated Hug-a-Tree, page 175), the feeling of reaching out from the fingertips with the arms elongated is important in order to maximize the work in the shoulder region and maintain resistance from the springs.

Imagery

Sitting on the arm chair feels like sitting on a throne. You should have a sense of being regal, of opening the arms wide in welcome. I use a different image for bringing the arms toward each other: pressing against a big balloon. Alternate the two images as you open and close the arms.

- ☐ Keep the back broad and the scapulae stabilized.
- ☐ Avoid thrusting the ribs forward as the arms go back.
- ☐ Maintain an elongated position with the arms without locking the elbows.

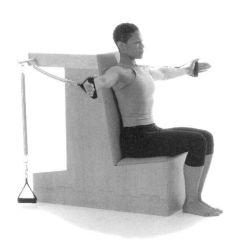

Inhale. Sit with the back against the chair and the legs together or hip-width apart. Hold the arms out in a T position with the elbows soft and palms facing forward.

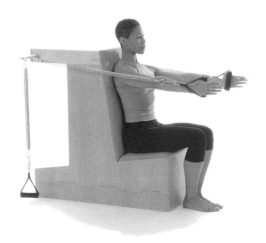

Exhale. Horizontally adduct the arms until they are in line with the shoulders and parallel to each other.

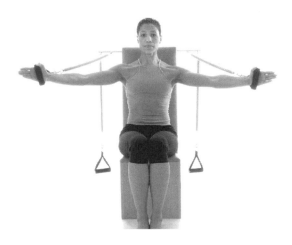

Inhale. Horizontally abduct the arms, returning to the starting position while keeping tension in the springs.

Circles

This exercise is an excellent way to promote shoulder control and mobility. Although the movement may appear to strain the shoulders, particularly as the arms lift overhead (which would be worrisome if any dysfunction, such as shoulder impingement syndrome, were present), this is not the case. The arms do not lift weight overhead (as they would with dumbbells); they resist the pull from behind, which in turn alters the muscle activation. In fact, during my rehabilitation after open rotator-cuff surgery on both shoulders, this series assisted me greatly in regaining range of motion without stressing the joint or musculature.

Imagery

Imagine that the arms are being lifted by a pulley attached to weights. The scapulae are the weights. As the weights draw down the back, the arms lift up. The ratio between the weights and the arms is finely balanced so that as the arms circle around the weights move slightly in and out like small pendulums, according to the movement. However, they always draw downward, maintaining a feeling of weightlessness in the arms.

☐ Keep the back broad and the scapulae depressed.
☐ Maintain abdominal engagement.
☐ Avoid thrusting the ribs forward.

Muscle Focus

- Latissimus dorsi
- Pectorals

Objectives

- To increase the range of motion in the shoulder joint
- To develop shoulder control
- To develop trunk stabilization

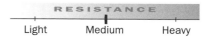

RESISTANCE
Light   Medium   Heavy

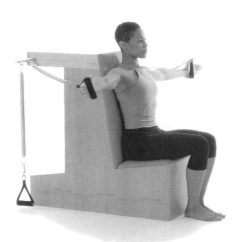

Inhale. Sit with the back against the chair and the legs together or hip-width apart. Hold the arms out in a T position with the elbows soft and the palms facing forward.

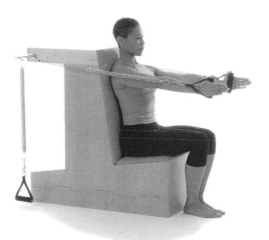

Exhale. Horizontally adduct the arms, drawing them together until they are in line with the shoulders and parallel to each other.

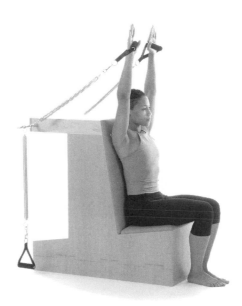

Inhale. Rotate the arms so the palms face down. Then lift the arms overhead and circle them around to the T position (starting position). Repeat this direction 5 to 10 times and then reverse the direction.

Salute

Muscle Focus

- Triceps

Objectives

- To strengthen the elbow extensors
- To develop horizontal adductor control of the shoulder

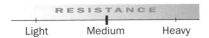

RESISTANCE

Light   Medium   Heavy

This exercise is very similar to the Reformer: Seated Salute (page 176), and like the other exercises in this series, serves as a good preparation for the more challenging reformer arm work (pages 177 through 181). Keep tension in the springs throughout the exercise while moving the arms on a slight diagonal, just above the line of the horizon. Typically the salute is performed with the elbows reaching out to the sides. However, to work the triceps more effectively, lower the elbows to shoulder height so that the arms are parallel to each other.

Imagery

As with the Reformer: Seated Salute, imagine the arms gliding along a ramp slightly above the horizon. The angle is slight so that shoulder elevation is not encouraged. Focus on the feeling of an infinite line. As a dancer, I learned the difference between a straight arm that ends at the fingertips and appears short and a soft line that appears infinite.

- ☐ Keep the back broad and the scapulae depressed.
- ☐ Direct the fingers forward throughout the movement.
- ☐ Avoid rolling the shoulders forward (internally rotating them).

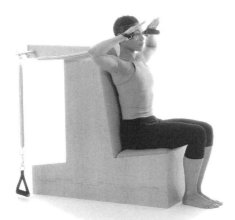

Inhale. Sit with the back against the chair and the legs together or hip-width apart. Place the hands in a salute position opposite the temples at eyebrow level, palms facing down.

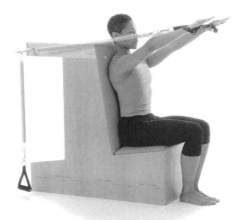

Exhale. Straighten the arms on a slight diagonal, maintaining a straight line upward from the shoulders.

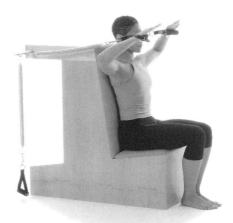

Inhale. Bend the elbows, keeping the fingers pointing in the direction of the movement. Return to the starting position, maintaining tension in the springs.

Biceps

I have added this exercise to the classic Pilates reper-toire on the arm chair because I wanted a biceps exer-cise that requires good trunk stabilization, particularly activating the back extensors, but is not hampered by tight hamstrings. The position of the body allows for more resistance than the Reformer: Seated Biceps (page 173) does, which is an advantage when the goal is to build muscle strength.

Imagery

Although the movement is similar to the seated-posi-tion biceps exercise on the reformer (page 173) and the same imagery regarding the movement of the arms applies, the trunk position in this exercise is different. It should feel like an intricate balancing act between the arms and trunk—as the trunk leans back and stabilizes, the resistance on the arms can be increased to the point where the trunk feels sus-pended from the arms.

☐ Keep the back extensors activated.
☐ Keep the arms parallel to each other and prevent the elbows from moving up or down.
☐ Avoid elevating the scapulae.

Muscle Focus
- Biceps

Objective
- To strengthen the elbow flexors
- To develop trunk stabilization

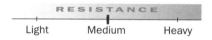

RESISTANCE

Light   Medium   Heavy

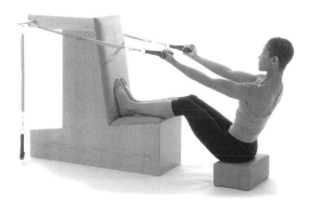

Inhale. Sit on a small box (or on the floor if you are tall), facing the chair with the feet against the chair back. Hold the handles with the arms straight out in front at shoulder height and with palms facing up.

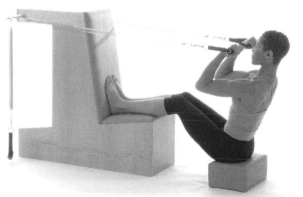

Exhale. Bend the elbows.

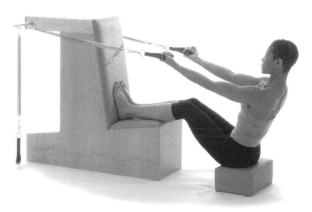

Inhale. Straighten the elbows to the starting position.

Rhomboids

Muscle Focus

- Deltoid posterior
- Rhomboids

Objective

- To strengthen the shoulder horizontal abductors and scapula adductors

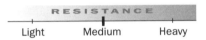

RESISTANCE

Light   Medium   Heavy

This exercise places the body and arms in a different position than in the reformer version (page 174). The arm position emphasizes internal rotation of the shoulder rather than the external rotation in the reformer version. Still, these two exercises have a great deal in common. In both, the position of the trunk is key to successful execution of the exercise. Also in both, I recommend first isolating the movement to shoulder horizontal abduction, and then later adding the scapular adduction and abduction. Doing so isolates and maximizes the glide of the scapulae rather than combining it with the movement of the glenohumeral joint.

Imagery

The movement of the arms resembles a rowing action, although the trunk, which provides a stable foundation for the movement, remains still. Despite this difference, the image of rowing a boat will assist in achieving the desired action.

- ☐ Keep the back extensors activated.
- ☐ Move the arms on a horizontal line.
- ☐ Keep the elbows high, reaching out and back.

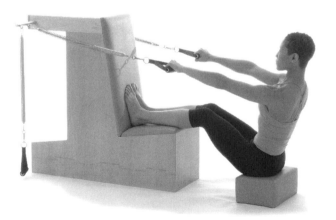

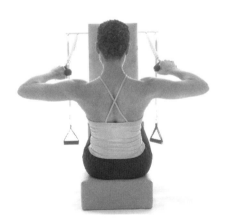

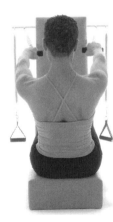

Inhale. Sit on a small box, facing the chair with the feet against the chair back, knees bent and legs together. Hold the handles with the arms straight out in front, opposite the shoulders, and with the palms facing down.

Exhale. Keeping the upper arms parallel to the floor, bend the elbows, pulling them out and back until they will not move any further without adducting the scapulae. (When you have perfected this movement in terms of form and muscle activation, you can add the adduction and abduction of the scapulae.)

Inhale. Straighten the arms, returning to the starting position.

CHAPTER 11

Magic Circle

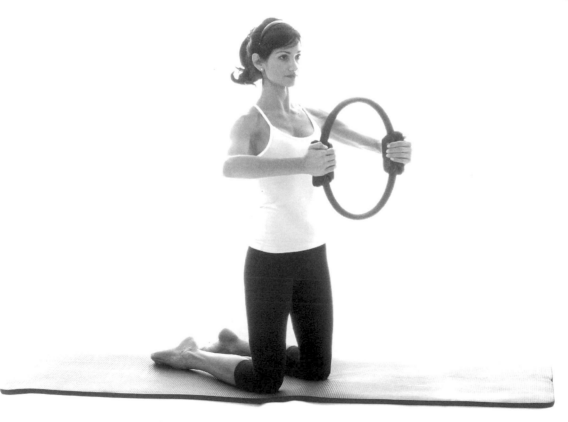

The number of aliases that exist for this simple ring reflects the wide variety of exercises that can be performed with it. It is the perfect travel companion, an ideal complement to the full-apparatus session, and an excellent piece to use in a mat work class to add challenge and variety.

The circle can be used simply to keep the body or a body part in alignment or in a desired position, such as holding it between the arms opposite the chest or above the head. Or it can be used to encourage the continuous activation of a certain muscle group; for example, holding it between the legs to help maintain adductor engagement. It can also be used to add resistance or heighten the level of coordination.

It often amazes me when I see some "new" device that works one or two muscle groups flood the fitness market and sell millions of units; often the magic circle works those same muscle groups and also does so much more. For instance, one popular piece of equipment is an inner-thigh apparatus that works the adductors—and that's it! The magic circle works the adductors just as well, but it also works the abductors, hamstrings, abdominals, back extensors, and arms. The secret is starting to get out, and now the magic circle is finally receiving its long overdue credit.

Many types of magic circles are now available in every conceivable packaging. Some offer more resistance than others; some are made of a super-light material and others are heavier. Choose one that suits your lifestyle and needs. In terms of resistance, err toward lighter rather than heavier. If you travel frequently and the circle is to become a travel companion, get the ultralight version. If it is to be used in a studio and will need to stand up to the demands of continuous use, get one that is made of the most durable materials, even if it is heavier.

Arms Bent

This is a fun, effective exercise to develop the chest muscles. Use the pumping action that is well-suited to the magic circle, and be aware of recruiting the pectorals on each pump. Keep the oval shape created by the arms consistent and the wrists firm as you squeeze the arms together.

Imagery

Although this image may seem a little graphic, try to bounce the pectorals with each pump. (This will work for both men and women, even though women typically have more to bounce!)

☐ Maintain ideal body alignment throughout.

☐ Draw the scapulae down the back.

☐ Perform small pumping movements.

Muscle Focus

- Pectorals

Objectives

- To strengthen the shoulder horizontal adductors

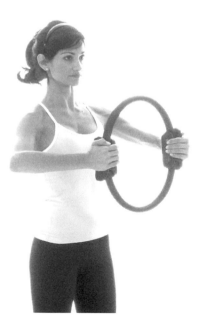

Inhale. Kneeling or standing upright, hold the circle directly opposite the sternum with the elbows slightly bent.

Exhale. Horizontally adduct the arms, pressing them together. Inhale. Maintain the tension in the circle and continue with small pumps.

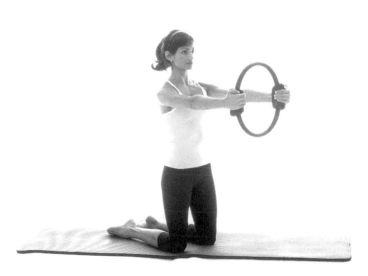

You can also perform this exercise with the arms straight, which adds length to the lever arm and further challenges the horizontal adductors of the shoulder.

Arms Overhead

Muscle Focus

■ Pectorals

Objective

■ To strengthen the pectoral muscles

This arm exercise is more difficult than it looks. Maintaining scapular depression and avoiding tension in the shoulders and neck is challenging enough. Adding the arm movement makes it even harder. The movement is so challenging that for most people this exercise is isometric—the arms remain still as they press together.

Imagery

This exercise never fails to evoke the image of a halo!

☐ Maintain ideal body alignment throughout the exercise.

☐ Draw the scapulae down the back.

☐ Lift the arms only as high as shoulder flexibility allows without elevating the shoulders.

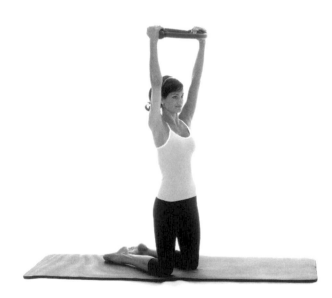

Inhale. Kneeling or standing upright, hold the circle with the arms reaching overhead.

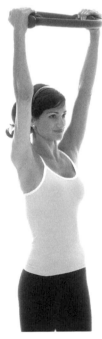

Exhale. Adduct the arms, pressing them together.

Inhale. Continue pressing the arms together, maintaining the tension in the circle. Return to the starting position.

Single-Arm Side Press

This exercise requires that you engage the shoulder adductors, particularly the latissimus dorsi, prior to the pumping action and keep them engaged throughout the sequence. Maintaining scapular stability and a constant slight bend in the elbow is important; the movement should occur in the glenohumeral joint.

Imagery

Imagine trying to pat the side of your leg, but the air is thick and gel-like and does not allow you to reach it. But you persist!

☐ Maintain scapular depression.

☐ Maintain ideal body alignment throughout the exercise.

☐ Avoid neck and shoulder tension.

Muscle Focus

▪ Shoulder adductors

Objective

▪ To strengthen the shoulder adductors

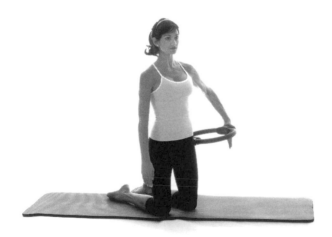

Inhale. Kneeling or standing upright, hold the circle in one hand and rest it against the side of the thigh directly below the hip joint. The elbow should be slightly bent and the shoulder slightly internally rotated.

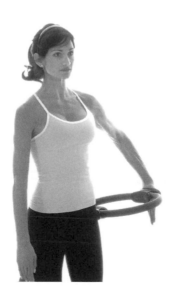

Exhale. Adduct the shoulder, pressing the hand toward the thigh.

Inhale. Maintain the tension in the circle and continue with small pumps. Return to the starting position.

Single-Arm Biceps

This is a simple yet effective biceps exercise. I added this to the repertoire years ago to provide a more comprehensive workout for the arms and upper body using the circle. Do this exercise slowly, holding the circle down for several seconds before allowing the arm to rise up.

Muscle Focus

■ Biceps

Objective

■ To strengthen the elbow flexors

Imagery

This always conjures up an image of Africa, where I grew up. I would see the people, particularly the women, carrying heavy loads on their heads, often balancing them with one hand. Their posture was perfect and strong as they walked gracefully, unencumbered by the enormous loads on their heads. This, to me, exemplifies the body in perfect balance.

☐ Keep the head centered.

☐ Press down with the ball of the hand, not the fingers.

☐ Find a comfortable place to rest the circle on the shoulder.

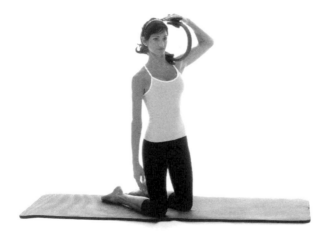

Inhale. Kneeling or standing upright, hold the circle in one hand and rest it on the shoulder directly above the joint. Bend the elbow and reach it out to the side.

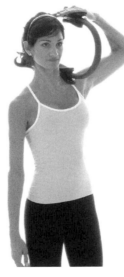

Exhale. Press the hand down toward the shoulder.

Inhale. Maintain the tension in the circle while returning to the starting position.

Seated: Above Knees

This is a straightforward, effective hip adductor exercise. However, you should view it as a full-body exercise, emphasizing the alignment of the trunk, head, pelvis, and feet. This exercise has several variations that you can perform by changing the position of the magic circle, including holding it below the knee and just above the ankles.

Imagery

The imagery for the entire series of magic circle hip adductor exercises, whether performed sitting, prone, or supine, is about the hip joints moving freely without affecting the solid alignment of the rest of the body. The feeling should be like the head of the femur moving in a soft gel or like a spoon stirring thick porridge.

☐ Find a comfortable location on the inner thighs to place the circle where it will not slip out.

Muscle Focus

▪ Hip adductors

Objective

▪ To strengthen the hip adductors

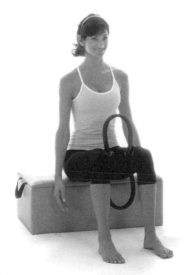

Inhale. Sit upright with the hips and knees at a 90-degree angle. Place the circle between the legs just above the knees, pressing it with the hip adductors.

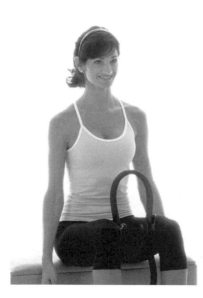

Exhale. Press the legs together evenly, adducting the hips.

Inhale. Maintain the tension in the circle and continue with small pumps. Return to the starting position.

Supine Knees

Muscle Focus

- Hip adductors

Objectives

- To strengthen the hip adductors
- To develop pelvic–lumbar stabilization

Although this exercise is geared toward strengthening the hip adductors, it requires good abdominal strength and exceptional pelvic–lumbar control. In addition, it is an optimal position in which to work the pelvic floor muscles.

If you suspect that you lack the abdominal strength needed for this exercise, try keeping the lower back flat on the floor instead of in a neutral spine position, even if this results in a slight posterior tilt of the pelvis. If the lower back starts rising off the floor into an arch (hyperlordosis), draw in the abdominal muscles deeper and lift the upper trunk into forward flexion. Place the hands behind the head and interlace the fingers to support the head in this position, like a hammock. If

this position still places stress on the back, perform the exercise with the feet on the floor.

Imagery

I like to imagine that the tailbone is a tail that lifts up between the legs, and as it lifts the sit bones are drawn together. Visualize this while hollowing the abdominals and squeezing the legs together. This helps to recruit the pelvic floor muscles and abdominal complex and deepens the work of the hip adductors.

☐ Maintain good pelvic–lumbar control and spinal alignment.

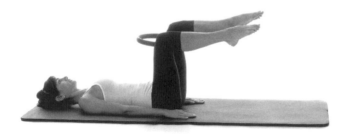

Inhale. Lie supine in a neutral spine position, with the hips and knees at a 90-degree angle (tabletop position). Place the circle between the thighs just above the knees.

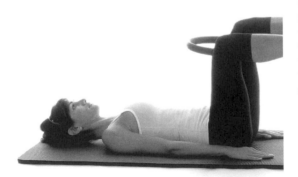

Exhale. Adduct the hips, squeezing the legs together. Maintain the tabletop position, with the hips and knees at a 90-degree angle and the shins parallel.

Inhale. Maintain the tension in the circle and continue with small pumps. Return to the starting position.

Like the previous exercise, this one strengthens the hip adductors and requires good abdominal strength and exceptional pelvic–lumbar control. Again, it has the benefit of providing an optimal position in which to work the pelvic floor muscles. However, because the legs are straight, the lever arm is longer, magnifying the work of the abdominals and hip flexors and demanding a very high level of control.

If the lower back starts rising off the floor into an arch, draw the abdominal muscles in deeper and lift into flexion of the trunk, placing the hands behind the head and interlacing the fingers. At the same time, lift the legs higher, closer to a 90-degree angle. I encourage experimenting with hip external rotation

as opposed to keeping the hips in a neutral position. Sometimes you can achieve a deeper contraction of the muscles and maintain better spinal support with the legs externally rotated (turned out). If this position still proves too challenging, bend the knees slightly.

Imagery

See Magic Circle: Supine: Knees (page 308).

☐ Maintain good pelvic–lumbar control and spinal alignment.
☐ Keep the legs at a consistent angle off the floor.
☐ Keep the neck and shoulders relaxed.

Muscle Focus

- Hip adductors

Objectives

- To strengthen the hip adductors
- To develop pelvic–lumbar stabilization

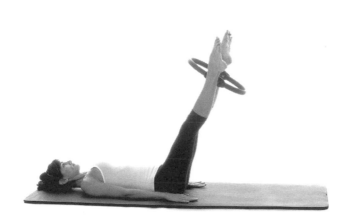

Inhale. Lie supine in a neutral spine position with the legs straight at a 60- to 90-degree angle to the floor. Place the circle between the legs, just above the ankles.

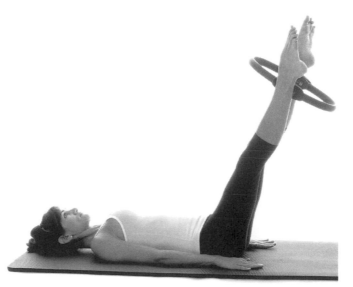

Exhale. Adduct the hips, squeezing the legs together.

Inhale. Maintain the tension in the circle and continue with small pumps. Return to the starting position.

Prone Knees Bent

Muscle Focus

- Hip adductors
- Hip extensors

Objective

- To strengthen the hip adductors and hip extensors

This exercise is exceptional for building strength in the hip adductors and hip extensors. Keeping the knees bent and lifting the thighs off the mat throughout the exercise maximizes the work of the hip extensors, using both functions of the hamstrings (knee flexion and hip extension). Avoid the tendency to tilt the pelvis anteriorly and hyperextend the lower back, which places stress on this area of the back. This is particularly pertinent when the hip flexors are tight or when the abdominals are not engaged sufficiently to counteract the anterior pull. In such cases, draw the abdominals in deeper and emphasize a posterior tilt of the pelvis by pushing the pubic symphysis forward. If necessary place a small cushion in the abdominal region to assist in preventing an anterior tilt of the pelvis.

Imagery

The body should feel like an archer's bow that has been pulled taut. As the feet lift higher toward the ceiling with each squeeze, the bow becomes more taut and the arc is accentuated.

- ☐ Extend the hips prior to squeezing the legs together, and keep them extended throughout.
- ☐ Maintain consistent 90-degree flexion in the knees.
- ☐ Keep the legs parallel as they squeeze together, as opposed to externally rotated.

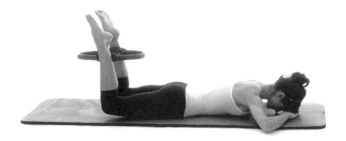

Inhale. Lie prone with the knees bent at a 90-degree angle and the thighs lifted off the mat. Place the circle between the legs and above the ankles (closer to the knee). Rest the forehead on the hands.

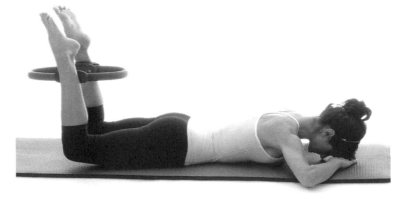

Exhale. Adduct the hips, squeezing the legs together.

Inhale. Maintain the tension in the circle and continue with small pumps. Return to the starting position.

Prone Knees Straight

Like the previous exercise, this one is exceptional for building strength of the hip adductors and hip extensors. Keeping the thighs lifted off the mat throughout the movement while contracting the adductors targets the hip extensors. Avoid the tendency to tilt the pelvis in an anterior direction. Although the knees are now straight, which releases the taut hip flexors, the lever arm has been lengthened, challenging the hip extensors and back extensors more and demanding a very high level of control, potentially placing more stress on the lower back.

Imagery

The image of the archer's bow (see Magic Circle: Prone Knees Bent, page 310) works well for this exercise too. In this case the feeling is one of elongating further into the bow shape with each squeeze of the legs.

☐ Extend the hips prior to squeezing the legs together, and keep them extended.

☐ Maintain strong abdominal work throughout the exercise.

☐ Keep the neck and shoulders relaxed.

Muscle Focus

- Hip adductors
- Hip extensors

Objective

- To strengthen the hip adductors and hip extensors

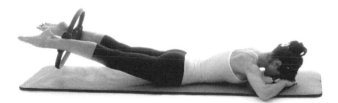

Inhale. Lie prone with the legs straight and the thighs lifted off the mat. Place the circle between the legs, just above the ankles. Rest the forehead on the hands.

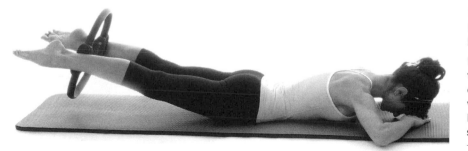

Exhale. Adduct the hips, squeezing the legs together.

Inhale. Maintain the tension in the circle and continue with small pumps. Return to the starting position.

Hamstrings

Muscle Focus

- Hamstrings

Objective

- To strengthen the hamstrings and hip extensors

One of my students came up with this excellent hamstring exercise years ago. Since then it has been refined and the element of hip extension has been added to it. A possible disadvantage of this exercise is that the knee moves within a very small range, if at all. However, if the goal is a small range of motion or an isometric contraction, then this will prove to be an advantage. I suggest orienting the pelvis toward a posterior tilt from the outset. That will counter the tendency to tilt it anteriorly, which often results in hyperextension of the lower back. Use a cushion under the abdominal region if necessary.

Imagery

Visualize the bow position you achieved in the Magic Circle: Prone Knees Bent and Prone Knees Straight exercises (pages 310 and 311), and add to that a hamstring curl that accentuates the arc shape. Maintain the bow shape with the working leg; the straight leg provides an anchor.

- ☐ Keep the thigh of the bent leg lifted off the floor throughout the exercise.
- ☐ Avoid externally rotating the working leg, and keep the thighs close together.
- ☐ Maintain abdominal activation throughout the exercise.

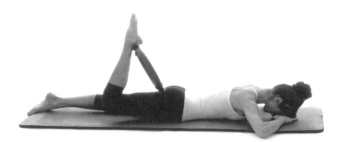

Inhale. Lie prone with one leg straight and the other bent at the knee. Lift the bent leg slightly off the mat. Place the circle below the gluteal muscle and behind the heel of the bent leg. Rest the forehead on the hands.

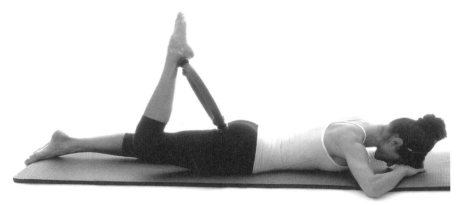

Exhale. Bend the knee further, pressing the heel toward the pelvis.

Inhale. Maintain the tension in the circle and continue with small pumps. Return to the starting position.

Swan

This swan exercise focuses on the upper and mid-back as opposed to the lower back. The lower back is often hyperactive, which inhibits the recruitment of the upper and mid-back muscles. Initially the legs should remain on the floor, uninvolved in the movement. Lifting the legs immediately activates the lower back and distracts from the focus of the exercise.

The posterior capsule of the shoulders figures prominently in keeping the arms aligned with the trunk. Ideally, the arms should line up opposite the ears. Make sure to keep the head aligned with the spine, avoiding the tendency to lift it to look straight forward rather than down and forward.

Imagery

This is a challenging back extension exercise that is wonderful to integrate into a mat work class. I like using the image of the halo (Magic Circle: Arms Overhead, page 304), even though the circle is not quite in the halo position. This image encourages the arms, head, and trunk to move as one unit.

☐ Adduct the legs throughout the exercise.
☐ Focus on elongation rather than height.
☐ Move the arms, head, and trunk as one unit.

Muscle Focus

▪ Back extensors

Objective

▪ To strengthen the back extensors and shoulders

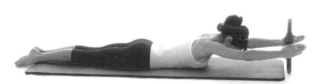
Inhale. Lie prone with the arms reaching overhead. Hold the circle in a horizontal position.

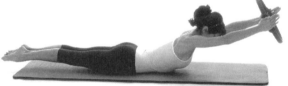
Exhale. Lift the upper body, pressing the arms together.

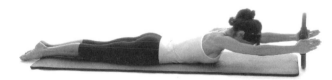
Inhale. Maintaining pressure on the magic circle, lower to the starting position.

313

CHAPTER 12

Sample Exercise Routines

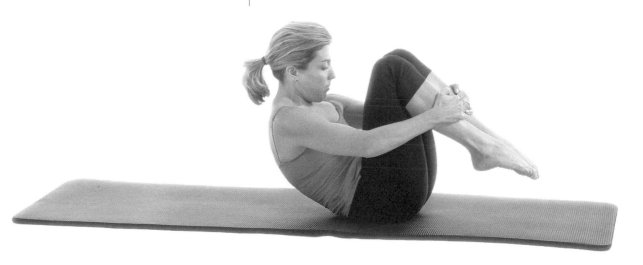

In this chapter I provide several sample routines for you to use in your Pilates practice. These will help you become acquainted with the exercises and learn how to sequence them effectively within the block system described in chapter 3. This in no way implies that the exercises *must* be practiced in the order I suggest in the following routines. I believe that being able to adapt to different situations is important. But using the block system offers a structure that promises a positive outcome and opens the door to myriad choices. For instance, when deciding which exercises to do for arm work, you can choose upper body exercises from a large pool of exercises in the arm work block that best suit your purpose at this time. The same goes for abdominal work, lateral flexion, back extension, and the other blocks. Practicing set routines (those offered here and others that you devise) is advantageous, so that they become second nature and imprinted in your muscle memory. The block system helps guide you in drawing the fine line between reinforcing movement patterns and allowing the work to become mundane and repetitious.

Sequencing Exercises

Once you have learned the exercises you should then incorporate them into a comprehensive, flowing routine. The mat work particularly lends itself to seamless transitions and unobstructed flow—one continuous movement from beginning to end. It starts with the first breath of the setup and continues to the final breath of the relaxation at the end.

I have been greatly influenced by years of dance and ashtanga yoga, as well as a familiarity with tai chi. These disciplines all share the quality of continuous movement. I call my approach to the mat work the *flow sequence,* and flow is the underlying quality in each exercise and the routine as a whole. Although maintaining the same degree of flow when working on the apparatus is more difficult, you should always experience a feeling of fluidity

and continuum, of deep concentration and inner focus. The quality of flow has many benefits. Apart from helping you feel good and look beautiful, it offers physiological benefits, such as heightening the cardiovascular effect, elevating the body temperature, and building muscular endurance, along with mental benefits, such as concentration and release of tension. This all culminates in a state I refer to as *meditation in motion.*

Creating transitions from exercise to exercise to make the sequence flow is a stimulating process. The transitions should be choreographed so that they become an integral part of the routine such that you avoid stopping, repositioning, and starting again, or when using the apparatus, lying down, getting up, placing the feet in the straps, taking them out of the straps, or adjusting the springs. Separate actions waste time and energy. Do keep in mind that although the transitions are important, they should not dictate the order of the exercises. The order must be determined by physiological principles, addressing the planes of motion, muscle groups, and safe progression. This is the premise of the block system.

The following guidelines will help you compile a session. The same guidelines apply to every session, whether it lasts 10 minutes or 60 minutes, whether it is done on the mat or on the apparatus, and whether it is fundamental or advanced. Keep in mind that to make a program effective and to see continued gains, you must gradually and consistently make the exercises more challenging. Effective cueing, using accessories such as rubber bands, modifying the exercises, adjusting the resistance, and introducing more difficult variations (with a similar muscle focus) can all help achieve this goal.

- Develop the session to progress from less demanding exercises to more demanding ones.
- Perform large muscle group exercises earlier in the session.

- Perform lower risk abdominal exercises earlier in the session.
- Keep programs progressive in the use of range of motion, resistance, complexity, and speed.
- Address as many muscle groups as possible during a session.
- Practice the various functions of the muscles: stabilization and mobilization.
- Incorporate all types of muscle contraction: isometric, concentric, and eccentric.
- Include all ranges of motion: flexion, rotation, lateral flexion, extension, and combinations of these.
- Balance the exercises according to the primary joints and their movements (such as hip flexion, hip extension, hip abduction, hip adduction, hip rotation).
- Emphasize a particular area based on individual needs while maintaining a good overall balance.
- Include appropriate more challenging exercises after an adequate warm-up.
- Add exercises that focus on balance and proprioception when appropriate.
- Work the mind and body together in harmony.

Individualizing a Sequence

Perhaps the most valuable quality of the Pilates method is its adaptability—it can cater to a broad range of people with differing needs. It is a solution for everyone, from those restricted in mobility to elite athletes. It can accommodate the young, elderly, fit, unfit, dancers, athletes, pregnant women, and the injured and rehabilitating. It is as beneficial for men as for women. I do not believe any other system offers such diversity and still challenges each person's capabilities to the maximum. Added to this is the calm, trusting, nurturing, and noncompetitive environment that is typical of most Pilates studios.

The extensive body of exercises, along with the choice of apparatus, allow the compilation of a program suited to each individual. The decision to introduce new exercises should be well thought out. Adding challenges is tempting, but new repertoire can be counterproductive if it is not appropriate. You must assess whether an exercise is of a suitable level, whether it will affect any injured areas adversely, whether it will help achieve a desired goal, and whether you (or your student) have adequate training and skills to perform it.

If you are a teacher designing a program, I encourage you to find out as much as possible about the individual you are working with. More important than what to do is what *not* to do, particularly in cases in which taking a certain tack may result in injury and even irreparable damage, such as when working with pregnant women or people suffering from back problems or osteoporosis, to name just a few. Become intricately familiar with the repertoire, be well educated in the science of human movement, know the body you are working with, and then be creative in developing options, never losing sight of the essence of the exercise. When in doubt, err on the side of caution, seek further professional advice (medical and otherwise), and most important, be safe, not sorry! When used as it was intended, Pilates can be the answer to anyone's quest for well-being.

Adapting Programs for Specific Populations

Specific populations is a general term that describes groups that have specific needs. There are two main groups: the first consists of people who may need to decrease the intensity of the work (elderly, injured, or rehabilitating), requiring modification of the exercises and the use of assists such as cushions, rubber bands, and springs. The second group consists of those who may need increased intensity (athletes, dancers, and gymnasts), requiring additional *overload* on the muscles and measures that make the exercises more complex. Both groups need specifically tailored programs, often with vastly different goals.

Even within the main groupings the goals may vary greatly. For instance athletes, dancers, and gymnasts often need *specificity training* in which they work on activity-specific skills and develop the neuromuscular system to improve performance. However, they may also need to improve general balance and enhance their overall conditioning program—in other words, they need *cross-training*. Pilates is exceptional for both forms of training.

It is beyond the scope of this chapter to provide exercise sequences for specific populations and modifications and variations for each exercise. However, by using the routines that appear in this book as a foundation, you can adapt them to your needs or those of your students.

Considering Safety

Whether you are doing mat work or working on the Pilates apparatus, safety is of paramount importance. In addition to following the general safety protocols for any exercise class—warming up, preparing the body for each action, monitoring heart rate and body temperature, and cooling down at the end of the session—you also need to know how to work safely with the full complement of Pilates apparatus. It is generally considered very safe equipment. It is *not.* In fact, it is potentially dangerous if not used correctly and with discretion, as the following story shows.

In 1989 I was in Australia, teaching and directing a dance department in a performing arts college where I had introduced a Pilates program. I had a Pilates studio at the college for my work with the students and some amateur and professional dancers and athletes. One morning I was teaching a young dancer, around 12 years old, doing mini roll-ups on the cadillac (page 211). She was a regular student and had done the exercise many times. She wanted to indicate something to me and let go of the push-through bar, which was attached to two springs. I was standing close by, and the bar flew into my mouth, crushing my four front teeth, sending me tumbling into the wall behind me, and knocking me out. I came around with my hand over my mouth, blood dripping out, and pieces of teeth in my hand.

Today all is fine, other than the fact that I have spent more hours in dentists' chairs over the past 17 years than I wish to recall. Was it anyone's fault? Probably not—just an unfortunate incident that illustrates the potential dangers of the apparatus. This apparatus was never intended for unsupervised mass use, yet given the exposure Pilates is now receiving and some of the modern trends in the way it is taught, this fact is often ignored. Good instruction and proper training are essential.

The features that make the equipment so beneficial to human conditioning also make it potentially harmful—there are springs, straps, and attachments all over the place. This equipment does not support the user; the user needs to support his or her body. Each exercise requires recruiting the body's stabilizers, which is one

Fundamentals to Take on the Road

If I told you about the many, and often odd, places I have practiced Pilates it would surely bring a smile to your face! I do an enormous amount of teaching worldwide, and I always take the fundamentals on the road with me. This usually consists of a mat and small accessories such as rubber bands and a magic circle (although the circle has become the cause of growing scrutiny during airport security checks). The beauty of Pilates is that you can compile a program for every occasion and any location as long as you follow the guidelines (see pages 316-317). Remember that consistency is the key, and if you let your Pilates practice lapse while you are traveling, all your hard work is diminished. Besides regular practice will keep you alert, in shape, and on top of your game at all times, even when sunning yourself on a beach in Hawaii!

reason this work is so functional and powerful. If you do not incorporate good stabilization, you risk not doing the movement correctly, or worse, the possibility of accident and injury.

Starting With Inner Focus

You are now familiar with both the philosophy and the exercises of Pilates and are ready to delve into your practice. I like to begin and conclude each session with a little relaxation or inner focus. If we commence the session with tension, that tension will compound as the body is challenged; then, rather than having a calming and rejuvenating effect and allowing you to achieve the goals of the exercises, the experience will be counterproductive.

A session on the apparatus often commences and concludes with a roll-down (page 24), which brings attention to alignment as well as serving as a path to inner focus, warm-up, and cool-down. After three to five roll-downs, I suggest a short warm-up on the mat before moving onto the apparatus. When doing the mat work, a session typically (though this is not required) begins and ends by going through a brief inner focus period in a sitting or supine position.

The following is a suggested outline for achieving inner focus when starting a mat work session.

1. Lie down on the mat in a supine position with the knees bent, legs parallel to each other and hip-width apart. Spread the feet comfortably on the floor. Place the arms by the sides of the body. Allow the spine to imprint into the mat.
2. Relax the feet, the back, and the neck.

3. Engage the adductors slightly to prevent the legs from splaying.
4. Imagine the pelvis floating in space with no forces pulling on it.
5. Visualize an elongated spine, relaxing the muscles of the back.
6. Reach the fingers toward the feet, gliding the scapulae down the back.
8. Elongate the neck, sensing the crown of the head reaching away from the body.
9. Relax the muscles of the face.
10. Be present in the moment, focus on the breath, and feel the lateral expansion of the chest on the mat.
11. Become aware of your body down to the last muscle fiber.
12. Engage the internal support system—you are now ready to move!

Mat Work Sequences

In the following section I provide three mat work routines: fundamental, intermediate, and advanced. Each routine builds on the previous one. Practice them by incorporating the principles in this book. Remember, the work is about quality, not quantity. Practice with integrity and make each movement the best that you possibly can. In the words of Joseph Pilates (in *Return to Life Through Contrology*), "Make a close study of each exercise and do not attempt any other exercise until you first have mastered the current one and know its routine down to the last detail without any reference to the text" (page 32).

Basic Mat Work Program

Exercises: 16; approximate time: 25 minutes

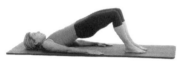

Pelvic curl, page 45

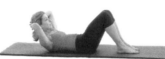

Supine spine twist, page 47

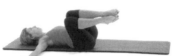

Chest lift, page 48

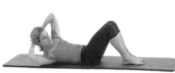

Chest lift with rotation, page 49

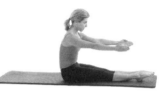

Roll-up, page 52

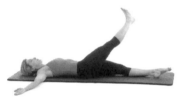

Leg circles, page 51

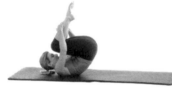

Rolling like a ball, page 54

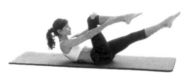

Single-leg stretch, page 56

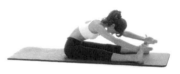

Spine stretch, page 63

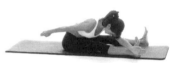

Saw, page 70

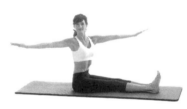

Spine twist, page 72

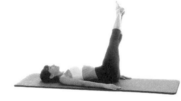

Corkscrew, page 73

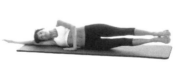

Side leg lifts, page 74

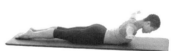

Basic back extension, page 76

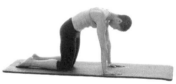

Cat stretch, page 82

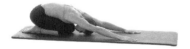

Rest position, page 81

Intermediate Mat Work Program

Exercises: 32; approximate time: 45 minutes

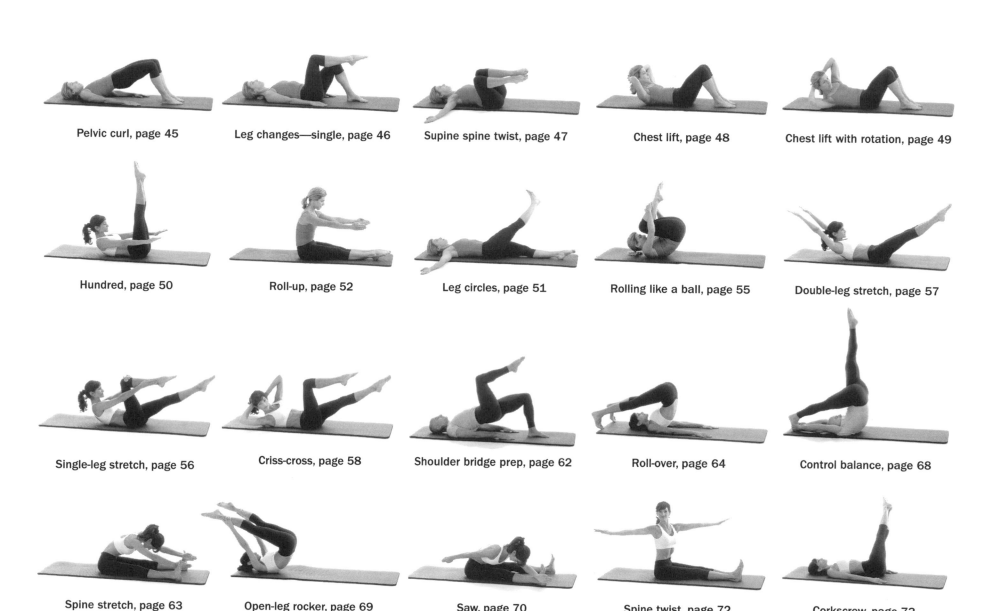

Pelvic curl, page 45

Leg changes—single, page 46

Supine spine twist, page 47

Chest lift, page 48

Chest lift with rotation, page 49

Hundred, page 50

Roll-up, page 52

Leg circles, page 51

Rolling like a ball, page 55

Double-leg stretch, page 57

Single-leg stretch, page 56

Criss-cross, page 58

Shoulder bridge prep, page 62

Roll-over, page 64

Control balance, page 68

Spine stretch, page 63

Open-leg rocker, page 69

Saw, page 70

Spine twist, page 72

Corkscrew, page 73

■ *(continued next page)* ■

321

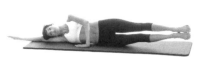

Side leg lift, page 74

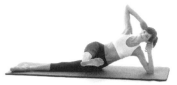

Side kick, page 75

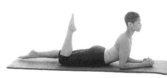

Single-leg kick, page 78

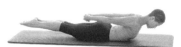

Double-leg kick, page 79

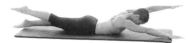

Swimming, page 77

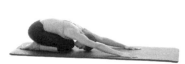

Rest position, page 81

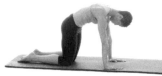

Cat stretch, page 82

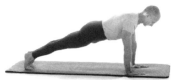

Front support, page 83

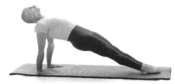

Back support, page 88

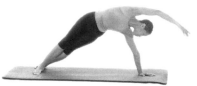

Side bend, page 96

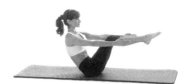

Teaser prep, page 100

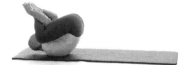

Seal puppy, page 105

Advanced Mat Work Program

Exercises: 44; approximate time: 60 minutes

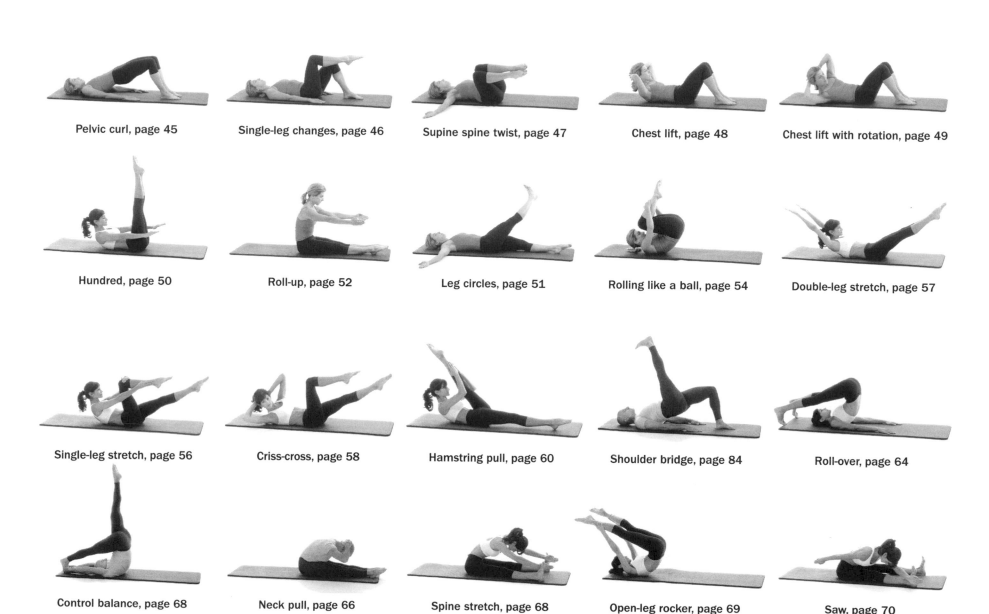

Pelvic curl, page 45

Single-leg changes, page 46

Supine spine twist, page 47

Chest lift, page 48

Chest lift with rotation, page 49

Hundred, page 50

Roll-up, page 52

Leg circles, page 51

Rolling like a ball, page 54

Double-leg stretch, page 57

Single-leg stretch, page 56

Criss-cross, page 58

Hamstring pull, page 60

Shoulder bridge, page 84

Roll-over, page 64

Control balance, page 68

Neck pull, page 66

Spine stretch, page 68

Open-leg rocker, page 69

Saw, page 70

■ *(continued next page)* ■

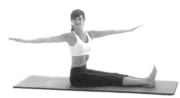

Spine twist, page 72

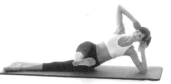

Side leg lifts, page 74

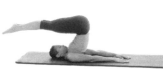

Side kick, page 75

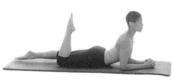

Single-leg kick, page 78

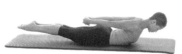

Double-leg kick, page 79

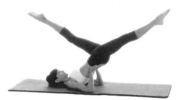

Scissors, page 90

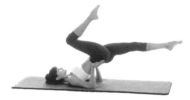

Bicycle, page 91

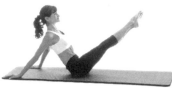

Jackknife, page 94

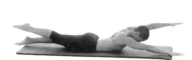

Hip circles prep, page 92

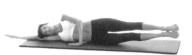

Swimming, page 77

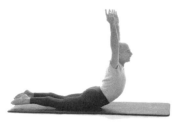

Swan dive, page 104

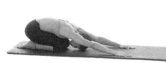

Rest position, page 81

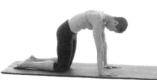

Cat stretch, page 82

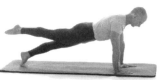

Leg pull front, page 85

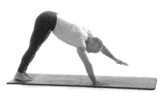

Push-up, page 86

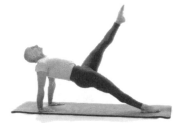

Leg pull back, page 89

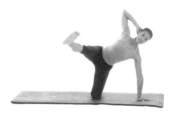

Kneeling side kick, page 93

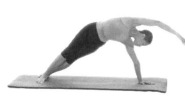

Side bend, page 96

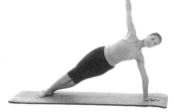

Twist, page 98

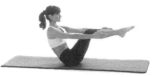

Teaser prep, page 100

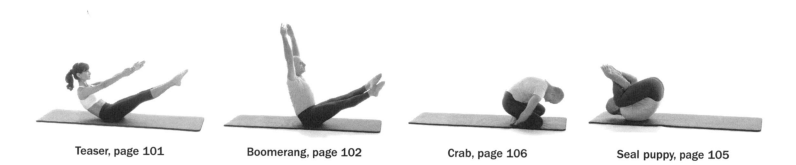

Teaser, page 101   Boomerang, page 102   Crab, page 106   Seal puppy, page 105

Apparatus Sequences

First and foremost when using any of the apparatus is safety. I cannot stress this point enough. Second, the session should be comprehensive, just as the mat work is. When working on the apparatus people sometimes do only a few exercises, often focusing on one area of the body. Remember, the apparatus are the tools we use, not the system itself. To reap all the benefits that Pilates offers, you must adopt the Pilates approach as well as the repertoire. I have always claimed that I would rather work out using conventional gym equipment with an instructor who uses a Pilates approach than work on Pilates apparatus with a Pilates instructor who does

not incorporate the principles of the work. The reason is simple: I know I will achieve better results in the first scenario. The block system ensures that each session you do is a Pilates session and not merely a few exercises done on Pilates apparatus.

I have offered three routines, one from each level, that can be used as frameworks to build on. In addition I have provided several alternative options, illustrating how the repertoire within each block can be interchanged. The possibilities are infinite, and as long as you adhere to the guidelines and principles in this book, you are guaranteed a positive outcome.

Fundamental Apparatus Program

Exercises: 30; approximate time: 60 minutes

OPTIONAL ▶

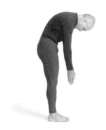

Roll-down, page 24

WARM-UP ▶

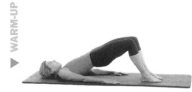

Pelvic curl (mat), page 45

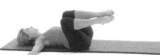

Supine spine twist, page 47

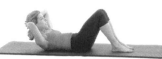

Chest lift (mat), page 48

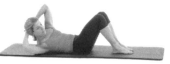

Chest lift with rotation (mat), page 49

FOOT WORK ▶

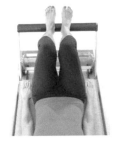

Parallel heels (reformer), page 112

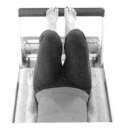

Parallel toes (reformer), page 113

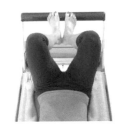

V-position toes (reformer), page 114

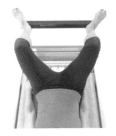

Open V-position heels (reformer), page 115

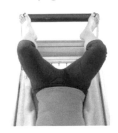

Open V-position toes (reformer), page 116

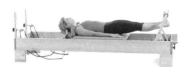

Calf raises (reformer), page 117

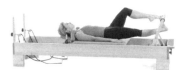

Prances (reformer), page 118

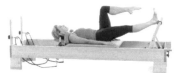

Single-leg heel (reformer), page 119

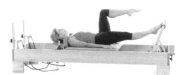

Single-leg toes (reformer), page 120

ABDOMINAL WORK ▶

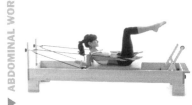

Hundred prep (reformer), page 123

HIP WORK ▶

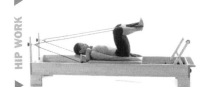

Frog (reformer), page 135

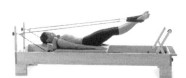

Down circles (reformer), page 136

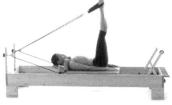

Up circles (reformer), page 137

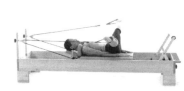

Openings (reformer), page 138

SPINAL ARTICULATION ▶

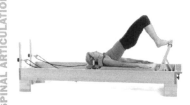

Bottom lift (reformer), page 142

Fundamental Apparatus Program

STRETCHES

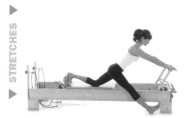

Hamstring stretch standing lunge (reformer), page 151

FULL BODY INTEGRATION

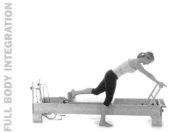

Scooter (reformer), page 155

ARM WORK

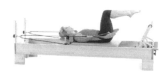

Extension (reformer), page 168 or (ped-a-pul), page 287

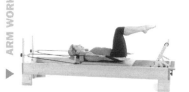

Adduction (reformer), page 169 or (ped-a-pul), page 288

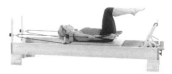

Circles (reformer), page 170 or (ped-a-pul), page 290

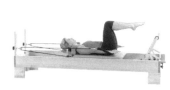

Triceps (reformer), page 171, or (ped-a-pul), page 289

LATERAL FLEXION AND ROTATION

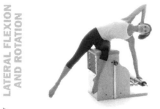

Side over (wunda chair), page 260 or (step barrel), page 279

BACK EXTENSION

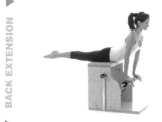

Basic swan (wunda chair), page 261 or Swan (step barrel), page 282

OPTIONAL

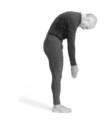

Roll-down, page 24

Intermediate Apparatus Program

Exercises: 31; approximate time: 60 minutes

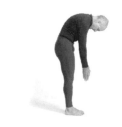

Roll-down, page 24

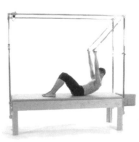

Roll-up (cadillac), page 210

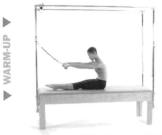

Mini roll-up (cadillac), page 211

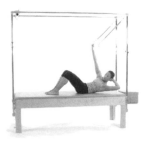

Oblique mini roll-up (cadillac), page 212

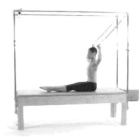

Roll-up top loaded (cadillac), page 214

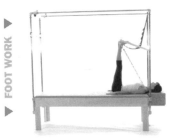

Double-foot positions—5 exercises (cadillac), page 207

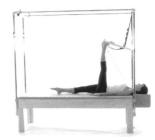

Calves and prances (cadillac), page 208

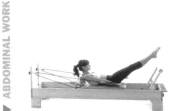

Single-foot positions—2 exercises (cadillac), page 209

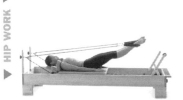

Hundred (reformer), page 124

Down circles(reformer), page 136

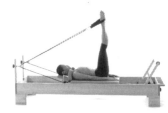

Up circles (reformer), page 137

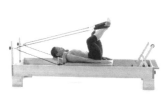

Extended frog (reformer), page 139

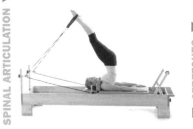

Extended frog reverse (reformer), page 140

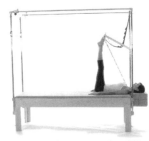

Short spine (reformer), page 146

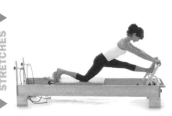

Hamstring stretch kneeling lunge (reformer), page 152

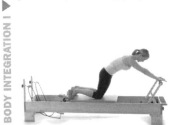

Knee stretch round back (reformer), page 156

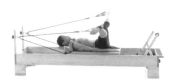

Knee stretch flat back (reformer), page 157

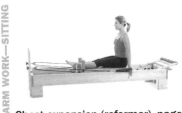

Chest expansion (reformer), page 172, or (arm chair), page 295

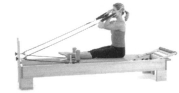

Biceps (reformer), page 173, or Hug-a-tree (arm chair), page 296

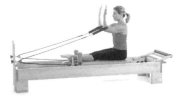

Rhomboids (reformer), page 174, or Circles (arm chair), page 297

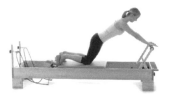

Intermediate Apparatus Program

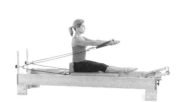

Hug-a-tree (reformer), page 175, or Salute (arm chair), page 298

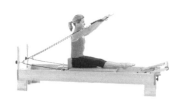

Salute (reformer), page 176, or Biceps (arm chair), page 299

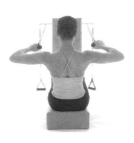

Rhomboids (arm chair), page 300

LATERAL FLEXION AND ROTATION ▶

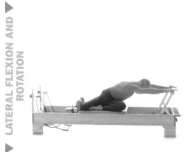

Mermaid (reformer), pages 198

BACK EXTENSION ▶

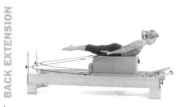

Breaststroke (reformer), page 202

OPTIONAL ▶

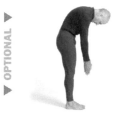

Roll-down, page 24

Advanced Apparatus Program

Exercises: 41; approximate time: 60 minutes

OPTIONAL
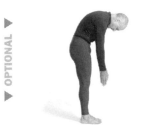

Roll-down, page 24

WARM-UP
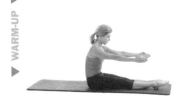

Roll-up (mat), page 25

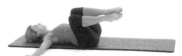

Supine spine twist, page 47

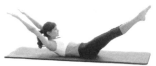

Double-leg stretch (mat), page 57

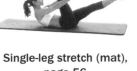

Single-leg stretch (mat), page 56

FOOT WORK
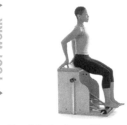

Criss-cross (mat), page 58

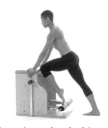

Double-foot positions—5 exercises (wunda chair), page 247

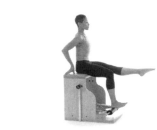

Calf raises (wunda chair), page 248

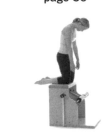

Single-foot positions (wunda chair), page 249

ABDOMINAL WORK

Cat stretch (wunda chair), page 251, Full pike (wunda chair), page 252

HIP WORK
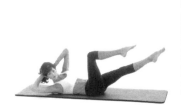

Hundred (reformer), page 124 or Coordination (reformer), page 125

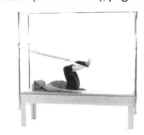

Frog (cadillac), page 216

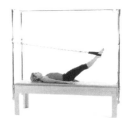

Hip circles (cadillac), page 217

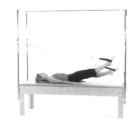

Walking (cadillac), page 218

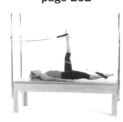

Bicycle and reverse bicycle (cadillac), page 219

SPINAL ARTICULATION
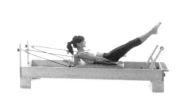

STRETCHES
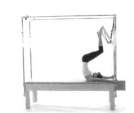

Tower (cadillac), page 222

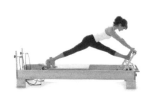

Hamstring stretch full lunge (reformer), page 153

FULL BODY INTEGRATION I
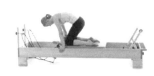

Reverse knee stretch (reformer), page 160

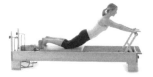

Down stretch (reformer), page 161

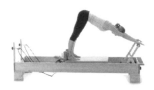

Elephant (reformer), page 162

Advanced Apparatus Program

ARM WORK—ROWING

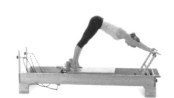

Up stretch (reformer), page 163

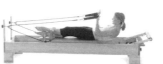

Rowing back I (reformer), page 182

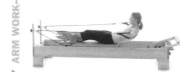

Rowing back II (reformer), page 184

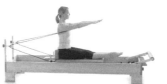

Rowing front I (reformer), page 186

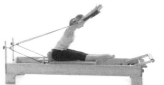

Rowing front II (reformer), page 188

LEG WORK

FULL BODY INTEGRATION II

LATERAL FLEXION AND ROTATION

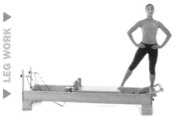

Single-leg skating (reformer), page 192, or Side split (reformer), page 191

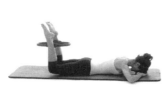

Prone knees bent (magic circle), page 310, or Supine ankles (magic circle), page 309

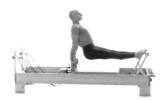

Balance control front (reformer), page 165

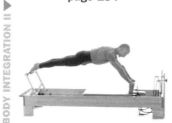

Balance control back prep (reformer), page 166

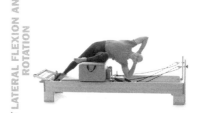

Side over (reformer), page 197, or (ladder barrel), page 268

BACK EXTENSION

OPTIONAL

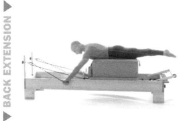

Pulling straps I (reformer), page 203, or Swan (ladder barrel), page 270

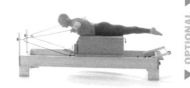

Pulling straps II (reformer), page 204

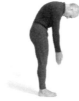

Roll-down, page 24

Now, as you embark on the journey of practicing Pilates you can look forward to the delightful and positive changes that lie ahead. Some people say that within 3 sessions you will *feel* different, within 10 sessions you will *look* different, and within 20 sessions you will *be* different. Certain changes—those relating to body awareness and alignment, muscle activation, the release of tension, rejuvenation, and inspiration—can occur immediately. However keep in mind that for significant physiological changes to take place, the muscles must be challenged consistently for at least six weeks. Joseph Pilates claimed, in *Return to Life Through Contrology,* that "if you faithfully perform [the] exercises regularly only four times a week for just three months . . . you will find your body development approaching the ideal, accompanied by renewed mental vigor and spiritual enhancement" (pages 18-19). Without consistency and discipline, profound changes are unlikely to occur. Pilates is not a cure-all potion. It is a well-designed system of physical and mental conditioning that, when practiced diligently, brings about the positive changes we strive for and the well-being that we deserve.

Discipline is a quality that is conveyed in each and every word that Joseph Pilates wrote, in his body language, in his teaching, in his being. For many, the practice of Pilates is the repetition of a series of exercises; for others it is a protocol prescribed by a physical therapist or a way to slim down. For many, it is the discovery of the wonders of a method that is experiencing unprecedented growth. I am not one to judge how or why a person should do Pilates. All I can convey are the intentions of Joseph Pilates and my personal experience.

Pilates was intended to be an approach to life, down to the finest detail of living, like bathing. I recently viewed newly discovered footage of Joseph Pilates, which at that point had been seen by very few people. Even after all these years of practicing the method, offering presentations about its history, researching the system, and reading Pilates' writings, as I watched these films I was amazed at the conviction of this person. He had ultimate belief in his system and a corresponding determination that it would be practiced universally. Yes, he actually demonstrates how to take a shower and wash every part of the body. It would be erroneous to ignore that he was strongly opinionated and had little respect for the medical community. It would be wrong to deny that he was an exhibitionist, egoist, reportedly an impatient teacher, and possibly a chauvinist who geared his method to be practiced mainly by men. It seems ironic that it is primarily women who have kept the flame alive all these years and still represent the vast majority of people practicing the method. Unfortunately much of the masculinity of the work has been shelved in the process. It is beginning to return, though, as more and more men teach and practice the work.

Still, we must recognize that Pilates was a "genius of the body" as George Balanchine supposedly called him. He embraced the power of the mind–body connection early on and viewed human movement as an intricate sequence of patterns, always seeing the human being as a whole. He was an unshakable idealist who believed that humankind deserved better. He created, arguably, the first home-gym equipment (the wunda chair) and spearheaded what is fast becoming one of the greatest surges in the history of the fitness industry. He furthered concepts that are only today being understood, embraced, and substantiated through research. Joseph Pilates was a man who was ahead of his time. He should be admired for his immeasurable contribution to society rather than idolized for things he did not do and for being someone he was not; this detracts from his genius rather than fortifying it. He was a human being, with vast knowledge and creativity that we can relate to even today, or perhaps more so today. He handed us a gift to enjoy and to enhance our lives.

In bidding farewell, I add my humble wish that we generously share our knowledge and life experience so that we may grow as individuals, as a community, and as the human race. And in so doing, through the practice of this powerful system, may we keep the essence of Pilates alive. Enjoy the adventure!

Selected Resources

Books

Calais-Germain, Blandine. 1993. *Anatomy of movement*. Seattle: Eastland Press.

Calais-Germain, Blandine, and Andrée Lamotte. 1996. *Anatomy of movement exercises.* Seattle: Eastland Press.

Cash, Mel. 1999. *Pocket atlas of the moving body.* London: Ebury Press Random House.

Conraths-Lange, Nicola.2004. *Survival skills for Pilates teachers*. Ann Arbor, MI: Logokinesis.

Corrigan, Brian, and G.D. Maitland. 1985. *Practical orthopaedic medicine.* Oxford, UK: Butterworth-Heinemann.

Dowd, Irene. 1981. *Taking root to fly*. New York: Dowd.

Dufton, Jennifer. 2003. *The Pilates difference*. London: Hamlyn.

Fitt, Sally S. 1988. *Dance kinesiology.* New York: Schirmer.

Franklin, Eric. 2002. *Pelvic power*. Hightstown, NJ: Princeton.

Friedman, Philip, and Gail Eisen. 1980. *The Pilates method of physical and mental conditioning.* Garden City, NY: Doubleday.

Gallagher, Sean P., and Romana Kryzanowska (editor). 2000. *The Joseph H. Pilates archive collection.* Philadelphia: Bainbridge.

Hessel, Jillian. 2003. *Pilates basics*. Emmaus, PA: Rodale.

Isacowitz, Rael. 2004. *Body arts and science international movement analysis work books: Mat, reformer, cadillac, ladder barrel and wunda chair, auxiliary.* Costa Mesa, CA: Author.

Iyengar, B.K.S. 1985. *The art of yoga.* London: Unwin.

Juhan, Deane. 1987. *Jobs body.* Barrytown, NY: Station Hill Press.

Kendal, Florence P., Elizabeth K. McCreary, and Patricia G. Provance. 1993. *Muscles: Testing and function.* 4th ed. Baltimore: Williams & Wilkins.

Kelly, Suzanne. 2005. *Pilates 4 kidzz*. Bloomington, IN: Authorhouse.

King, Bruce. 1991. *Rule of the bones: Exercise theory and program for correct body usage.* New York: Bruce King Foundation for American Dance.

Kounovsky, Nicholas. 1971. *The joy of feeling fit.* Mattituck, NY: Amereon House.

Lingauer, Gabor. 2002. *Muscle doctor*. Victoria, Canada: Trafford.

Myers, Thomas P. 2001. *Anatomy trains.* London: Harcourt.

Netter, Frank H. 1989. *Atlas of human anatomy.* Summit, NJ: Medical Education, Ciba-Geigy.

Pilates, Joseph H. 1945. *Return to life through contrology.* Reprinted 2003. Miami: Pilates Method Alliance.

Pilates, Joseph H. 1934. *Your health: A corrective system of exercising that revolutionizes the entire field of physical education.* Reprinted 1998. Incline Village, NV: Presentation Dynamics.

Robinson, Lynne. 2004. *The body control Pilates pregnancy book.* London: Pan Books.

Tardent, Helen. 2005. *Beautiful pilates.* Camberwell, Australia: Penguin.

Thompson, Cem W. 1989. *Manual of structural kinesiology.* 11th Edition. St. Louis: Times Mirror/Mosby.

Journals

Betz, Sherri R. April 2005. Modifying Pilates for clients with osteoporosis. *IDEA Fitness Journal.*

Fiscella, Catherine. May 2005. *The lumbar spine. IDEA Fitness Journal.*

Isacowitz, Rael. June 2005. Successful cueing for Pilates. *IDEA Fitness Journal.*

Joseph, Regina. January 2006. Closing the gender gap. *PilatesStyle.*

Kaplan, Ruth. Spring 2005. Pilates without borders. *PilatesStyle.*

Videos and DVDs

Fletcher, Ron. *Ron Fletcher Workshop Tape.* The Ron Fletcher Company.

Isacowitz, Rael. 2003. *Rael Pilates System 7, 17 and 27.* Carlmarsh III Productions.

Gentry, Eve. 1991. *The Eve Gentry Technique.* Institute for the Pilates Method.

Liekens, Bob, Alycea Ungaro, and Peter Fiasca. 2003. *Classical Pilates technique.* Classical Pilates Inc.

Pilates, Joseph H. *Demonstrating the principles of his method with Clara, students and friends, 1932-1945.* From Joseph and Clara Pilates personal collection. Attained by Evelyn de la Tour and bequeathed to Mary Bowen. Mary Bowen made it available to the Pilates community.

Trier, Carola. 1989. *Carola shares . . .* A Dadmehr Production.

Web Sites of Interest

Balanced Body: www.pilates.com.

Body Arts and Science International: www.basipilates.com.

Body Control UK: www.bodycontrol.co.uk

California Therapy Solutions: www.californiatherapysolutions.com

Dynamic Chiropractic: www.chiroweb.com

Pilates Method Alliance: www.pilatesmethodalliance.org.

Physician and Sports Medicine: www.physsportsmed.com

Scoliosis: www.scoliosis.com

Scoliosis World: www.scoliosis-world.com

Somatics on the Web: www.somatics.com

Index

Index

About the Author

Rael Isacowitz, MA, is the founder of Body Arts and Science International (BASI), an international organization devoted to Pilates education since 1989. Recognized as a contemporary approach to the works of Joseph Pilates, this teacher-training program is active in many countries around the globe. As a leading expert in the Pilates method, Isacowitz has close to 30 years of experience practicing and lecturing in universities, clinics, and studios worldwide. With a rich background as a dancer, athlete, yogi, and Pilates practitioner, Isacowitz brings to his teaching unparalleled expertise combined with a passion for his work.

In collaboration with Balanced Body, the largest Pilates equipment manufacturer in the world, Isacowitz designed the concept for a new line of Pilates apparatus and has been featured in numerous publications in several languages all over the world. His DVD series has won several awards and was *Health Magazine's* Pilates choice for 2006. He served on the board of the Pilates Method Alliance and has been a driving force in several initiatives advocating educational standards in the Pilates community. He continues to support this organization and others in various countries, striving to set industry guidelines and maintain the integrity of Pilates.

Isacowitz received his teaching credentials (DipPE) and bachelor of education degree in Israel at the prestigious Wingate Institute of Physical Education, where he was later invited to join the faculty. Isacowitz went on to complete his master of arts degree in dance at the University of Surrey, England. He lives with his wife and son in Southern California, close to On Center Conditioning, the Pilates studio he extablished in 1991 that serves as the headquarters for BASI. He blends his passion for Pilates with his insatiable love for surfing, wind surfing, skiing, and living life to the fullest.

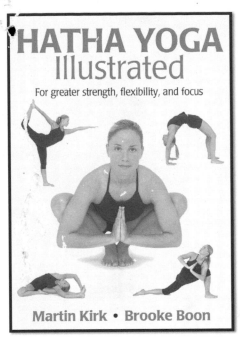
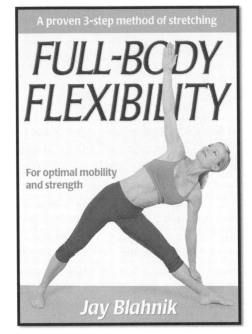